FUNDAMENTALS
OF RADIOLOGY

FUNDAMENTALS OF RADIOLOGY

Third Edition

Lucy Frank Squire, M.D.

Professor of Radiology, Downstate Medical School,
State University of New York, Brooklyn, New York

Consultant in Radiology, Massachusetts General Hospital,
Boston, Massachusetts

Drawings Modified from Well Known Paintings are by Francis Cunningham

A Commonwealth Fund Book
Harvard University Press
Cambridge, Massachusetts and London, England

First edition entitled *Fundamentals of Roentgenology*.

Copyright © 1964 by the Commonwealth Fund

Second and third editions entitled *Fundamentals of Radiology*.

Copyright © 1975, 1982 by the President and Fellows of Harvard College

10 9 8 7 6 5 4 3 2

Library of Congress Cataloging in Publication Data

Squire, Lucy Frank
    Fundamentals of radiology.

    "A Commonwealth Fund book."
    Includes index.
    1. Diagnosis, Radioscopic.   I. Title.   [DNLM: 1. Radiography.
WN 100 S774f]
RC78.S69   1982   616.07'572   81-20268
ISBN 0-674-32925-2   AACR2

Printed and bound in the United States of America
by Vail-Ballou Press, Inc.

Preface

In undertaking the writing of this textbook, I have been concerned with providing not a compendious reference work in which one might hope to find "the roentgen signs by which diseases are diagnosed," but rather an instruction manual which would help students learn how to *look at* x-ray films. The student will find that radiology affords him a memorably graphic means of correlating and retaining material of all kinds learned in other disciplines. It is important, therefore, for every graduating physician to know how to examine a radiograph and to be able to derive certain kinds of information from it. He should recognize the shadows produced by some of the commoner types of pathologic change, relating those shadows to the pathology in a logical way and with modest confidence. As the late Dr. Felix Fleischner suggested, basic facts will be continually reviewed throughout a lifetime of practice by the physician who learns in medical school how beautifully and logically imaging procedures document pathophysiology.

The young practitioner finds that he can best discuss his own patients' films with the radiologic consultant if he has learned in medical school to expect pathology to relate to roentgen shadows. He must recognize in the radiologist another consultant in the whole-patient study, and not an oracle issuing incomprehensible diagnostic statements. He will be a better physician if he understands enough about roentgen shadows to want to discuss and rediscuss the details of the films on his patients with the experts who have made and interpreted them, until both are satisfied that imaging methods have been applied ideally to the problem at hand.

In preparing a third edition of this book I have made a number of major changes. Obsolete and redundant illustrations have been deleted, and material has been added to introduce the student to some of the newer imaging modalities (sonography, computerized tomography, and certain isotope studies). Chapter 15 has been extensively revised again to encompass changes in our understanding of renal and biliary diagnosis and to give the student at least a basic feeling for the choice of procedures in the diagnostic workup of a number of common medical problems. Unknowns to test the student's advancing expertise, on the other hand, have been reduced in number, since so many are available to him now in the collaterally published *Exercises in Diagnostic Radiology* series (W. B. Saunders). Several of these workbooks were revised and updated in 1981.

It is my earnest hope that the need for more readable study materials for medical students will be recognized by teacher-writers in other fields. Today's harassed medical students are finding it more and more difficult to study from standard reference works. I hope that in the next several decades teachers and medical publishers, working together, will undertake to prepare programmed materials that are both instructive and, because they are also entertaining, unforgettable.

Lucy Frank Squire

1 West 72nd Street
New York, N.Y. 10023

Acknowledgments

This book was written originally with the help of a grant from the Commonwealth Fund. William Cornwell and Thomas Callear, editors of *Medical Radiography and Photography*, made available to me previously published illustrations as well as extensive files of unpublished prints of radiographs at the Eastman Kodak Company in Rochester, N.Y. These compose a very large part of the material in the book, and all credits to the original contributors appear in an appendix at the end. Alice Russell and Rosemary Terry of the Eastman Kodak editorial staff spent many hours helping me to locate, organize, and identify those materials.

Dr. Bernard Epstein contributed the laminagrams the students have found so helpful. Dr. Henry Jaffe graciously allowed me to reuse the beautiful color plates in the bone chapter. Dr. Morton Bosniak and Dr. Alec Megibow generously provided the superb CT scans in Chapters 14 and 16. Dr. George Leopold and Dr. Barbara Gosink very kindly agreed to supply the sonograms in Chapter 14, and I am much indebted to them. Dr. Joshua Becker, Dr. Serge Dallemand, Dr. Gwendolyn Hotson, Dr. Bernard Suster, and Dr. Nathanial Solomon, all members of the harmonious department in which I work, helped me to locate new material and provided critical help with the new sections in the book, for which I am affectionately grateful. Shelley Eshleman, medical illustrator, executed the newer diagrams, and her expertise is much appreciated. Jacqueline Parenti, with the greatest good humor, shouldered the monstrous task of committing the manuscript to a word processor to facilitate editing changes.

Finally, I have worked closely with Susan Hayes, Assistant Director at the Harvard University Press in charge of Production and Design, in planning this third edition. Her intelligence, efficiency, and idealistic (yet practical) sense of the obligation of textbook publishers to student readers in a period of inflation gave me the courage I needed to rework the book, and I am very much obliged to her.

L.F.S.

Contents

To Dr. Richard Schatzki
with grateful appreciation
for his inspiration
and example

FUNDAMENTALS OF RADIOLOGY

This volume is published as part of a long-standing program between **Harvard University Press** and the **Commonwealth Fund**, a philanthropic foundation, to encourage the publication of significant and scholarly books in medicine and health.

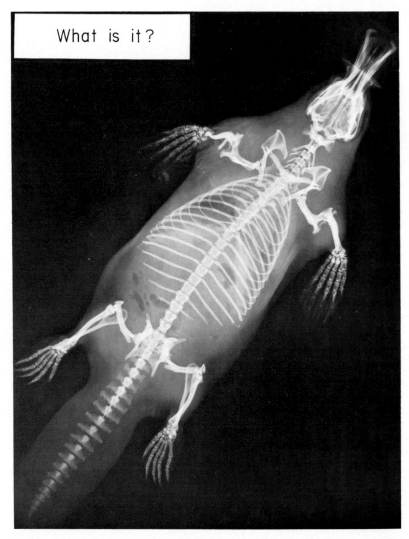

Figure 1-1. Its name is *Ornithorhynchus anatinus*, and you have never seen an x-ray portrait of it before. Nevertheless, there is one creature and one only in the animal kingdom which could give this x-ray appearance, and you can reason out its identity.

CHAPTER 1 Introduction and Basic Concepts

As you probably already know, x-rays are produced by bombarding a tungsten target with an electron beam. They are a form of radiant energy similar in several respects to visible light. For example, they radiate from the source in all directions unless stopped by an absorber. Like light rays, a very small part of the beam of x-rays will be absorbed by air, whereas all of the beam will be absorbed by a sheet of thick metal. The fundamental difference between x-rays and light rays is in their range of wavelengths, all x-rays being shorter than the wavelength of ultraviolet light. The useful science of radiology is based on this difference, since many substances which are opaque to light are penetrated by x-rays. It was this attractive property which caught the attention of Professor Roentgen of the University of Würzburg on a cold November night in 1895 when he first observed certain physical phenomena he could not explain.

Roentgen had been experimenting with an apparatus which, unknown to him, caused the emission of x-rays as a by-product. Accustomed to the darkened laboratory, he observed that whenever the apparatus was working, a chemical-coated piece of cardboard lying on the table glowed with a pale green light. We know now that fluorescence, or the emission of visible light, can be produced in a variety of ways by complex nuclear energy exchanges. But in 1895 Roentgen recognized at first only the fact that he had unintentionally produced *a hitherto unknown form of radiant energy which was invisible, could cause fluorescence, and passed through objects opaque to light*. When he placed his hand between the source of the beam and the lighted cardboard, he could see the bones inside his fingers within the shadow of his

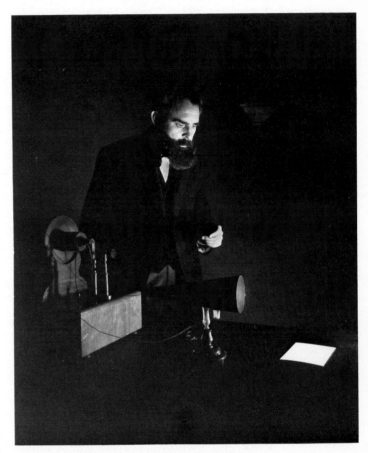

Figure 1-2. Staged version of the discovery of the roentgen ray.

hand. He found that the new rays, which he named x-rays, penetrated wood. Using photographic paper instead of a fluorescing material, he made an "x-ray picture" of a hand through the door of his laboratory.

1

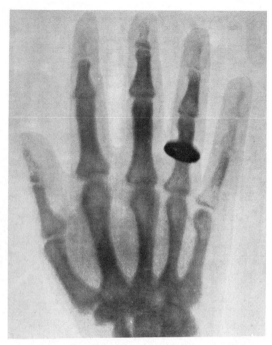

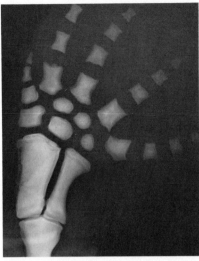

Figure 1-4. Actually, not a hand. Guess what it might be. (Note: Throughout this book you will find rhetorical questions and unanswered propositions. Sometimes they will be found answered in the text immediately following; sometimes, if you read straight along, you will find the answer several pages later buried in the text or incorporated into the legend of a related illustration. It is my intention to help you learn by reasoning.)

Figure 1-3. Radiograph of hand with ring made in Roentgen's laboratory on January 17, 1896. This is also how Roentgen's hand appeared as a shadow on the fluorescing paper.

Six years later the first Nobel Prize in physics was awarded to Roentgen for his discovery, and by then this remarkably systematic investigator had explored most of the basic physical and medical applications of the new ray.

The idea of being able to see through opaque objects caught the public fancy all over the world, and a great deal of nonsense was written on the subject in many languages within the first decade after its discovery. There is a fascinating file of cartoons and articles in the Library of Congress documenting this fever. It was even predicted that the mind would be explored by the radiologist, but in time others seem to have preempted that field.

Are you quite sure you can imagine exactly what Roentgen saw when he first observed that he could "see through his hand" with the help of the new ray? In order to grasp this clearly, you must first understand the important difference between what one sees fluoroscopically (Figure 1-3) and what you see today in an x-ray film of the hand, such as the one in Figure 1-4. You should call this a *radiograph*, not an "x-ray."

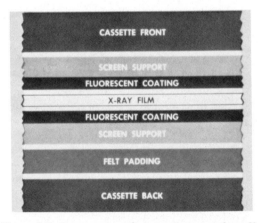

Figure 1-5. Cross section of a cassette, or modern film holder. The x-ray film in use today consists of an acetate sheet coated on both sides with photographic emulsion, and the cassette is constructed so that cardboard fluorescent screens are applied in contact with each side of the film. In this way light rays reinforce the photochemical effect on the film of the x-rays themselves.

When light hits photographic film, a mysterious photochemical process takes place in which metallic silver is precipitated in fine particles within the gelatin emulsion, rendering the film black when it is developed chemically. Places on the film which are not exposed to light remain clear. When a "positive" paper print is made of this "negative" film, the values are reversed: the black, silver-bearing areas prevent light from reaching the photosensitive paper, while clear areas in the film permit the paper to be blackened.

The x-ray film you will see in medical school is equivalent to the negative film you may have worked with in your own photographic darkroom. X-rays, like light rays, precipitate silver in a photographic film, but they do so much less rapidly than light. A patient cannot be expected to hold still long enough for films to be made using x-rays alone, and too much exposure to radiation is both dangerous and technically undesirable. Therefore, an ingenious reinforcing technique has been worked out using a special film container, or *cassette.*

The cassette contains a fluorescent screen which is activated by the x-rays and in turn emits light rays which reinforce the photochemical effects of the x-rays themselves on the film. In this way the silver-precipitating effect of the x-rays combined with that of the light rays they generate work together to blacken the film. When an object interposed between the x-ray beam source and the cassette has absorbed the rays, no light activation of the fluorescent screen will take place; neither x-rays nor light rays will reach the film, and no silver will be precipitated.

In Figure 1-6 a woman's left hand has been placed over the cassette and exposed to a beam of x-rays. Notice that the film not covered by any part of the hand has been intensely blackened because very little of the beam was absorbed by the *air,* which was the only absorber interposed there between x-ray tube and film. The fleshy parts of the hand (or *soft tissues,* as they are called by the radiologist) absorbed a good deal of the beam so that the film appears gray. Very few x-rays reached that part of the film directly under the *bones,* because bones contain large amounts of calcium. All *metals* absorb x-rays to an extent depending on atomic number and thickness. No x-rays at all were able to pass through the gold ring, and the film underneath it was not altered photographically.

What Roentgen saw, on the contrary, was the

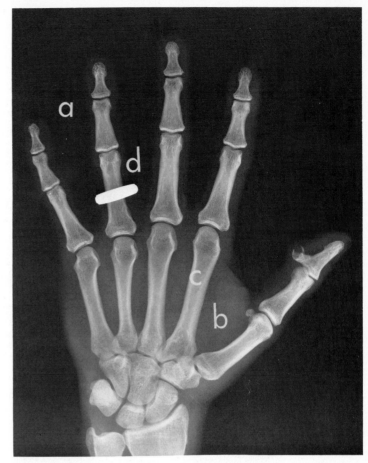

Figure 1-6. Modern radiograph of a hand. (*a*) Blackened area where only air is interposed between beam and film. (*b*) Soft tissues absorb part of the beam before it reaches the film. (*c*) Calcium salts in bone absorb even more x-rays, leaving film only lightly exposed and relatively little silver precipitated in the emulsion. (*d*) Dense metal of ring absorbs all rays; no silver is precipitated. (Note: This, like all x-ray illustrations in textbooks and periodicals published in this country, is a doubly reversed print, so that what you see here is what you will see whenever you hold a film of the hand against the light.)

reverse of all the light-dark values you have been looking at in the film of the hand. X-rays reached the coated cardboard in abundance all around his hand so that the *background* fluoresced vigorously, while the shadow of his hand emitted less light and appeared gray-green. The cardboard underneath the bones of his fingers appeared darkest of all, since it received almost no activating rays. (Compare Figure 1-3.)

Figure 1-4 is not a human hand but a whale's flipper reduced photographically.

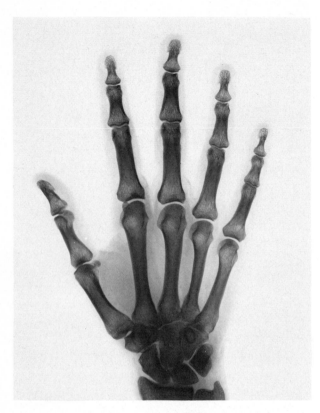

Figure 1-7. Positive print of a radiograph of the hand, made by singly reversing the values. This is also approximately as the hand would look on the fluoroscopic screen.

You would be disappointed if you visited a *conventional fluoroscopy room* because you would see little or nothing unless you had adapted your eyes to darkness for some time beforehand. Fluoroscopic light is very faint unless it is amplified electronically. Today almost all fluoroscopic rooms are equipped with such "image intensification" machines, much more costly than conventional fluoroscopes, but functioning in a lighted room and affording better detail with less radiation exposure to the patient.

You may not see much fluoroscopy in your lifetime, but you will see many thousands of x-ray films. For this reason I suggest that you make a practice of thinking in terms of the white and black values that relate to the usual x-ray film as you saw them in the hand in Figure 1-6. Think of dense objects as white and of those more easily penetrated as gray or black. All the illustrations in this book are printed like Figure 1-6, and you will find that most American journals and books print x-ray illustrations in this way. When you have occasion to study from British and Continental journals, you will find that positive prints are often employed (see Figure 1-7).

While it is essential to understand which are the more dense (or *radiopaque*) substances and which the more transparent (or *radiolucent*) ones, your concern, even as you first begin looking at radiographs, should not be only with density. One often makes quite reasonable and useful deductions from the *form and shape* of roentgen shadows. If you figured out that Figure 1-1 was, and could only be, a radiograph of a duck-billed platypus, you have experienced the sort of educated guessing one uses all the time in radiology. One guesses imaginatively and then subjects one's own guess to a rigorous logical analysis based on roentgen and medical data. Putting together expected density and expected form, you will soon find that you can predict the appearance of the radiograph of an object or structure.

Begin, then, by applying imagination and judgment to a variety of nonmedical objects. Try to predict the type of shadow that would appear on the film if you x-rayed (1) a coin, flat and then on edge; (2) a paper cup, empty and then containing a teaspoonful of buckshot; (3) a closed wooden box containing a watch; (4) an electric heating pad; (5) an egg.

Figure 1-8 is a radiograph of a woman's purse. Although the cloth from which the purse was made offered almost no obstruction to the x-rays, anything made of metal inside it, including the frame of the purse, absorbed the rays and left a white profile on the film. You will be able to identify from their outlines alone a paper clip, a bobby pin, a safety pin, a pair of rimless spectacles, coins, a lipstick case, two locker keys (overlapped), a nail file, and a metal pencil. You can almost construe the girl: a poverty-stricken, myopic individual who is taking two lab courses but wears makeup. One might, of course, be mistaken as to the state of her finances: folding money, even in pounds sterling, would be quite radiolucent.

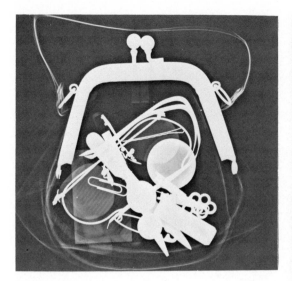

Figure 1-8

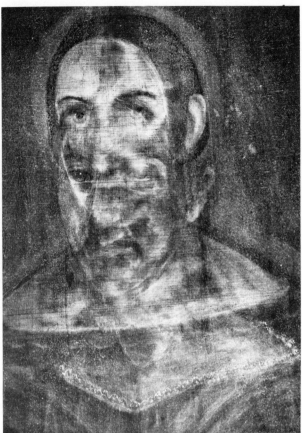

Figure 1-9. Radiograph of a portrait in oils painted over an earlier portrait. Only the woman with the pale eyes was visible on viewing the painting.

Pure metals are relatively radiopaque and so are their salts. Consequently, so also are the mixtures of oil and brilliantly colored metallic salts responsible for the whole field of oil painting. The radiography of paintings and other works of art is a fascinating and technically useful branch of the science. Frauds, inept reconstructions, masterpieces painted over by amateurs may sometimes be detected by x-ray studies.

In Figure 1-9 two painters have used the same canvas, or, dissatisfied with his portrait of the man whose eyes appear as the lower pair, the same painter may have done the portrait of the woman with the light eyes and severely dressed hair, covering over the earlier portrait. Only the lady was visible as one looked at the painting.

Variations in the precise metallic composition of artists' colors used at different times in history may help in the identification and dating of such works of art. The pigments in use since about 1800 have been made of the salts of metals with much lower atomic numbers than the older pigments and for that reason will x-ray quite differently.

Thus a modern forgery of an old master, no matter how adroit a copy, will have an entirely different radiograph from the original. On the other hand, a copy made by a pupil of the master or another artist of the same school, painting at about the same time in history with the same hand-ground, earth-mineral colors, could be expected to x-ray in about the same way.

The characteristic use of brushstrokes, which, even better than his signature, often stamps the work of a great artist, may also help to identify a concealed painting covered over by a lesser artist. You would be able to imagine the radiograph of a contemporary canvas with the vigorous, heavy brushstrokes of Van Gogh showing through, for example.

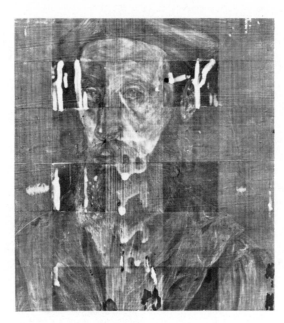

Figure 1-10

Remember, too, that any radiograph of a painting represents the summation of not only the various paint densities but the x-ray shadows of the canvas itself and the supporting structures. The wooden frame on which the canvas is stretched will cast some shadow, and if there are any nails in the wood they will appear in the radiograph also. Figure 1-10 shows a radiograph of a painting supported on wooden strips. The curious white areas are wormholes which have been filled with whitelead. The x-rays have been completely absorbed, you notice, by the white-lead *casts* of the wormholes, and under them no x-rays have reached the film to blacken it. The white areas on the film are actually, therefore, *shadow-profiles* of these white-lead casts. Remember this! It has an important parallel in barium work in medical x-ray studies of the gastrointestinal tract.

The industrial uses of x-ray are many and important. Flaws, cracks, and fissures in heavy steel can be shown by x-raying big equipment or building materials. Especially powerful machines are needed for this sort of work, ones which will produce a more penetrating beam of x-rays of very short wavelength, often called "hard x-rays." X-rays of long wavelength, or "soft x-rays," are used to study thin or delicate objects. Very soft x-rays are used to study tissue sections of bone 1 or 2 microns in thickness (microradiography), while very hard x-rays are used to penetrate deep into the body and destroy malignant tumor cells (radiation therapy). In between these two extremes fall the wavelengths which are used in medical x-ray diagnosis.

The *electromagnetic spectrum* is a scaled arrangement of all types of radiant energy according to wavelength. Within the range used in diagnostic radiology, the x-ray technician is trained to select and use the particular wavelength suited to the density and thickness of the part he is filming. He does this by varying the kilovoltage of his machine: the higher the kilovoltage, the harder or more penetrating the beam of rays produced. He can also vary the amount of radiation in the beam by altering the milliamperage used, and, finally, he can control the time of the exposure. Thus, for instance, for a thin object like the hand he uses a soft beam for a short time, and for a dense object like the head, a hard beam and a long exposure.

6

Radiodensity as a Function of Thickness

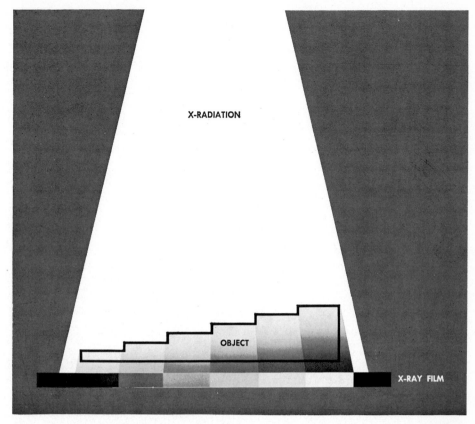

Figure 1-11. *Radiodensity as a function of thickness of the object.* Here the object to be filmed is of homogeneous composition and has a stepwise range of thickness. Gray shading indicates degree of absorption of the x-rays.

Thickness Kept Constant While Composition Varies

Having reasoned through all this, you must consider in greater detail the *relative radiodensities* of various substances and tissues. In order to do this most easily, let us eliminate thickness completely for the moment. Consider an imaginary row of 1-centimeter cubes of lead, air, butter, bone, liver, blood, muscle, subcutaneous fat, and barium sulfate. Can you arrange them in the order of their radiodensity, decreasing from left to right?

If they were all pure elemental chemicals, you certainly could arrange them in order by looking up their atomic numbers. Only one of them is quite so simple as that, and a judicious guess will surely place first to your left as most dense the cube of lead, with an atomic number of 82. Are you hesitating between bone and barium sulfate? Barium has an atomic number of 56, and calcium in the bone cube has an atomic number of 20. However, bone is not even pure calcium salt. It has a functioning physiologic structure with holes and spaces to accommodate body fluids and marrow. It is composed of an organic matrix into which the complex bone mineral is precipitated. All such organic substances will reduce the radiodensity of the cube of bone, and it would consequently have even less radiodensity than a similar cube of packed bone dust. The cube of barium sulfate must be placed next to the lead cube, therefore, and after it, the cube of bone.

7

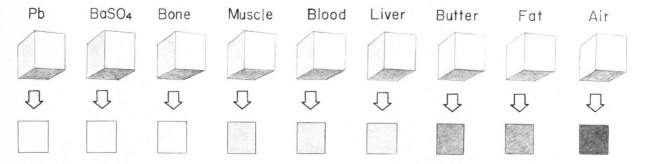

Figure 1-12. Thickness kept constant while composition varies.

As to the most radiolucent of all, you can have no trouble with that: surely you will have put the cube of air far to the right, at the opposite end of the scale from the lead. The film under the air cube will be black, since the sparse scattering of air molecules offers almost no obstacle to the rays. The square of film under the lead, unaltered because no rays penetrated the cube to reach it, will be clear white, while that under the bone will show a tinge of gray.

Butter and subcutaneous fat have very similar x-ray densities. They are extremely radiolucent and must be placed next to air in the scale we are considering. Neither butter nor fatty tissue is homogeneous, since one is never quite free of water and the other contains both circulating fluids and a supporting network of fibrous connective tissue. Their squares on the radiograph would be almost the same very dark gray.

In between the three very dense cubes and the three very lucent ones there remain to be arranged the three cubes of blood, muscle, and liver. These will all x-ray an almost identical medium gray, and you can remember that all moist solid or fluid-filled organs and tissue masses will have about the same radiodensity, greater than fat or air but considerably less than bone or metal. Thus the muscular heart with its blood-filled chambers could be expected to x-ray as

you see it on the chest film, a homogeneous mass much denser then the air-containing lung on both sides of it, but showing no differentiation between muscular ventricular wall and blood within the ventricle.

Remember that in the above discussion of relative radiodensities, we have kept thickness and form constant, as well as such technical factors as kilovoltage and time of exposure. I have planned this deliberately so that you might more easily build a working concept of the relative densities of different tissues. In practice, the radiologist adjusts the technical factors to accentuate these differences. Upon this useful spectrum of differing radiodensities of human tissues is based the whole field of medical radiography.

Once these considerations are learned, radiology becomes an exercise in logical deduction and an absorbing habit of mind. More important for you, it is also a delightful extra dimension in learning, a sort of custom-tailored illustrative tool related to nearly everything you will study in medical school. If you wish, you can use it to help you learn from the first day you begin to study anatomy, through your courses in physical diagnosis, pathology, medicine, and surgery, as a means of comprehending and remembering medical facts.

How Roentgen Shadows Inform Your Eye as to Form

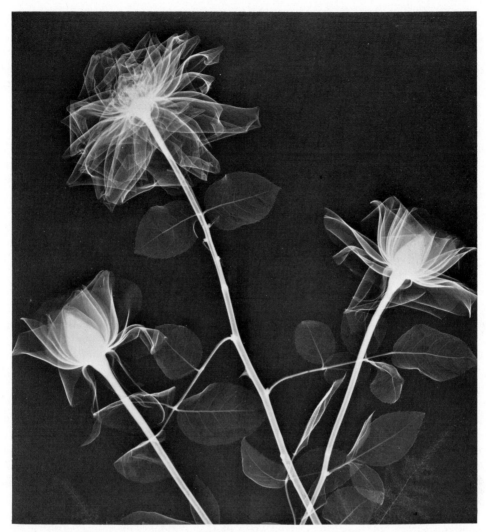

Figure 1-13

Consider now the contribution of *form*. Figure 1-13 is a radiograph of three roses, which we can use as an example of the basic logic of the roentgen shadows of complex objects. Flowers require only a very soft beam, of course, because they are both thin and delicate. A glance will tell you that one rose is full-blown and the other two more recently opened. You can deduce a great deal of information from the form, outline, shape, and structure of roentgen shadows. This is so true that in time you will learn to recognize with confidence the *identity* of certain shadows in medical radiographs because of their shape or form.

Now study the density of various parts of a single petal and compare the radiodensity, or whiteness, of the petals with that of the leaves. The leaves look less dense than the flowers and stems. Notice, too, that the veins within each leaf are denser than the rest of it. Veins of leaves have, of course, a structure independent of the cells composing the flatter part of the leaf. Stems are thicker and they also convey fluid. In both medical and nonmedical radiographs you can anticipate added density, in general, wherever there is fluid.

Radiographs Are Summation Shadowgrams

Another reason for the denser appearance of the petals compared with the leaves in Figure 1-13 is that they do not lie flat against the film but are curved and folded and overlap one another. This gives you a clue to a very important facet of radiologic interpretation. A sheet of any uniform composition, if it lies flat and parallel to the film, will have a uniform x-ray density and cast a homogeneous shadow. If it is curved, however, those parts which lie perpendicular to the plane of the film will radiograph as though they were much more dense.

This is perfectly simple. X-rays pass through a complex object and render upon the film not a picture at all but a "composite shadowgram," representing the sum of the densities interposed between beam source and film. Thus a sheet of rose petal which lies perpendicular to the film, or in the plane of the ray, is equivalent to many thicknesses of petal laid one upon another and, quite logically, is much more dense than a single sheet lying flat. Find the leaf which is turned on edge.

Curved sheets, considered geometrically, arrange themselves into groups of planes, if you will, and should be so considered in imagination when you are interpreting an x-ray film. Of course, in nature, and consequently in medicine, the curved plane is common and the symmetrical plane rare. In the radiograph of any curved-plane structure, therefore, learn to think in terms of those parts of it which are *relatively parallel to the film* and those which are *roughly perpendicular to it.*

Observe, finally, that the shadow of the stem of the rose in Figure 1-13 has a form you will find characteristic of any *tubular structure* of uniform composition. The margins are relatively dense because they represent long, curved planes radiographed tangentially, and the center area between them appears as a darker, more radiolucent streak. Rose stems are not truly hollow as one looks at them with the naked eye, but the central core, like that of tubular bones, is filled with a structure having less radiodensity. Hence that stem looks hollow and tubular on the film, just as a hollow tube containing air would look.

By this time you have several important principles clearly in mind, although you have learned them largely from examples. *First,* you know that x-rays are radiant energy of very short wavelength, beyond light in the electromagnetic spectrum, and that they penetrate, differently according to their wavelengths, substances opaque to light.

Second, you know that a beam of x-rays penetrates a complex object like the hand in accordance with the relative radiodensities of the materials which compose the object. You know that it produces on the film a composite shadowgram representing the sum of those radiodensities, layer for layer and part for part. You know that radiodensity is a function of atomic number and of thickness.

Third, you have realized that the parts of an object may become recognizable as to form, and their structure deduced, according to whether they are constructed most like solid or hollow spheres, cubes, or cylinders, or like plane sheets lying flat or curved upward away from the film.

Because I believe that the working of problems and puzzles will greatly increase your enjoyment of this book, I have included some in every chapter. They are geared to the chapter in question both in subject matter and in difficulty. In general, they are presented with a few details about the patient, and you should imagine yourself the intern or practicing physician in charge of that patient. Often, especially in the early chapters, you are asked not for a diagnosis but rather for an impression of variation from the normal of a particular structure. You will see that this will help you to gauge as you go along just how roentgen shadows can be reasoned out and used as a mnemonic device in learning medicine. I think it will also persuade you that you know more and can reason better than you had realized (a comforting thought). The answers are provided in Appendix A at the back of the book, and the Unknowns are numbered 1-1, 1-2, 1-3, etc., 2-1, 2-2, 2-3, etc., in relation to the chapter in which they appear.

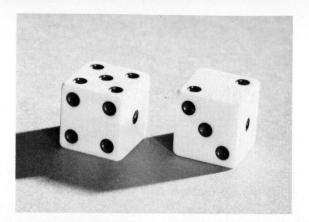

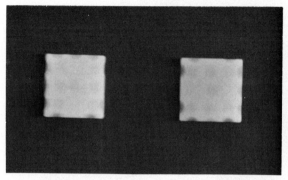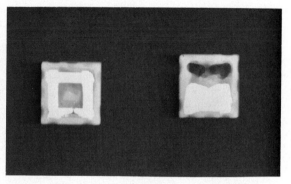

Figure 1-14 (*Unknown 1-1*). Sometimes the radiologist figures in criminology as an adjunctive source of information. The lucky throw you see in the innocent-looking pair of dice in the photograph was actually not luck at all but planned economy. Below are two radiographs, one of a pair of loaded dice and one of a pair of unloaded dice for which they could be switched. It is simple enough to decide which are the loaded dice, but can you figure out precisely what has been done to them?

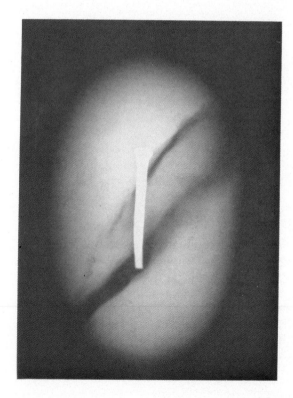

Figure 1-15 (*Unknown 1-2*). This is not a familiar object, and though you can figure out what its structure is from this, its radiograph, you will be very gifted indeed if you can say where it was when found.

CHAPTER **2** An Invitation to Think
Three-Dimensionally

Changes in Roentgen Shadows When You Change
Your Point of View or the Technique Used

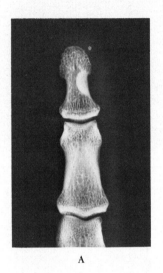 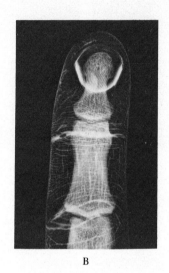 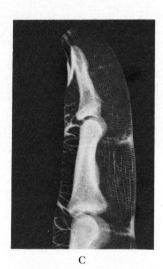

A   B   C

Figure 2-1

These three radiographs of a finger illustrate at once how important it is for you to learn to think in three dimensions about x-ray shadows. Note that the soft tissues in A are seen as a faint uniform gray outline encompassing the bones. In B and C, however, the skin with its wrinkles and folds as well as the crevice between the cuticle and nail all seem to become visible. This is because they have been coated with a creamy substance containing a metallic salt.

Actually, the skin itself is no more visible than it was before, but the radiopaque cream collecting on its patterned, irregular surface forms a visible coating which marks the position of the skin. A and B were made in the *frontal projection;* C is made from the side and is called a *lateral view.*

Although A probably looks very flat to you

and B and C give an illusion of depth, you will have realized that you can look at a medical x-ray film and *think about it three-dimensionally* even though you do not see it that way. The radiograph is a composite shadowgram and represents the added densities of many layers of tissue. One must think in layers when looking at any radiograph.

The most striking contrasts in radiodensity exist in the region of the chest, where air-filled lungs (radiolucent) on both sides of the muscular fluid-filled heart (relatively opaque) occupy the inside of a bony cage (a fretwork of crossed radiopaque strips). It is practical, therefore, to discuss the chest first in this book and to outline for you a system by which you can study chest radiographs.

12

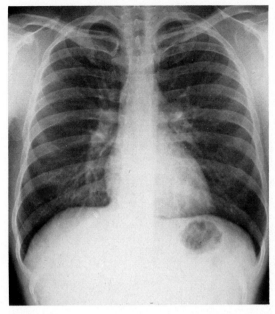

Figure 2-2A

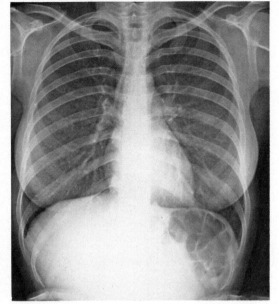

Figure 2-2B

The Routine Postero-Anterior (PA) Film

In Figure 2-2A imagine the structures through which the x-ray beam has passed from back to front: skin of the back; subcutaneous fat; lots of muscle encasing the flat blades of the scapulae, vertebral column, and posterior shell of the rib cage; then the lungs with the heart and other mediastinal structures between them; the sternum and anterior shell of the ribs; pectoral muscles and subcutaneous fat; breast tissue and, finally, skin.

Note the additional crescents of density that are added in Figure 2-2B, where the x-rays have had to traverse the female breast in addition to all the other tissue layers. Below the shadow of the breast and above that of the diaphragm the film is blacker where more rays have reached it.

One of the problems which will worry you as you begin looking at chest films will be how to put them up on the light boxes against which they are viewed: since they are transparent, you can look through them from either side. *Always place them so that you seem to be facing the patient.* Naturally this is only possible with PA and AP views.

X-ray films are usually marked by the technician to indicate which was the patient's right side, or, in the case of films of the extremities, whether it was his right or left leg, for example. In chest films one can usually be somewhat independent of the marker because the left ventricle and the arch of the aorta cast more prominent shadows on the left side of the patient's spine. Always view a chest film, then, so that the patient is facing you with his left on your right, and remember that when one says "left" in speaking of a finding on the film one invariably means the *patient's* left. When you read "the right breast is missing" you are going to check, automatically, the breast shadow to your left.

Most of the chest films you see will have been made with the beam passing in a sagittal direction "postero-anteriorly," the x-ray tube behind and the film in front of the patient. This is the standard PA chest film, and films of all kinds are called PA views *if the beam passes through the patient from back to front.* It has become customary to make a PA chest film of any patient who is able to stand and be positioned.

13

PA and AP Chest Films Compared

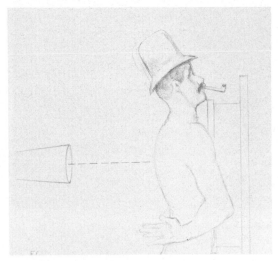

Figure 2-3. A (above left): Posteroanterior beam produces a PA chest film, the conventional view you see most often. B (above right): Anteroposterior beam produces an AP film. Note that the film is named for the direction the beam takes through the patient. (Drawings after Cézanne.)

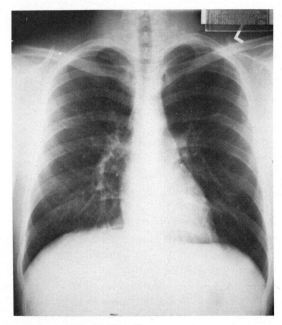

Figure 2-4A. PA chest film.

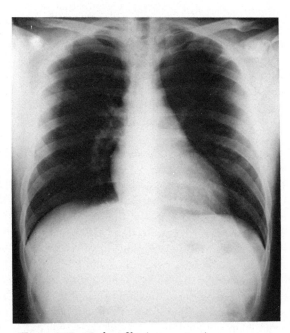

Figure 2-4B. AP chest film (same patient).

Less satisfactory but often valuable AP films of the chest are made when the patient is too sick to leave his bed. The patient is propped up against his pillows and the film is placed behind him, the exposure being made with a portable x-ray machine at the foot of the bed. Thus the ray passes through the patient "antero-posteriorly." You will be seeing such portable AP films of your very sick patients, and although they do not compare in quality with the PA films made with better technical facilities in the x-ray department, they do offer important information about the progress of the patient's disease. Sometimes a patient who cannot stand is not too sick to be taken in his bed to the x-ray department and filmed AP with the equipment available there, a better film being obtained in this way than is possible with the portable unit. Fluoroscopy can only be carried out in the x-ray department.

An AP film is not precisely comparable with the standards for normal which your eye will have set up for you based on the larger number of PA films you see. This is because the divergence of the rays enlarges the shadow of the heart, which is far anterior in the chest, and the position of the patient leaning back makes the posterior ribs look more horizontal. This is all particularly true at the shorter tube-film distances used in portable radiography.

The Lateral Chest Film

After the standard PA film, the next most common view of the chest is the "lateral." It is marked with an R or an L *according to whether the right or the left side of the patient was against the film.* Note how the ribs all seem roughly parallel, some pairs superimposed by the beam, forming a single denser white shadow. Mark how far the vertebral column projects into the chest. Large segments of lung extending farther back on either side of the spine are superimposed on it in the lateral view. You may not be able to tell whether you have a right or left lateral in your hand if the technician has forgotten the marker.

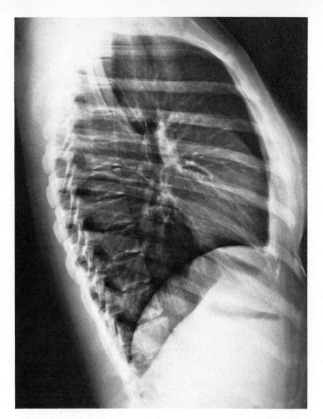

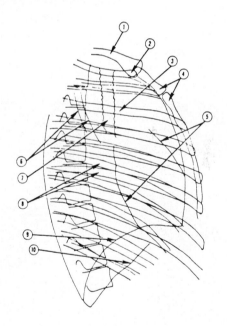

Figure 2-5 (above). Right lateral chest film.

Figure 2-6 (below). Labeled tracing of Figure 2-5: (1) clavicle, (2) medial end of the first rib, (3) pair of third ribs superimposed, (4) manubriosternal junction, (5) anterior and posterior surfaces of the heart, (6) scapulae, (7) air in the trachea, (8) pair of sixth ribs not superimposed, (9) and (10) right and left diaphragms.

15

The Lordotic View

Here is a patient who was admitted to the hospital with a persistent cough, one episode of blood-streaked sputum, weight loss, and a daily fever. The routine PA chest film in Figure 2-7 is not strikingly abnormal at first glance, but there was a strong clinical suspicion of pulmonary tuberculosis, so a special projection called a *lordotic view* was made. Here because the patient stands leaning backward in exaggerated lordosis, the horizontal beam of AP x-rays foreshortens the chest by penetrating it at such an oblique angle that the anterior and posterior segments of the same ribs are superimposed. The result of this maneuver is, of course, to project the clavicles upward so that by looking between the ribs one can much more effectively visualize the lung tissue of the apex. Note that this case is a good exercise in the use of *bilateral symmetry* in examining films made with a sagittal beam. Now one is able to see that there *is* a fluffy white shadow in the upper part of the left lung, best seen in the second interspace. Note that there is nothing like it in the same interspace on the other side. Analysis of the patient's sputum confirmed the diagnosis of tuberculosis.

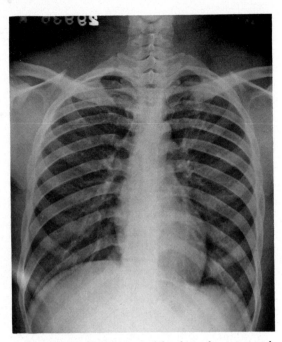

Figure 2-7. Standard PA view of the chest of a patient with cough, fever, weight loss, and hemoptysis.

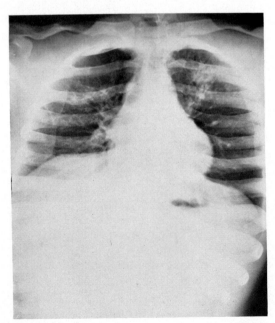

Figure 2-8. Special lordotic view of the chest of the same patient.

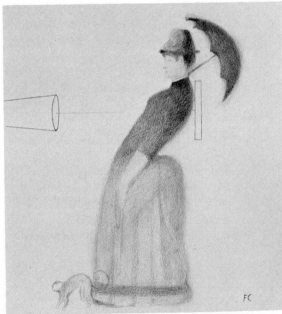

Figure 2-9. Position in which Figure 2-8 was made.

16

The chest film in Figure 2-10 offers you an opportunity to test your progress in three-dimensional thinking. It has an obvious artifact of metallic radiodensity. The shape of the metal object suggests it might be a bullet. This, in fact, is a film made on a soldier wounded in the Sicilian campaign during World War II. He was invalided out to a hospital, where the surgeons observed what you observe. They requested, as you are about to do, a lateral view to determine the location of the bullet. It might, of course, be in any of the structures whose roentgen shadows superimpose in this view on the origin of the fifth rib.

The importance of localizing a bullet is illustrated by the cross-section drawing. If the bullet is lodged in the spinal cord or the trachea, or in one of the major vascular structures at this level, there may be less hope of saving the patient. In point of fact, the bullet was located harmlessly in the anterior mediastinum, had not injured any vital structure, and was removed without incident. (For the lateral view see Figure 2-12, next page.)

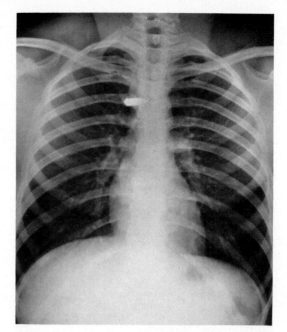

Figure 2-10

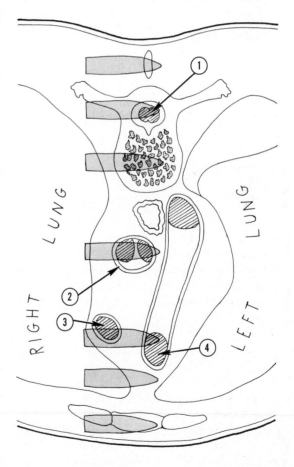

Figure 2-11

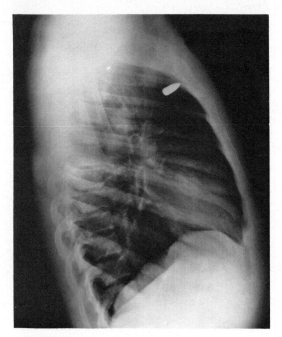

Figure 2-12

At about this point you will begin to say to yourself, "How am I going to know which views are important for me to understand and learn to use?" If, in the course of your training in medicine, you can familiarize yourself with the chest structures and their shadows *as seen in the standard PA and lateral views,* you will have built yourself a very useful and satisfying tool, and you should have no trouble in doing so. Do not feel confused or defeated if occasionally you see a chest film which looks like nothing you have ever seen before. Some of these will be in fact films of grossly abnormal chests. Others, however, will turn out to be films made by special or rarely used x-ray projections and procedures with which you are not yet familiar. You should rely comfortably on your acquaintance with the standard views, but not be incurious or resistant to the possibilities of other modes of examination.

There are all sorts of ingenious obliquities of projection and many fascinating special procedures in the armamentarium of the radiologist which you will want to know about. Two of them, the posteroanterior obliques of the chest, are sometimes used in studying the heart. Detailed study of the ribs is obtained by obliques made anteroposteriorly with a Bucky diaphragm, as will be discussed later. Others, designed for visualizing a particular structure in a particular way, also offer anatomic information not otherwise available. Sometimes these views or procedures are carried out at the discretion of the radiologist and on his initiation. At other times you will ask for them specifically or, better yet, discuss with a radiologist the advantages of their being used in the study of your patient's particular problem.

You can never know precisely where a foreign body is located from a single radiograph. A film made at right angles to the first is essential, and minute metallic foreign bodies in the eye are localized very accurately by a refinement of this procedure. Fractured bones can appear to be in good position, end to end, in one film, although a second film made at right angles shows that the fragments are separated and do not align. Often the taking of such supplementary lateral films is a routine matter. At other times you will have to ask that they be taken on your patients. Always ask for a right lateral chest film if you think the lesion is on the right, so that the structure to be studied is as close as possible to the film. In most clinics in this country a chest series includes a PA chest film and a *left* lateral. Can you decide why?

18

Body-Section Radiographs or Tomograms

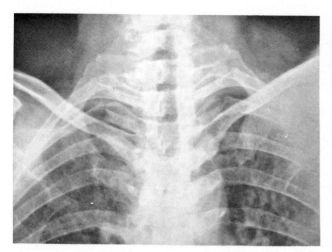 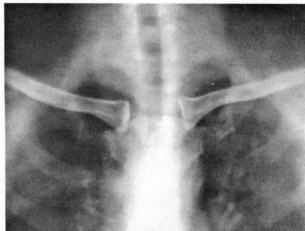

Figure 2-13A   Figure 2-13B

The two films in Figure 2-13A and B were made of the same patient. A, on the left, is an ordinary PA radiograph; B is a special-procedure film called a "body-section radiograph." This type of study is going to be very useful to you throughout this book and will help you to visualize better the shadows which must be added together to make up the usual x-ray film. It is important, therefore, to understand how body-section radiographs are made.

Imagine that a frozen cadaver is sawed into *coronal* slices about 1 inch thick and that you then make a radiograph of each slice. Each film will have on it only the shadows cast by the densities of the structures in that slice. There will be no confusing superimposition of the shadows of structures from other slices to trouble you. How much simpler it would be, for example, to be able to study the manubrium and medial halves of the clavicles if they were not superimposed upon the shadow of the thoracic spine as they are in the standard PA chest film. On the next few pages you will find some radiographed slices of such a cadaver to study. They are arranged in order from front to back, the very first slice having been omitted. (It included the anterior chest wall, rib cartilages, and sternum.) You will find it helpful to refer back to these slices as you learn the x-ray appearance of various organs and structures.

Notice how well you can see in Figure 2-13B the shadows cast by the clavicles where they join the manubrium.

Body-section studies (like those in Figure 2-13B above) effectively slice the living patient so that you can study the shadows cast by certain structures free of superimposed shadows. The term body-section radiograph is a general one and there are different types of sectioning studies, the techniques of which depend upon the result desired, this is, the shadows intended for study and those one wishes to distort. You will hear the terms laminagram, tomogram, and computerized tomogram. All are body-section studies. On first acquaintance they will all look blurred and confusing to you, but in this book you will be shown many paired studies so that you have the usual x-ray film in the same projection for comparison. Whenever you are puzzled by one of them, try coming back to the cadaver slices to get your bearings, remembering that *only the structures in one plane will be in focus in the section study*. Remember too that the thickness of these particular cadaver slices may not match perfectly the chosen plane of the section study you happen to be looking at, since the pivot point determining the plane of a body-section study is calculated arbitrarily for a certain distance in centimeters from the surface of the chest.

19

Coronal Slices of a Frozen Cadaver Radiographed

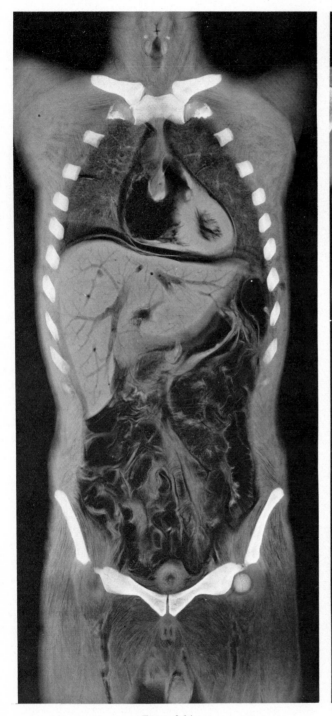

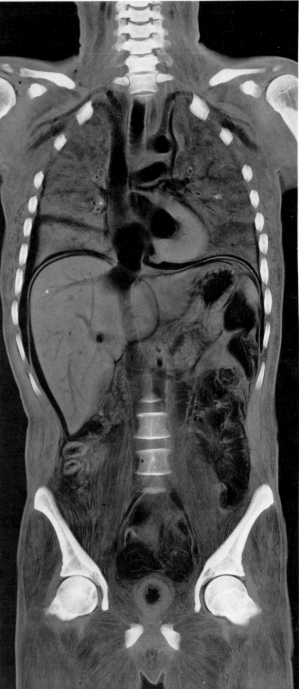

Figure 2-14

Figure 2-15

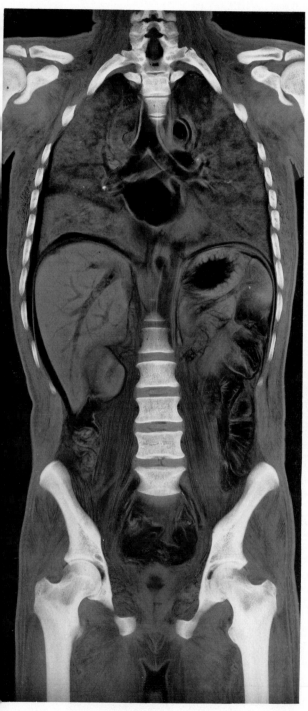

Figure 2-16

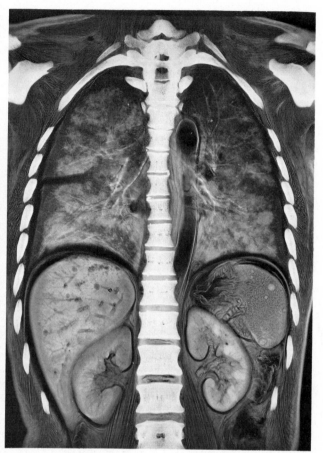

Figure 2-17

Figures 2-14 to 2-17. Radiographs of a series of coronal slices of cadaver, arranged from front to back. Identify the following:

Junction of manubrium and clavicles
Superior vena cava (empty and filled with air)
Fundus of the stomach
 (Each of the above locates the level of the slice, just as a
 body-section study would identify the level of the slice by
 including certain structures and excluding others.)
Symphysis pubis
Empty cavity of the left ventricle
Trachea, carina, and major bronchi with the air-filled left
 atrium immediately below them

Note the change in shape of the liver from section to section.

Tomograms Give You Radiographs of Slices
of the Living Patient (here in the coronal plane).

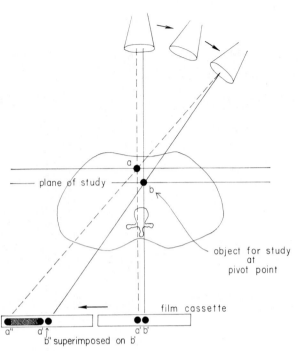

Figure 2-18. Tomogram for a coronal slice.

Technically this is done by *moving both the x-ray tube and the film around the patient during the exposure.* They are moved about a pivot point calculated to fall in the plane of the object to be studied. In this way the shadows of all the structures *not* in the plane selected for study are *intentionally blurred* because they move relative to the film. Thus, in the diagram (Figure 2-18) the object to be studied, *b*, will be "in focus" on the film, while the shadow of an object at *a* will be magnified, blurred, and distorted to lie between *a'* and *a"* on the film. Only the structures in the plane of the pivot point will be recognizable (as in Figure 2-19C); the shadows representing organs in front of or behind it are distorted in such a way that shape and form are no longer recognizable and the blurred images are easy for your eye to ignore.

B

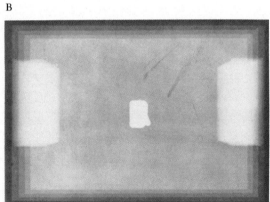

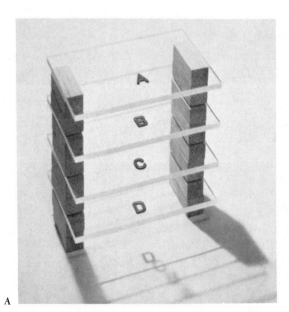

A

Figure 2-19. Demonstration of the effect obtained with body-section studies. A: Series of plastic shelves each holding a lead letter superimposed vertically. B: Conventional radiograph superimposes the shadows of the letters. C: Body-section study at level of "C" shows that letter clearly but distorts and blurs the others.

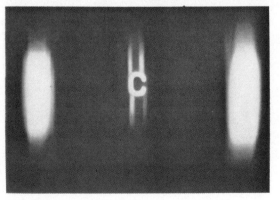

C

Computerized Axial Tomography

Currently an exciting new procedure is evolving in radiology, the "cat" scan (CAT, CT, CTT, EMI—all synonyms). This was first developed in England specifically as an adjunct to the radiologic investigation of intracranial problems. Its unique value lies in the fact that by adding computer techniques to tomography, for example of the brain, gray matter can actually be differentiated from white matter.

The practical clinical application did not occur until 1973. Up to that time the plain-film radiographic density of all intracranial contents was identical and no resolution of interfaces could be expected between parts of the normal brain, tumor, hemorrhage, or fluid in the ventricles. Now, in patients with head injuries, for example, subdural hemorrhage can be detected by CT as different from brain tissue, without the use of more complex or invasive diagnostic methods. You would not be able to function in your practice of clinical medicine without a sound understanding of general radiology and the way in which it has been expanded in usefulness through computerized tomography.

You can begin by understanding how computerized tomography differs from ordinary tomography, which we have just discussed on the opposite page. If you conceive of the body as a three-dimensional complex of miniature 1-millimeter cubes of tissue, then any body-section slice (for example a cross section in the transaxial plane of the body) can be considered as *a mosaic of cubes one cube thick. Remember that the convention says you are always looking at the lower face of the slice from the patient's feet.* In the simplified example of one design of CT scanner above (Figure 2-20), an electronic detector moves continuously in an arc of 180 degrees around the patient while receiving the transmitted x-ray beam emerging from the slice. The detector continuously converts the information it receives into amplified electrical pulses, which are recorded and stored in a computer. These pulses vary in intensity in proportion to the degree of *attenuation* or *absorption* of the x-ray beam through that particular diagonal line of cubes. The electronic detector device is one hundred times more sensitive to the absorption differences of tissues than conventional x-ray film is known to be.

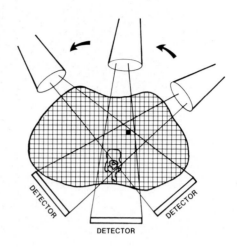

Figure 2-20. Computerized tomography.

Thus if the one cube shown near the center of the mosaic slice above contains a good deal of calcium, the part of the beam passing through it is partially absorbed (attenuated) each time it is recorded by the detector-computer. The uncalcified tissue cubes around it absorb very little of the beam by comparison, and the detector converts those portions of the beam into much more intense pulses for the computer to record.

The computer then calculates the *average* absorption of each of the cubes that make up the slice (among them our hypothetical calcium-containing cube). The resulting average numbers can be printed on paper. This composes a map of the densities of all the cubes constituting the slice, and when those numbers are reproduced on a screen as dots, the brightness of which conforms to the density of the cube of tissue it represents, it will resemble the known cross-sectional slice of the human body. Computerized transaxial tomography thus provides us with slices of the living human body expressed in terms of density much more discriminatory than those of ordinary radiographic images.

23

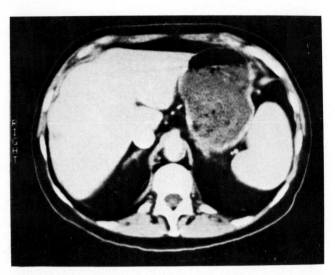

Figure 2-21. CT scan of the upper abdomen.

You are looking up from the patient's feet at a map of the densities in the slice through the patient's liver, which looks very much like a radiograph of an axial slice of patient would look (sections of rib and vertebral body are dense white as they would look in a radiograph if one were able to x-ray a cross-section slice of the living patient). The straight line, black above and gray below, is a *fluid level* of contrast material (dense) in the stomach with air (lucent) above it. Since the patient is lying on his back on the table we *see* the fluid level.

The gray round object just anterior to the body of the vertebra is the aorta. This image is telling you that the cluster of cubes in the mosaic which represents the cross-sectioned aorta is denser than the fat surrounding it, but not so dense as the bone in the vertebral body posterior to it.

You will be seeing many more computerized tomograms as we go on from chapter to chapter in the book whenever they are of particular use as an adjunct to radiologic diagnosis.

Now try your hand at the following unknowns as a review of the reasoning behind the various types of imaging you have been considering in this chapter.

The end in view in showing you these two unknowns is to see whether you can figure out precisely what was being radiographed.

Since each of the individual average numbers the computer produces represents the density of a particular cube of the mosaic slice from which it was made, it is easy to imagine a hypothetical slice like the one in Figure 2-20 with a single dense calcium-containing cube or cluster of cubes surrounded by much less dense ones.

These density numbers are related to the attenuation coefficient values of the cubes they represent in contrast to that of water—taken as zero, an arbitrarily assigned value. Thus materials having attenuation coefficient values greater than water (like our calcium-containing cube) will have *positive* CT numbers (expressed in *Hounsfield units*, after one of the inventors of CT). Those with densities less than water will have *negative* CT numbers. Examples: air is −500 and bone +500. Fat, protein, and body fluids lie somewhere in between.

The density numbers are assigned a specific shade of gray or color for viewing on a screen (TV monitor) and permanent images are obtained by photographing the screen. In Figure 2-21 you see such a photographic record of a computerized tomogram taken through the abdomen.

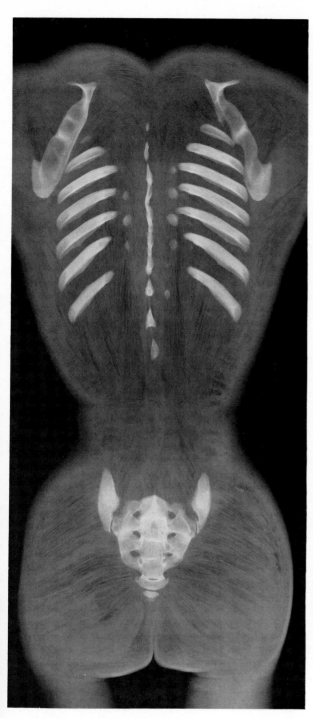

Figure 2-22 (*Unknown 2-1*).

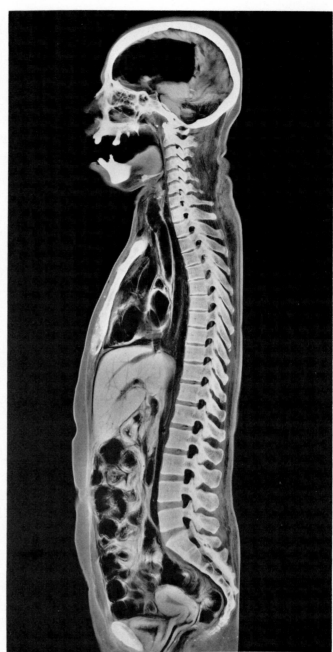

Figure 2-23 (*Unknown 2-2*).

CHAPTER 3   How to Study a Chest Film

Hardly anyone ever reads the preface to a book, but if you read mine, you know that the goal of this book is twofold: to help the medical student understand x-ray shadows as an aid to learning in the other disciplines, and to equip him with a basic knowledge of the reasons for the roentgen appearance of some of the common disease conditions he will meet as a physician. It is my hope that those who study this book will develop a habit of mind in which every shadow on the radiograph arouses the responsive question, "*Why* does it look like that?"

One glance at a chest film is often enough to "see" a very striking abnormality. Having seen it, the observer must reason out its structural identity, seldom quite so obvious, and attempt to deduce the nature of it in accord with his knowledge of the patient's illness. While the single-glance approach has its value, it is full of danger to the patient, because the presence of a very obvious abnormality tends to suppress psychologically your search for more subtle changes. And the subtler changes are quite often more important to the patient than the obvious ones.

Let us say that you correctly interpret the shadow of a large mass in the lung on Mr. B's chest film (Figure 3-2A) as being consistent with the cancer you thought he might have when you examined him. You will have failed him if you neglect a deliberate quest for any possible secondary involvement of his bones, since quite a different program of treatment may then become appropriate. Figure 3-2B illustrates the point by showing in more detail, with a more penetrating x-ray beam, the extent of his bone destruction.

The system generally employed by the radiologist is to *look at* various structures in a deliberate order, concentrating on the anatomy of each while excluding the superimposed shadows of other structures. Even as an exercise in intellectual discipline, this is not as difficult as it

sounds. Prove it to your own satisfaction by trying to *look at* one clavicle or one rib on any of the chest films in this chapter, thinking of its normal anatomic proportions and excluding other shadows overlying it which you know are not part of the bone you are studying.

The best way to be systematic about studying any film is to adopt a definite order in which you look at the structures whose shadows appear there. For a chest film you will *look at* the bony framework and then, just as deliberately, *look through it* at lung tissue and the heart.

Begin with the scapulae. Then look at the portions of humerus and shoulder joint often visible on the chest film. Inspect the clavicles, and then finally study the ribs, quickly but in pairs from top to bottom. When you can, always compare the two sides for symmetry. The spine and sternum are, of course, superimposed upon each other and upon the dense shadows of the mediastinal structures in the PA view so that, at the kilovoltages used for lung study, little of the beam penetrates and the film remains unexposed down the midline.

Remember that the technique used for chest films has been designed for study of the lung: what you see of the bones is incidental. Ideal techniques for studying these same bones will be quite different. In a PA chest film, for example, the scapulae and posterior ribs are as far as possible from the film. Therefore they are enlarged and distorted to some extent. In addition, on the chest film the scapulae have been intentionally rotated to the sides as much as they can be by placing the hands on the hips, palms out, with the elbows forward. Try it. In the PA view of the chest this maneuver prevents the superimposition of the scapular shadows upon the upper lung fields, and only the medial margin of the scapula will be seen overlapping the axillary portions of the upper ribs. Decide whether the scapulae were properly rotated in Figure 3-1.

26

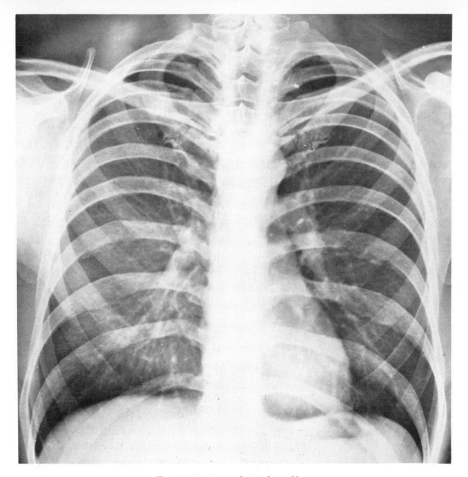

Figure 3-1. Normal PA chest film.

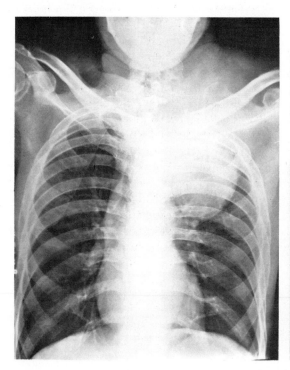

Figure 3-2. A (left): PA chest film of Mr. B, admitted with cough, chest pain, hoarseness, and a fist-sized mass in the left supraclavicular region. B (below): Detail study of the thoracic inlet made AP with a more penetrating beam. Left posterior first rib and parts of the first two thoracic vertebrae have been destroyed by tumor.

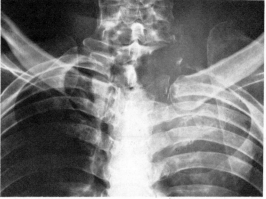

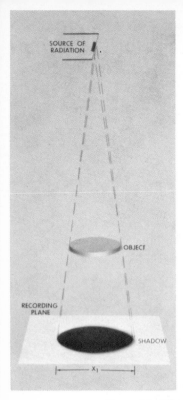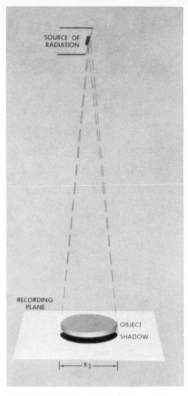

Figure 3-3. Effect of projection in enlarging the roentgen shadows of objects far away from film.

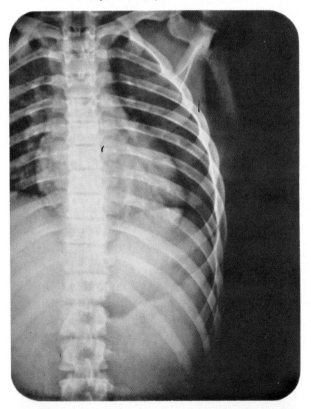

Figure 3-4. AP view of the chest made with the posterior ribs close to the film. The heart, far from the film, is projected and looks larger than normal.

Do not discount the factor of projection in altering the appearance of structures far away from the film. You need not be confused by such changes, however, once you are familiar with them. In Figure 3-3 you have a diagram illustrating the effect of projection, in which you can equate the "object" with the scapula in any AP and PA chest film. You can equate it also with the anteriorly placed heart in the AP film, Figure 3-4. Note that the heart in this film appears to be larger with less sharp margins than the hearts in the PA chest films you have seen up to now. Note also the slight difference in the width and shape of the posterior interspaces compared with those on the usual PA film.

The routine chest film measures 14 by 17 inches, and its cassette film holder is placed with the long dimension vertical. In broadchested persons little of the *shoulder girdle* and *humerus* will be seen, but in slender, smaller individuals you may actually have all of the shoulder and most of the upper arm to study. Figure 3-5 is a radiograph of the shoulder made AP. Figure 3-6, next to it, is a photograph of the bones of the shoulder so that you can look back and forth. Notice how you seem to see the coracoid *through* the spine of the scapula because they superimpose, just as you see the head of the humerus and the acromion additively.

The man in Figure 3-7 had fallen from a horse and had his arm immobilized in plaster (*a,a*), which you see more densely wherever the ray came through it tangentially. Since there are several fractures and several fragments, this is what is called a *comminuted* fracture. Note the folds and wrinkles in the plaster and the point in the axilla where the cast ends (*b*).

The woman in Figure 3-8 could not comb her hair or tie her apron strings without intense pain in her shoulder. She had tenderness over the insertion of the supraspinatus tendon and, as you see, she has *calcification* in that area and around the shoulder joint—dense white shadows not present on any of the x-rays of normal shoulder

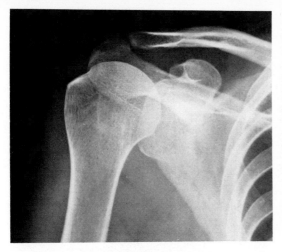

Figure 3-5. Identify: clavicle, acromioclavicular joint, head and greater tuberosity of humerus, glenoid, acromion, and coracoid process.

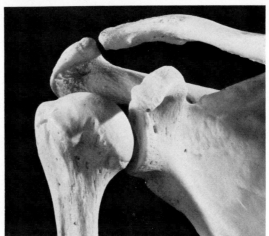

Figure 3-6. Photograph of the bones of the shoulder.

you have seen so far. These findings (b) are typical of "bursitis" or calcific peritendinitis of the shoulder.

Note the dense white triangular shadow medial to the midhumerus (a) in Figure 3-8. It is common in radiology and is called an "overlap shadow." It is created in this instance by the *added densities* of heavy breast and soft tissues of the upper arm. The confusion arising from the unexpected density of the shadow at a will

be easy for you to resolve if you remember that *thickness* as well as *composition* determines radiodensity. Although fat, skin, and muscle ought to be less radiodense than bone, the shadow cast by a thick mass of these tissues will approach that of bone as you see it in this figure. Note, on the other hand, that a small amount of air imprisoned in the axilla is black on the film, probably because it was a long pocket of air x-rayed end-on.

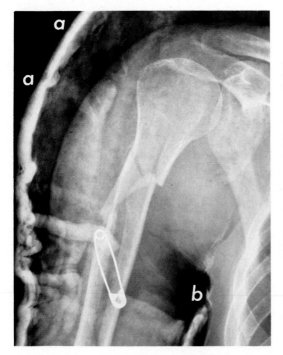

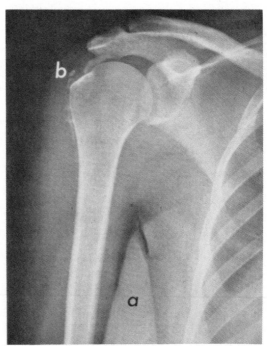

Figures 3-7 (left) and 3-8 (right). Two patients with shoulder pain.

Systematic Study of the Rib Cage

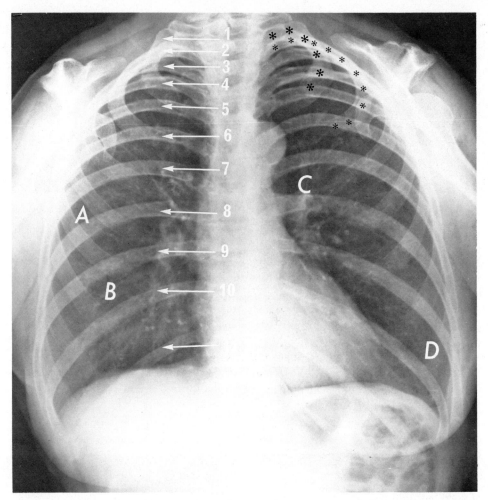

Figure 3-9. Counting and identifying ribs and rib interspaces is an important part of the systematic chest film survey. (See text for instructions.) Note, incidentally, that the breast shadows in this patient come well below the level of the diaphragm and do not obscure the lower lung field; in many female patients they do.

Using the bilateral symmetry of each pair of ribs in Figure 3-9, and beginning at the origin of the first rib at its junction with the first thoracic vertebra, trace each rib as far as you can anteriorly to the beginning of the radiolucent (and hence invisible) costal cartilage. The ribs are useful to the radiologist because he locates an abnormal shadow by its proximity to a particular rib or interspace on a film he is describing. Anyone reading his written report can identify in this way the precise shadow he was discussing. Thus A in Figure 3-9 could be described as lying in the seventh interspace on the right close to the axilla (that is, the outer third of the space between the posterior halves of the right seventh and eighth ribs). If you do not locate it there, count again, for you are probably getting lost in the overlap tangle of ribs 1, 2, and 3. To avoid this, identify carefully the first rib by finding its anterior junction with the manubrium and following this rib *backward* to the spine. Then count down the posterior ribs. B would be said to be located in the ninth interspace on the right. Note that the word "interspace" always implies the space between *posterior* segments of adjoining ribs unless the anterior is specified. Try your hand at designating the location of C and D, covering the left half of this figure and the spine with all its numbers. (Have you noticed anything peculiar about this film? Is there anything missing?)

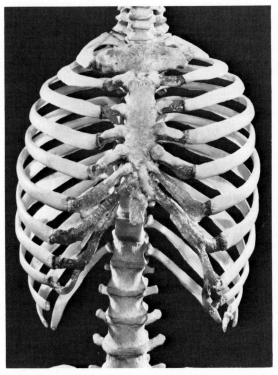

A

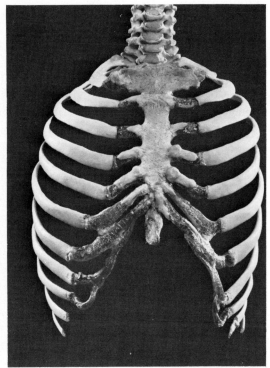

B

Figure 3-10. The bony thorax photographed in a way to help you visualize chest films three-dimensionally. Imagine the location of the diaphragm in each figure—then turn the page. B and C were photographed with the thoracic cage stuffed with black velvet.

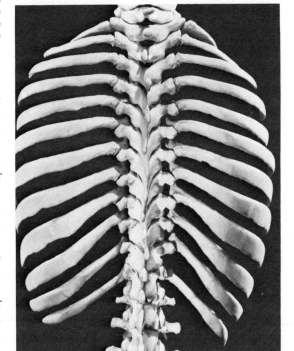

C

The *ribs* confuse everyone beginning to look at chest films. The miracle is that one can discern anything useful about the heart and lungs through such a crosshatched pattern of shadows. Three-dimensional thinking will be easier if you try to concentrate first on the posterior halves of the ribs and then the anterior. In Figure 3-10B and C the same thorax was photographed from the front and from the back after the cavity had been stuffed with black velvet to give you the illusion you seek in trying to study the posterior ribs while excluding from your mind the anterior ones.

Warning! Remember to think in terms of *coronal* slices and the summation shadows they produce, as in the cadaver in Chapter 2. The *transaxial* shadows usually used in CT are useful, too, in three-dimensional thinking, and we will return to them presently.

Rotation Produces Confusing Shadows

Because of their curiously curved shape, the shadows of the two *clavicles* will appear symmetrical on the chest film only if there is no rotation of the chest. In a perfectly true PA film the beam passes straight through the midsagittal plane. The arms and shoulders of the patient are arranged symmetrically, and the technician checks for rotation and corrects it before making the exposure. Turned even a few degrees, the clavicles will exhibit a remarkable degree of asymmetry. This fact will prove very useful to you, because a glance at the clavicles will tell you whether or not the beam has passed through the sagittal plane and whether you are therefore looking at a true PA or AP film without rotation.

Even slight rotation is undesirable in a chest film, because the heart and mediastinum are then radiographed obliquely and their shadows appear enlarged and distorted. If you think of the mediastinum as a disc of denser structures

flattened between the two inflated lungs and normally x-rayed end-on in a PA chest film, it is easy to see how rotation of this disc will produce a wider shadow. If it were a valid finding, enlargement of the heart or widening of the mediastinal shadow would be an important piece of roentgen evidence for disease. One has to be able to disregard apparent enlargement due to rotation, therefore, and the best clue to rotation is asymmetry of the shadows of the two clavicles. Learn to watch them, mentally noting their symmetry or lack of it, in your systematic survey of the chest film.

Now look back at Figure 3-9. Did you notice that there were no clavicles? The patient was born without them and is an ideal subject on whom to learn to count ribs. Compare this with any normal chest film and observe that you can mentally subtract the shadow of the clavicle when you want to in order to study or count the first three ribs.

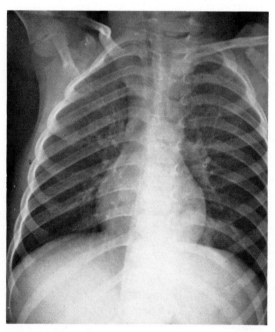

Figure 3-11. Chest film made when the patient was accidentally somewhat rotated. Note marked asymmetry of the clavicles.

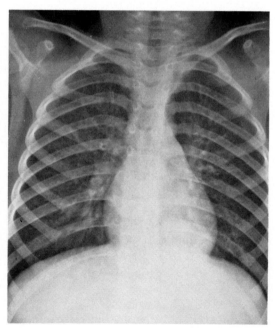

Figure 3-12. Same patient refilmed precisely PA.

Problems in Studying Ribs and Clavicles

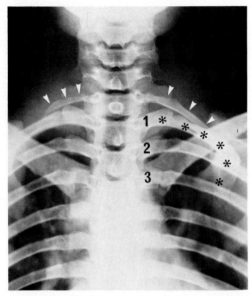

Figure 3-13 (*Unknown 3-1*). If you think the ribs are correctly labeled here, how do you account for the structures indicated by white arrows?

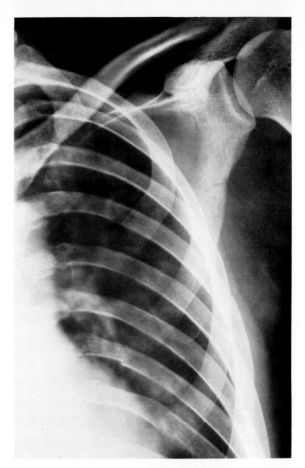

Figure 3-14 (*Unknown 3-2*). This patient has been filmed after an automobile accident. Which rib is fractured?

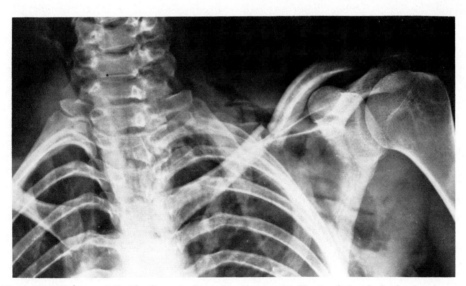

Figure 3-15 (*Unknown 3-3*). The figure is obviously not a true PA film (medial end of right clavicle seen overlying fourth interspace) for the very good reason that the patient was in a great deal of pain. Study the bones, using normal shoulder girdle in Figure 3-14 for comparison. Then study the soft tissues outside the chest cage around the shoulder girdle, also comparing those in Figure 3-14. How do you account for the dark streaks?

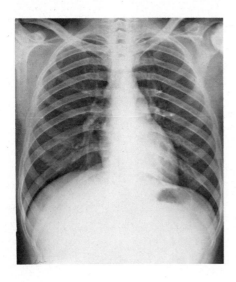

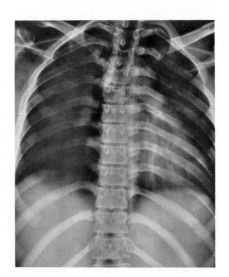

Figure 3-16 (left). Regular chest film made PA at 6 feet with the patient standing.

Figure 3-17 (right). AP film of the chest exposed for study of the spine. Patient lying down. Bucky diaphragm used. Ideal exposure for a chest film today is somewhere in between these two and allows faint visualization of the intervertebral spaces through the heart.

The thoracic spine is not well seen in the chest films you have been looking at because its density added to those of the mediastinal structures and sternum together absorb almost all the rays and few reach the film to blacken it. This is true of the techniques commonly used for studying the lung. Seeing detail through very dense parts of the body requires a different technique. More penetration can be achieved in several ways. One is by increasing the exposure factors (kilovoltage, milliamperage, and time) to produce a beam of x-rays of shorter wavelength, so-called harder rays. A film made in this way is often called an "overexposed film," intentionally overexposed in order to increase the penetration of dense structures.

Unfortunately, when x-rays impinge on matter of any kind, secondary x-rays are generated which radiate in all directions as from many point sources of light. This is called "scattered radiation" and is, of course, added photographically to the primary beam, additionally blackening the film. Since there are thus multiple sources of radiation, a blurred and distorted image is produced. Moreover, increasing the exposure factors to produce a harder and more penetrating beam also increases the amount of scattered radiation. Thus, a simple overexposed film will usually be lacking in contrast and sharpness.

Scattered radiation can be eliminated by an ingenious device called the *Bucky diaphragm.* Interposed between the patient and the film, it is a flat grid composed of alternate very thin strips of radiolucent and radiopaque material (wood and lead, for example). Only the most perpendicular rays pass through the lucent strips. The oblique rays, representing most of the scattered radiation, strike the sides of the lead strips and are absorbed.

If the interposed grid is motionless, of course, the lead strips will appear on the film as fine white lines. To prevent this, it is only necessary to move the grid across the film all during the exposure; no lines will appear.

You will find that in an obese patient, or in any patient whose spine, mediastinum, skull, or heavy long bones must be studied by x-ray, Bucky-technique films will have been made automatically by the technician. Every film of the abdomen which you will see will have been made in this way also.

The PA chest film in Figure 3-16 was made expressly for the purpose of studying the lung. Figure 3-17 was made AP (so that the spine toward which the study was directed would be close to the film), and a Bucky diaphragm and the appropriate exposure technique were used to produce it. Notice how well you can see the structure of the vertebrae with their interposed

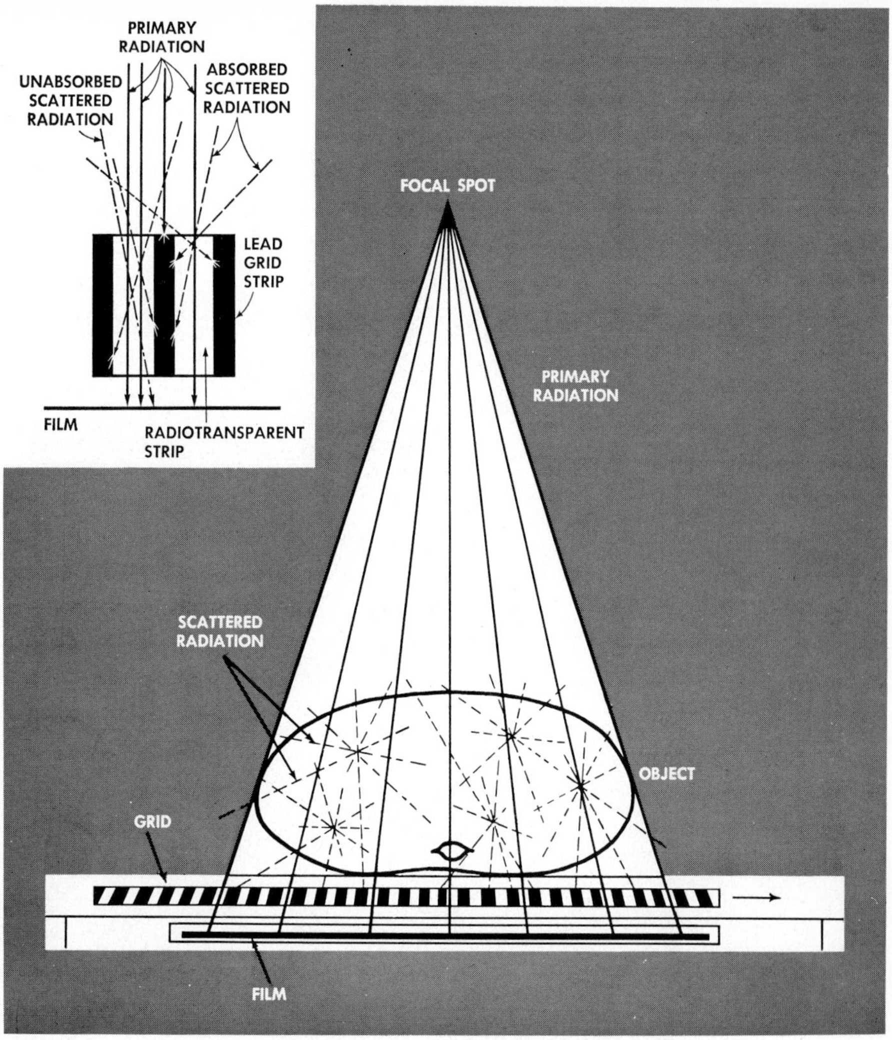

Figure 3-18. The Bucky diaphragm, plus increased kilovoltage and time, give the desired increased penetration and clearer detail to radiographs of thick parts of the body (see text).

cartilaginous discs, which should be just visible in a routine chest film. Note also that here you can see the ribs below the diaphragm, scarcely visible in most regular chest films. This film would be useless for studying the lung, all the delicate detail being lost.

Just as the lung detail is "burned out" with these techniques, so also are the soft tissues of the chest lying outside the thoracic cage. Having completed your survey of the bones, you should now *look at* these soft tissues, studying breast tissues, supraclavicular areas, axillae, and the tissue along the sides of the chest. You will be able to study them in any film exposed for study of the lungs, and soft tissues often give you important information about the patient. Are his soft tissues scanty, indicating perhaps that he has lost weight? Are the normally symmetrical triangles of dark fat in the supraclavicu-

lar region disturbed in any way? Look back at Figure 3-2A and at Unknown 3-3. Always be sure to check whether there are two breasts; a chest film showing one missing breast often means that the patient is being studied for recurrence of cancer, and attention should be directed toward bones and lung field for evidence of metastases. The lung field under a missing breast appears a little darker than the other lung field because of the missing breast and pectoral muscles removed at the time of the mastectomy. Look forward a few pages, identifying the female patients, and see if you can find one with a breast missing on the left.

So much, then, for the first step in studying a chest film: a systematic survey of the bones and soft tissues. You are now ready to look past the bones at the shadow of the lung itself.

CHAPTER 4 The Lung Itself

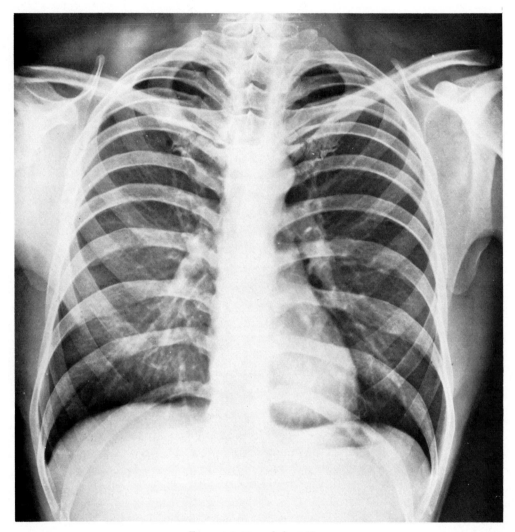

Figure 4-1. Normal chest film.

Look now past all those distracting shadows of the ribs and soft tissues at the roentgen images which belong to the lung itself. Because of its contained air the normally expanded lung is largely radiolucent, as we have said, but nevertheless you do see in Figure 4-1 traceries of branching gray linear shadows. What precisely are they? You can reason it out.

Reflect first that logically any structure of greater radiodensity suspended in the middle of a radiolucent structure like the lung will absorb some of the x-rays and cast a gray shadow on the film, a patch of film where less silver has been precipitated.

If this structure is spherical and of uniform composition, it will cast a round shadow. If the

36

surface of the mass is knobby and irregular, knobs will be present in the outline as in Figure 4-2. If the suspended dense structure is cylindrical, like a blood-filled vessel traversing lung substance, a tapering linear gray shadow results, and if the vessel branches, the shadow will be seen to branch.

When a vessel passes through the lung in a direction roughly parallel to the film (and perpendicular to the ray), its tapering and its branching will be accurately rendered on the PA film. But if it passes through the lung in a more nearly sagittal direction, it will then line up with the beam, absorbing more x-rays so that its shadow will appear as a dense round spot. The situation is analogous to the rose leaf on edge in the first chapter. You can find such end-on vessels in Figure 4-1, or in any chest film.

That the normal "lung markings," as the radiologist calls these linear shadows, are indeed vessels and not bronchi and bronchioles is also quite logical. The bronchial tree, being air filled and thin walled, casts little or no shadow when it is normal. It is practical, therefore, to think of the normal lung markings as wholly vascular.

The tracheobronchial tree may be *rendered visible*, of course, with relatively harmless radiopaque fluids instilled via a tracheal catheter into the lung of a living patient, who later coughs up or absorbs and excretes the opaque substance. This procedure, called *bronchography*, is carried out under local anesthesia to depress the cough reflex and provides important information about patients with bronchiectasis.

Figure 4-2. Mass suspended in air-filled lung casts a shadow recording its knobby outline.

Figure 4-3A. The tracheobronchial tree coated with opaque material, a bronchogram. Vessels filled with blood are only faintly seen.

Figure 4-3B. Regular chest film. Air column in trachea, but rest of tracheobronchial tree not visible at all. Note faint vascular shadows.

Figure 4-2

Figure 4-3A

Figure 4-3B

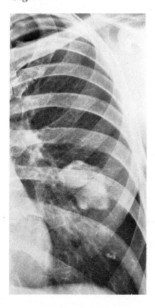
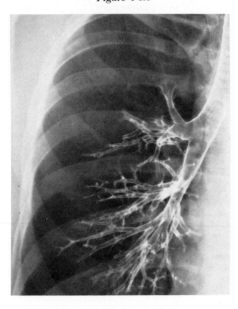
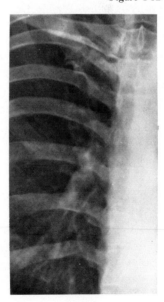

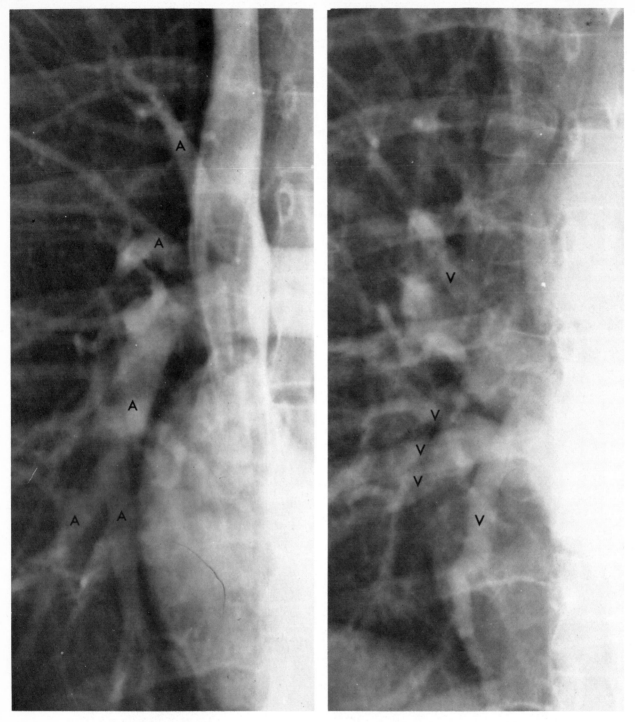

Figure 4-4

Figure 4-5

The *vascular tree* within the lung may also be further opacified in the living patient, so that the vessels are more clearly seen than they are on the plain chest film. Radiopaque fluid miscible with blood may be injected quickly into an antecubital vein or through a filament catheter, so that a particular volume of blood passing back through the right heart to the lungs is "seen" as a series of dense white "casts" of the cardiac chambers and the pulmonary vessels in sequence. Multiple rapid-filming devices or x-ray movies are used to record the passage of the visible "bolus" of blood from the heart to lungs, back to the heart, and out to the body tissues. Figure 4-4 shows an opaque-filled bolus of blood coming into the right heart from the superior vena cava and out into the lung via the *pulmonary arteries*. Figure 4-5, a film made a second or two later, shows the *veins* filled. Note their more horizontal course. The arteries now contain only blood and cast only faint shadows.

38

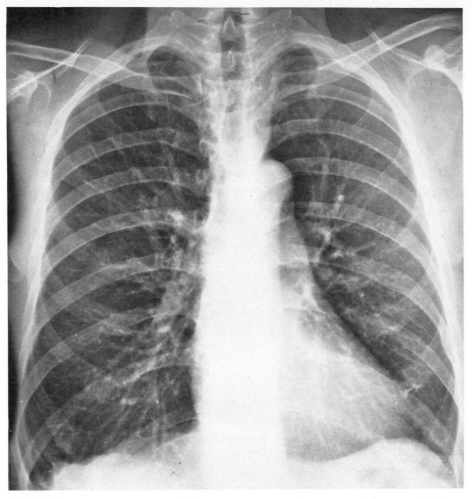

Figure 4-6. Normal chest film. Note how difficult it is to be sure which are arteries and which veins on this "plain film" without added contrast material.

Much less dramatic but nonetheless important information is available from any simple PA chest film as you study the vascular shadows in the lung marked only by the blood they contain. Notice first that the largest vessels at the hilum of the lung cast the heaviest and widest shadows, just as you would expect. This Medusa-like tangle of arteries and veins on either side of the heart shadow is referred to by the radiologist in his reports as the "hilum" or "lung root." The right hilar vessels seem to extend out farther than those on the left, but this is only because a part of the left hilum is obscured by the shadow of the more prominent left side of the heart. Measured from the center of the vertebral column, the vessels will be found to be symmetrical except for the slightly higher takeoff of the left pulmonary artery, which hooks up over the left main bronchus rather abruptly (Figure 4-7). For this reason the left hilum on any normal chest film is a little higher than the right.

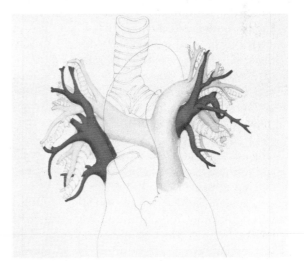

Figure 4-7. The anatomical composition of the hilum. The aorta has been rendered as though transparent. Tracheobronchial tree indicated with cartilage rings; arteries light and veins dark.

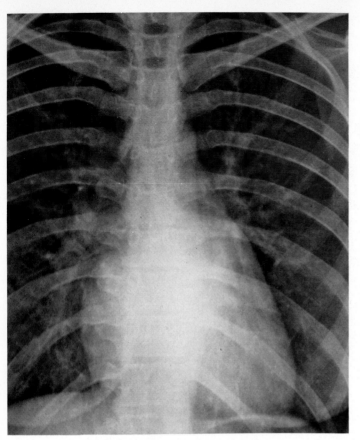

Figure 4-8. Engorged hilar root shadows in mitral stenosis. Note upper lobe vessels which are enlarged in mitral disease. Compare with Figure 4-1.

Compare the normal hila in Figure 4-1 with a few abnormal hilar shadows. The lung root may be enlarged because of engorgement of its *veins*, for example, in any condition in which there is obstruction to the return of oxygenated blood from the lung to the left side of the heart. Such a condition exists in acute left heart failure after a myocardial infarction. More chronically the same situation exists in rheumatic heart disease with mitral stenosis, where the gradual narrowing of the mitral valve results in back pressure in the pulmonary veins. Figure 4-8 shows the appearance of the hilum in moderately advanced mitral stenosis. Note the enlargement of the lung root and its obviously fat and tortuous branches, compared with the slim, straight vessels in Figure 4-1.

Dilatation of the *arteries* in the hilum will also become familiar to you in types of congenital heart disease in which an abnormal opening in the septum reroutes blood from the left chambers back into the right chambers and to the lesser circulation, thus overloading the right heart and pulmonary arteries. A patent ductus

arteriosus with a shunt of blood from the aorta to the pulmonary artery, and septal defects between the atria, commonly give this picture. Figure 4-9 shows an example of the marked hilar arterial engorgement seen in congenital heart disease of this type.

There is often actually some enlargement of both veins and arteries, and it is not usually possible for you to say from the plain radiograph which vessels predominate. In judging the appearance of the hilum in the patient whose film you see for the first time, you will decide simply that you are looking at vascular trunks of normal caliber or that they are enlarged. However, it is a constantly diverting game of logic to reason out whether veins or arteries probably account for most of the enlargement of a thickened root shadow, and in any well-studied cardiac patient you will probably have no difficulty in doing so.

The vascular trunks of the hilum normally branch and taper out into the lung field in all directions. They are so fine in the far peripheral lung close to the chest wall that you can scarcely see them. If you mask off between two pieces of paper first the hilum and medial half of the lung

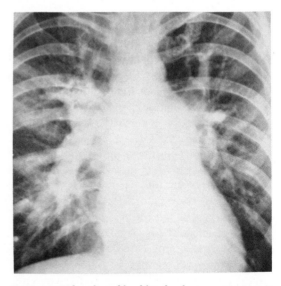

Figure 4-9. Hila enlarged by dilated pulmonary arteries in a patient with interatrial septal defect. Normal quantity of blood returning to the right atrium from the vena cava is augmented by blood shunted through the defect from the left atrium. This results in recirculation of blood through the lungs, overload of the pulmonary circulation, and dilated arteries.

40

and then the lateral half, you will be struck by the decreased number of trunks laterally. But this will not surprise you when you recall that the lung is much thicker medially where it bounds the mediastinum than at its lateral extremity, and that there are many more vessels superimposed on each other in the medial half of the lung field on the radiograph. If you similarly divide the lung field on the x-ray film into upper and lower halves, you can see at once that there are many more branching vascular trunks in the lower half of the lung than there are in the upper half. This too is a function of thickness, and to think three-dimensionally about the vascular tree within the lung at this point is to recall the pyramidal shape of the lung with its broad base against the diaphragm and its apex coming to a point under the arch of the first rib.

You will be disturbed from time to time by the juxtacardiac portion of the lower right lung (the right cardiophrenic angle). Many vascular trunks overlap there in the PA view because those for the anteriorly placed middle lobe are superimposed on those for the posteriorly placed lower lobe. One is easily misled into supposing there to be some increased density in this area, when in fact none exists. You can prove this to your own satisfaction by reviewing in films on this page and preceding ones the appearance of the portion of the right lung lying just above the diaphragm and to the right of the heart. Observe that even in normal films (see Figure 4-1) the area looks more heavily traversed by vessel trunks than you expect it to be. Part of the difficulty is the visual trick your eye plays; you are probably comparing the lung on the two sides of the heart, but because of the shape of the heart, the lung tissue just beyond the left border of the heart is not actually comparable to the problem area on the right which we have been discussing. The point is easily proved by measuring from the midline: the truly comparable part of the left lung field lies closer to the midline, obscured by the shadow of the heart itself. In Figures 4-10 and 4-11 you have abnormal and normal cardiophrenic angles to compare.

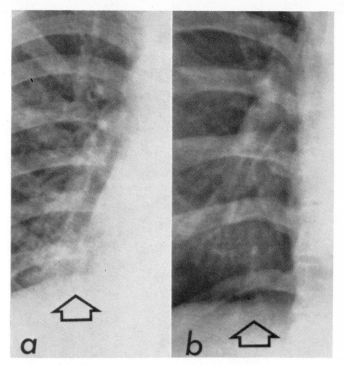

Figure 4-10. Right cardiophrenic angle, a section of the lung field often difficult to assay because of the large numbers of vessels superimposed. In *a* a fluffy density is filling in the area which is seen to be clear in the normal, *b*. Man in *a* had pneumonia.

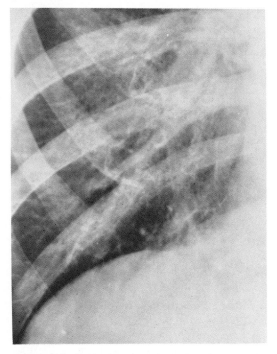

Figure 4-11. Cardiophrenic angle and lower right lung field in mild cardiac failure. The shadows of the engorged veins in the hilum superimposed on those of the arteries give a matted, thickened look to the hilum and lung field. Note Kerley's B-lines—horizontal, laterally placed linear or beaded densities which represent engorged lymphatics or thickened interlobular septa in which those lymphatics lie.

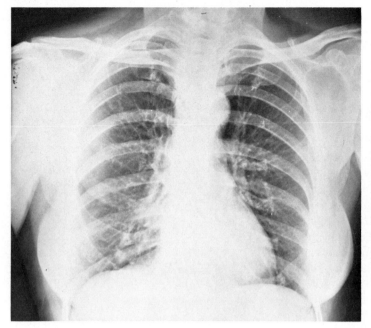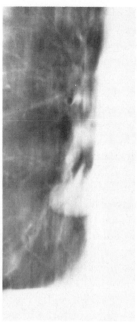

Figure 4-12 (left). Ill-defined thickness in the lower part of the right hilum in a patient with cough and bloody sputum, proved on body-section study, Figure 4-13 (right), to be a smooth round mass below a clearly normal right pulmonary artery. Finding at surgery: benign adenoma.

Often enlargement of the hilum is not vascular in nature. There are many *lymph nodes* in the hilum and mediastinum, lost among the heavier shadows of vessels and normally too small to be seen. They may enlarge, however, and become visible, either singly or in groups (when they respond to an inflammatory process in the lung, for example, or are secondarily invaded by tumor.) They may be seen as overlapping round shadows, or when they are matted together, they may cast a confluent shadow as you see in Figure 4-12.

Primary tumor masses occurring near the hilum are common. If you are thinking three-dimensionally about the lung root on the radiograph, you will also realize that tumor masses in the peripheral lung tissue in front of or behind the hilum may cast shadows which superimpose on that of the hilum in the PA chest film. Figures 4-12 and 4-14 are examples of this sort of problem. In Figure 4-12 the mass is just below the right hilum, and in Figure 4-14 it is either behind or in front but superimposed on a true left hilar mass of tumor-invaded nodes. A variety of special procedures will help to distinguish the nature of such masses. Bronchography will determine whether they relate to the bronchus or simply displace it, and angiocardiography will give you the same information about the major vessels. Body-section studies are immensely useful as well, and you should think of those in the illustrations used here as radiographs of a slice of the patient made through the level of the hilum in the coronal plane.

Hilar enlargements due to tumor tend to be rounder and smoother in outline and are more frequently unilateral. Masses which prove to be clusters of enlarged nodes, you will find, tend to look like what you would expect if you radiographed a bunch of grapes, with many overlapping round shadows. Vascular hilar enlargements, on the other hand, taper into the lung field and are almost invariably bilateral. You are going to see exceptions, of course, but these very rough generalizations will provide you with a temporary working rule. Remember too that you must expect to see hilar enlargements which are *combinations* of tumor and nodes (as in 4-14) or vessels and nodes. The place of plain tomography and computerized tomography in analyzing such masses will be discussed in the chapter on the mediastinum.

42

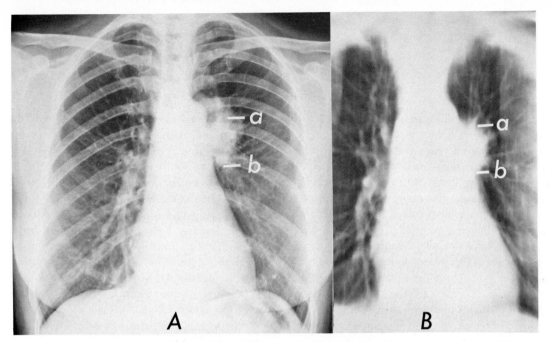

Figure 4-14. A: Left hilar mass, normal right hilum. Note that the body-section study, B, was made through the hilum. It shows a cluster of enlarged nodes in the hilum, (*a-b*), but it excludes the upper part of the original shadow in A, overlapped on that of the nodes and representing the primary tumor behind or in front of the hilum. Thus the abnormal shadow on the plain film is actually two densities overlapping. A lateral film might help; additional body-section studies would show at what level the primary mass lay.

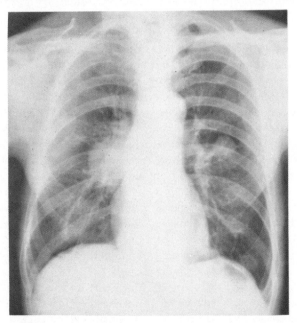

Figure 4-15. Mass superimposed on the hilum. Patient is a male; heavy pectoral shadows may simulate breast shadows. Rounded "hilar" mass is crossed by normally tapering vessels and is probably behind the hilum. Left hilum extends laterally a little farther than one expects it to and may conceal a second mass superimposed partly on the aortic shadow. Close to the left hilum in the mid left-lung field (seventh interspace and overlapping the eighth rib) there is a rounded shadow outlined by normal lung around it. The medial posterior portion of the right seventh rib is missing. (All findings were proved due to tumor.)

43

Limitations and Fallibility

Finally, remember that sometimes a very innocent-looking hilum is not actually normal and may conceal among its vascular shadows tumor-involved nodes not yet large enough to be seen on the films. Retrospective studies of the films in large groups of patients who were found to have tumor-involved hilar nodes at surgery have shown a number of perfectly normal-appearing hilar shadows. The radiologist can do nothing about this except to report that your patient *seems* to have normal hilar shadows, and both you and he have to consider that the presence of involved but normal-sized nodes would make a difference in the treatment of the patient. You will hear a good deal more in subsequent chapters about what I shall call the *fallibility of the method*, by which I mean areas in which you must anticipate some unreliability of the roentgen examination, some quite unavoidable failure of the x-ray studies to give you the information you need about your patient. You learn the limitations of other modes of inquiry constantly in medical school, and you must be aware that despite its great usefulness the radiographic inquiry also has some limitations, even in the hands of the most expert interpreter. When he can help you solve a specific problem, the radiologist will do so. When he knows he cannot help you, *or that a simple negative report is likely to be misinterpreted as a clean bill of health for the structure in question*, it is his obligation to warn you of the fact. It is this type of problem which, more than anything else, makes it imperative that you not rely entirely on the written report but supplement it with a personal conference with the radiologist while viewing the films yourself.

The first "false negative" film you see on a patient of your own will convince you that intelligent film reporting is dependent upon some knowledge of the patient's problem. Without that information the radiologist cannot truly serve the best interests of the patient, cannot offer you a written report for your records which is framed around the difficulties of a particular human being with a particular set of symptoms.

Contemporary medical practice is a collaborative affair for medical students as well as for their instructors in clinical work, and medical students must not feel hesitant about approaching someone in the department of radiology for an explanation of shadows which puzzle them or for the physiologic implications of a particular roentgen finding. A relationship of mutual trust, good-fellowship, and devotion to the evolution of new ideas must be developed and fostered between radiologist and physician-in-training. The younger people, because of their more recent study of allied fields, are often in a position to contribute to the refreshment of knowledge of the more mature.

Look, for example, at Figures 4-16, 4-17, and 4-18, which are called "wedge arteriograms" and represent an exciting approach to one aspect of pulmonary physiology, feasible in the living patient and contributing important information about his small pulmonary arteries which was once not obtainable without lung biopsy. A fine catheter is passed from an arm vein through the right chambers of the heart out along the pulmonary artery. It is wedged into one of the smaller lung vessels in a portion of the lung free of overlap from the shadows of mediastinum or scapula. Pressure readings are made, and then a small amount of radiopaque fluid is injected as the film exposure is being made. Figure 4-19 shows the normal appearance of the smallest vessels of the arterial bed in the lung periphery. Some of these are vessels too small to cast any shadow well-defined enough to study on the plain film (compare Figure 4-1). Yet the pressures on the right side of the heart and in the main pulmonary arteries must reflect the status of these small vessels, the distensibility of their walls, the structure of their intima, and their characteristic branching, whether normal, decreased, or increased.

Obtaining and then analyzing studies of this sort in the course of the workup of the patient are clearly collaborative procedures between you and the specialists you entrust with the problem, and the same philosophy ought to apply to more routine procedures.

Pulmonary Arteriography

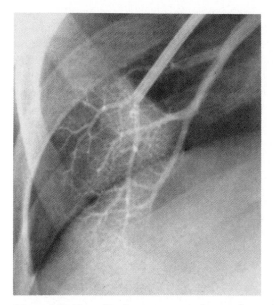

Figure 4-16. Normal wedge arteriogram showing the capillary bed in the lung.

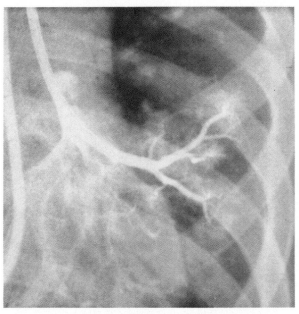

Figure 4-17. Patient with pulmonary hypertension. From the narrowing of small end-arteries and sparse branching this has been called the "pruned tree" arteriogram. Pulmonary flow is reduced 50 percent.

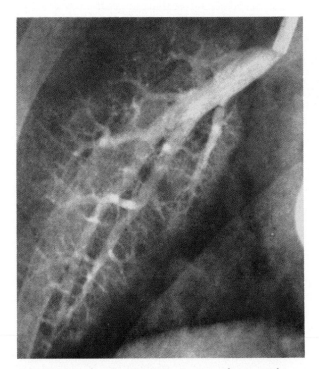

Figure 4-18. Wedge arteriogram on a patient with interatrial septal defect and a left-to-right shunt so extensive that the pulmonary flow was increased to 470 percent of the systemic flow.

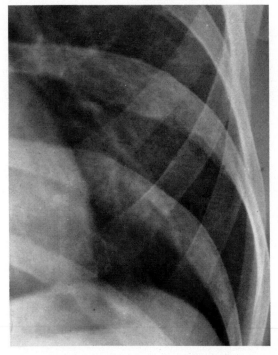

Figure 4-19. The nonopacified normal peripheral lung for comparison. Now you are looking at the terminal vessels with blood in them but no contrast material, as you see them regularly on routine chest films.

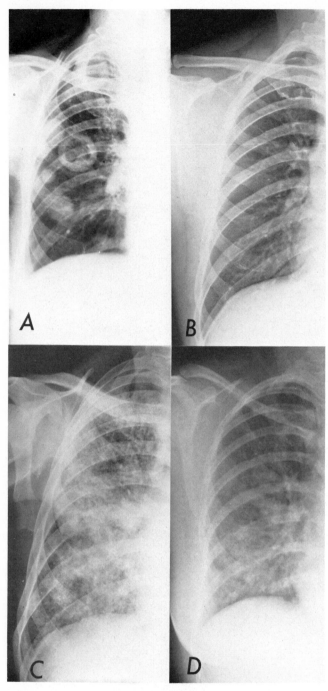

Figure 4-20. (See text.)

Solitary and Disseminated Lesions in the Lung

Imagine now the *alveolar portion of the lung* folded like a conical cuff around three sides of the hilum. You have looked at the peripheral lung when it was normal and seemed completely radiolucent in the lateral third of the PA film, where it is not superimposed on hilar trunks. What shadows will be added, then, if the vascular tree is normal but the alveolar lung is sprinkled with minute tumor nodules, patches of pneumonia, or small areas of collapse, or where it is threaded and reefed in by scar tissue from old infections or flooded with interstitial fluid?

Look briefly over the eight lung fields on these two pages and then come back to the text. Are there any normals? Which ones seem to have changes in the lung so widespread that you think at once of some generalized process involving *all* lung tissue? Which show fewer than six isolated areas of abnormality?

Now consider them one by one. In A, several round shadows hang in an otherwise normal lung, their margins smooth and sharp, since they are surrounded by well-aerated lung tissue on all sides. One of them appears circular with a darker central area because it has a hollow, air-filled cavity inside it. (More x-rays pass through this part than through the shell tangentially.) The radiologist may not be able to tell you whether these are tumor nodules growing in the lung or granulomas expanding similarly; he *can* help you to assess the probabilities for one or the other diagnosis on the basis of their appearance, their growth rate from film to film over a period of time, and the clinical story.

B, the right lung of the patient seen in E, is normal and can be used as a norm for studying the others.

Both C and D show innumerable patches of increased density which, on the original film, involved both lungs. (G is the left half of D.) Unfortunately, many different conditions produce a picture similar to these two films. Some are common, others rare. From the film alone, without any knowledge of the acuteness of the patient's illness or of his occupational background, or even of the tentative clinical diagnosis, you cannot guess at the most probable diagnosis. You can describe the abnormal shadows—no more.

However, when you know that the man in C had inhaled beryllium salts in a fluorescent-lamp factory over a period of time, you *can* say that his chest film shows shadows just like those seen in autopsy-proved cases of berylliosis where myriads of small granulomas and a lacework of scar tissue produce such roentgen shadows in the lung. On the other hand, if you know that the woman in D and G was pulled out of the water several hours ago, half drowned, her film becomes intelligible because this is a picture often seen after such mishaps. Many small areas of collapse from inhaled water and bronchial secretions produce this sort of patchy density. In addition, from the violent struggle in the water there is usually some pulmonary edema with extra fluid in the interstitium of the lung about the vessels and extensive hemorrhage.

Any chest film is only a point on a curve in the course of the patient's disease. *Change* from film to film in a day or a week or a year often alters the whole spectrum of diagnostic possibilities considered on viewing the original film. You may still not be able to be sure what the patient has, but you can then be sure of a good many things that he has not. To know that the man in C had shown the changes you see there for several months before this film was made, and that his lung picture did not change appreciably before he died, would strongly affirm your conviction that he had a chronic lung injury, probably related to his known industrial exposure. The half-drowned woman got well in a few days, and you could predict she would. In fact, H shows her left lung two days after G. Slightly enlarged vessel shadows seem the only remaining abnormality.

In case you have not been able to find anything wrong with E, look again at the ninth interspace. This solitary nodule had not changed since a chest film one year before, and at surgery it proved to be a benign tumor. In F the entire lung is sprinkled with minute areas of a density rightly suggesting calcium and representing the healed scars of an old infection, unchanged for many years. It has been estimated that such lesions must be at least 2 millimeters in size to be visible by x-ray.

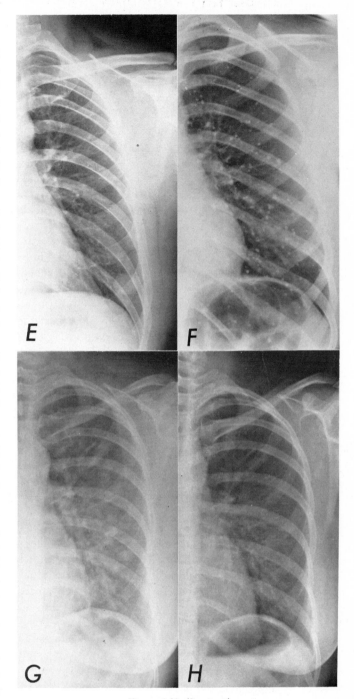

Figure 4-21. (See text.)

Important Concepts about Radiology and the Interpretation of Films

The preceding page spread was not intended to confuse you but to give you an idea of some of the types of *disseminated lesions* in the lung parenchyma which you will be seeing, and to impart a feeling for the problems you and the radiologist may have to face in interpreting the shadows cast by such lesions. To be sure, some shadows in the lung are easier to interpret than others, and it is important for you to realize early in your study of radiology that there are many times when no diagnosis can be made with certainty from the films. There are many other times when the radiologist can be definite about his diagnostic interpretation of the films and will insist in the best interests of the patient. There are, in fact, some conditions in which the appearance of the radiograph is to be trusted as a diagnostic clue even more than the opinion of the pathologist based on a single biopsy specimen. A well-informed, modern pathologist will agree that his opinion is not necessarily the final answer and that his contribution to the whole patient's study must be fitted into the pattern formed by all other diagnostic evidence.

If you remember in looking at radiographs that an abnormal shadow consistently present on two or more films must have been produced by an area of abnormality in the patient's tissues, but that sometimes the form and shape of that shadow give definite clues to its nature and sometimes they do not, you will be able to keep in good focus the problems of interpreting such shadows. You will be seeing roentgen shadows of all kinds in this book, some of which can be interpreted sensibly in only one way (example: the presence of congenitally duplicate structures). Other roentgen shadows, like those on the preceding page spread, might be cast by any one of several different abnormal processes going on in the patient's tissues, and one can interpret them only up to a point.

The knowledge acquired by a radiologist who reads films several hours a day for ten years, who habitually checks affirmative statements against clinical, surgical, and autopsy findings, and who regularly reads the periodicals covering new work in the field, makes it possible to recognize most of the types of shadows about which one may be definite. That experience also teaches one not to guess about the significance of many other types of shadows. There is absolutely no excuse for diagnostic guessing at any time. On the other hand, a frank guess plainly *labeled* as such may be a useful device for examining the whole diagnostic problem, just as a working clinical diagnosis is a guess in the sense of a feasible possibility.

In sum, your best procedure in medicine is to assay the patient's problem on the basis of a good history and a careful physical examination, and then to order such radiographic procedures as are pertinent to your working diagnosis. If subsequently you find film shadows in keeping with it, you will have affirmed to some extent your initial feeling about the patient's disease process. If no abnormal roentgen findings are present, you may have to revise your impression—or you may feel strongly enough to retain it, temporarily at least. If repeated diagnostic studies of all kinds refute your impression, you will, in time, have to revise your working diagnosis.

The one thing you must not do is attempt to make of radiology a card-sorting device on which you lean more and more in order not to have to make up your mind about a differential diagnosis on the basis of the history and physical examination alone. Nothing can take the place of a careful historical record and a thorough physical examination. Allowing yourself the slack discipline of looking at x-ray films before you have studied the patient will create in you a sense of dependence on these procedures which is out of proportion to their importance. You cannot hope to develop the invaluable tool that a brilliantly taken history and physical can become if you use the x-ray to guide your hand instead of to check its accuracy.

On the other hand, after you have ordered and examined films on your patient in accordance with your working diagnosis, if the radiologist raises the possibility that the patient may have a condition you had not considered, he is trying to help you with a labeled guess based on his experience in viewing films. It may be a simple matter for you to refute that possibility by another procedure or test.

I should like to recommend that you consciously choose, in medical school and later, a realistic and mature attitude toward the art and science of radiology (for it is both science and art). Medical students are prone to adopt attitudes which do not help them to profit by the aid radiologic data can be to them in learning. One of these attitudes is expressed by the person who says, "It is all a mystery, impossible to understand; the radiologist see things I cannot hope to see." This is patently defeatist, as I hope I have already proved to you. You may not see as much as the radiologist, but with his help you can indeed see the abnormal shadows which are present and you can relate them to the patient's disease. It goes without saying that to do so is an accretional process and that the more determinedly sensible your approach is, the more you will learn.

Another dangerous attitude you should avoid is the one which demands diagnostic labels prematurely. It is rigidly unimaginative, for example, to say, "Pneumonia as a process in the lung should always look the same on the x-ray film." Of course it does not; why would it? The process the pathologist sees at autopsy varies from patient to patient, in both gross and microscopic findings, even though he labels them all "pneumonia." The disease process varies in accordance with the type of patient who is playing host to the disease, his physiologic responses, his capacity to resist, his age when he contracts the disease, the treatment which has been administered to him, the presence of coincidental disease processes. Why, then, would not the radiograph reflect such variation?

It does indeed, and while one must remember that it does so vary, one may at the same time be comforted by the fact that it usually varies within certain fairly well described limits. Thus the radiologist becomes accustomed to a spectrum of shadows for any given disease process, and the more experienced he becomes, the more accurately he will interpret those shadows in the light of the patient's clinical picture. For example, the radiologist recognizes the *changes* in a pneumonic process at various stages of healing and will often be able to advise the clinician that the process is healing at an expected rate or alert him to the fact that the healing is being unaccountably delayed and that the reason for this may be of vital importance. He recognizes the fact that pneumonia expresses itself in the lung in one way in an infant and very differently in an old man who has the leftover scar traces of many similar infections in his lung and perhaps a compromised blood supply. In general, the infant recovers clinically and his chest film clears very rapidly, while the old man takes longer to throw off the process and his chest film may be expected to show changes lingering on for some time. Invariably the radiograph is recording a phase of the pathologic process, since it is a factual shadowgram, so that the very fact that "pneumonia does *not* always look the same" is of importance to you, the clinician.

In *Life on the Mississippi* Mark Twain describes the confusion he experienced while an apprentice pilot. He endured a learning process which required him to recognize the appearance of the riverbank by day and by night, with the water at different levels, at different times of the year and in different kinds of weather. As a pilot he had to know the landmarks up one side of the river and down the other, a total of several thousand miles of bends and turns to be memorized, together with the soundings of a river bottom which was constantly changing. If you have not read it, do, because the contrast between the purely rote memorizing, of which it is an excellent example, and the type of rational learning you can apply to so much of medicine will give you courage. Some have felt that diagnostic radiology was a tallying process, innumerable characteristic roentgen pictures to be learned by memory. It is not, and I hope that this chapter will have enlisted your interest in the fascinating intellectual procedure involved in putting together the story of the patient, what you hear through the stethoscope, and what you see in the chest film.

The philosophic digression you have just read was necessary at this point in order to orient you toward the proper handling of roentgen data. Do not let it prevent your being aware of how much you already know about analyzing a chest film. You know, for example, from this chapter that the hilum and normal lung markings are mostly vascular. You have realized that changes in the size and tortuosity of these shadows may reflect vascular changes related to either heart or lung disease. You have set up a system for studying these structures deliberately in a certain order. You recognize that vascular engorgement in the hilum may be arterial or venous or both, and that only experts can tell which. You know that when there is evidence of inflammation in the lung, hilar engorgement will probably represent both vessels and swollen lymph nodes. You are going to look very carefully at the hilar shadows of any patient who you believe has a lung tumor, but you will remember that early in the disease an innocent-appearing hilum may conceal tumor-positive nodes which will become apparent only when they grow large enough.

You know that the normal lung parenchyma is very radiolucent itself and that the normal lung markings are the vessels which traverse it. You have seen a few examples of parenchymal lung disease where tumor, inflammation, scar tissue, or abnormally increased interstitial fluid increased the absorption of x-rays and cast disseminated shadows on the film, gray-white spots superimposed on the vascular tree.

You have, I hope, accepted the fact that sometimes differing conditions may cast shadows so similar that no positive diagnosis can be made from the films alone. In these patients it becomes a team effort by all the doctors concerned to fit together clinical findings of all sorts, including the radiographic evidence, in order to settle on a working diagnosis. At other times the experience of the radiologist in looking at similar films of patients with about the same signs and symptoms will enable him to be more definite in his interpretation. Serial films in the course of an illness ought to be reviewed constantly and should be reinterpreted if necessary in the light of new developments in the overall clinical picture.

50

Review Unknowns

Unknown 4-1 (no figure). It is eleven o'clock at night. You receive a telephone report that an admission chest film on a patient you have just examined shows the shadow of a straight pin overlying the dark shadow of the air-filled trachea. The patient, a woman in for elective foot surgery tomorrow, talked comfortably when you were with her. What should you do?

Unknown 4-2 (Figure 4-22). A 23-year-old medical student gives you a two-week history of cough, fever, weight loss, and bloody sputum, but he was able to go to classes today. Figure 4-22 shows a detail of his right midlung field. He tells you that an insurance chest film was entirely negative three months ago. Compare what you see here with the eight lung fields you have just studied. What sorts and shapes of abnormal shadows do you see? How would you be inclined to interpret them in terms of pathologic changes which might cast such shadows? Weighing all factors (history, possible pathologic condition, and roentgen appearance), which of the following very general catagories of lung disease do you think most probable in this patient:

Acute inflammation one day old
No disease
Subacute inflammation one month old
Chronic lung insult related to employment
Metastatic tumor spread in the lung

Unknown 4-3 (Figure 4-23). Routine checkup on well patient. (Past history withheld.)

Unknown 4-4 (Figure 4-24). By a careful and systematic search determine whether this man's chest film is normal.

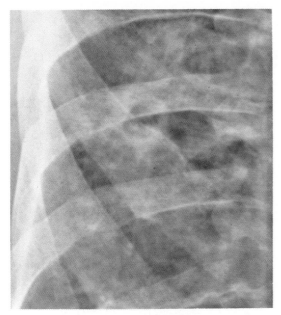

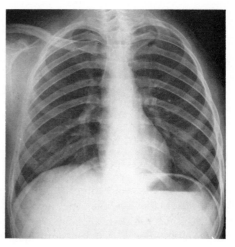

Figure 4-23 (*Unknown 4-3*).

Figure 4-22 (*Unknown 4-2*).

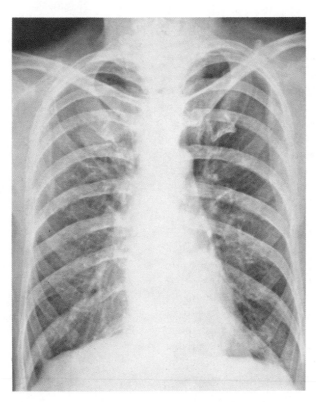

Figure 4-24 (*Unknown 4-4*).

CHAPTER 5 The Roentgen Signs of Lung Consolidation —Air Space Disease

Consolidation of a Whole Lung

By massive lung consolidation I mean, for practical purposes, that a whole lung, a whole lobe, or at least one entire bronchopulmonary segment is solid in that it is almost entirely airless. The solid part will cast a uniformly dense shadow on the film, of approximately the same density as the heart shadow, and its projection shadow will relate to the shape of the part involved. Although this sounds as though a theoretical situation were being proposed, the fact is that in everyday radiologic practice shadows of this kind are common. Hardly a day passes in a big general hospital without there turning up, for example, a radiograph in which by a logical analysis of the abnormal shadows on the chest film one can recognize a consolidated lobe in a patient with clinical lobar pneumonia. Likewise a shadow which can only represent a solid right upper lobe may be recognized in a patient already suspected of having lung cancer. To learn first the roentgen appearance of whole-lung consolidation and then that of consolidation of only one lobe is the orientation of this chapter.

In Figure 5-1 you have diagramed for you the roentgen findings you must anticipate when one or the other *whole lung* becomes solid but does not change in size or shape. Begin by noticing that in A the normal heart shadow is thrown into relief by the normally aerated lung on either side of it. So also the two domed diaphragmatic shadows covering the liver and spleen are seen in relief because there is air in the lung above them. The stomach bubble under the medial half of the left diaphragm may be seen in the standing patient as the shadow of radiolucent air imprisoned in the fundus of the stomach above a horizontal fluid level. When present, the stomach bubble effectively locates the level of the diaphragm.

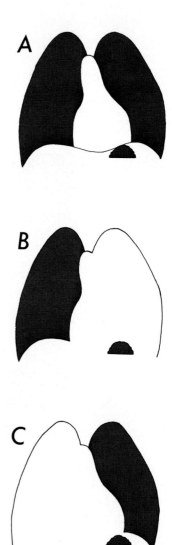

Figure 5-1

52

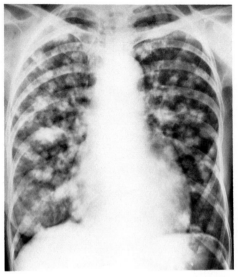

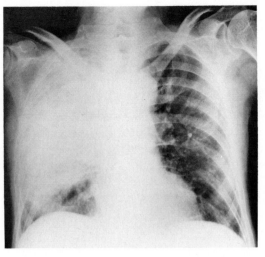

Figure 5-3

Figure 5-2

Now suppose that the entire left lung becomes consolidated, as in B. The heart, mediastinal structures, and dense lung are all of the same density now and their shadows merge into one, so that the left side of the heart profile disappears. They also merge with the shadows of the spleen and left lobe of the liver, and the outline of the left diaphragm is therefore lost, its location indicated only by the rays which reach the film through the air in the stomach. Look back at the cadaver sections in Chapter 2 to check these relations of stomach, spleen, and diaphragm.

If the left lung remains normal and the right solidifies, the chest film will look like C. The liver, right lung, and heart being nearly identical in density, their shadows now merge.

Disappearance of profiles or interfaces normally seen, then, on a chest film of this sort implies solid change in the lung next to them because the usual air/solid roentgen interface no longer exists. It is interesting to realize that even a lung which is riddled with small disseminated nodules of tumor will still contain enough air to behave like a well-aerated lung in respect to profiles. The patient in Figure 5-2 proved at autopsy to have both lungs generously sprinkled

with tumor nodules; yet you do see the heart shadow and both diaphragms because of the air in alveoli around the disseminated lesions.

Contrast with it Figure 5-3, in which pneumonia consolidating the entire upper part of the right lung but sparing the lower part results in loss of the upper part of the mediastinal and heart shadows, but preserves those of the right diaphragm and liver.

Any consolidation against the mediastinum will result in loss of a part of the mediastinal border, therefore, and any consolidation of the base of the lung will erase the shadow of the diaphragm or a segment of it. Because the heart is in the anterior half of the chest, consolidation which erases the border of the heart must, of course, be located in the anterior part of the lung; so you will not be surprised the first time you observe for yourself that although the diaphragmatic shadow on one side is absent and the lower part of the lung on that side appears dense, the border of the heart is seen clearly through it, thrown into relief by juxtaposed air-filled *anterior* lung. When you see this you will reason accurately that the lower lobe, in contact with the diaphragm, is solid, while the rest of the lung is normal.

53

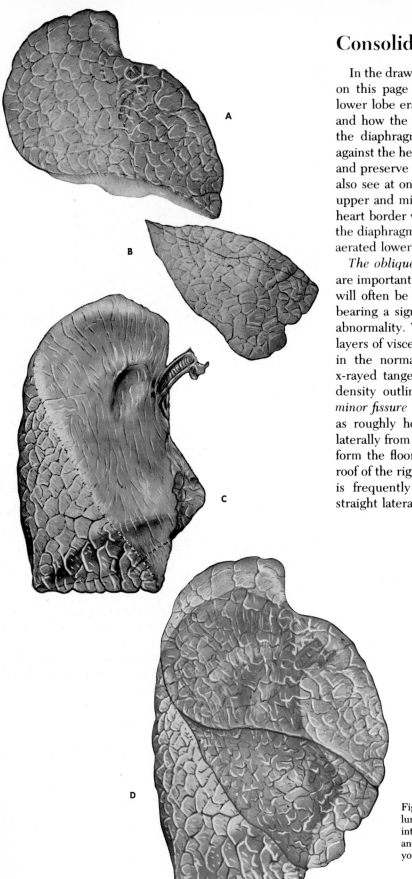

Consolidation of One Lobe

In the drawings of seemingly transparent lung on this page you can see exactly why a solid lower lobe erases the shadow of the diaphragm and how the upper lobes, which do not touch the diaphragm, apply themselves, full of air, against the heart in the anterior part of the chest and preserve its profile in the PA film. You can also see at once how, with consolidation of the upper and middle lobes on the right, the right heart border would disappear but the profile of the diaphragm would be preserved by the well-aerated lower lobe.

The oblique planes of the two major fissures are important to remember, since their location will often be visible to you in the lateral view bearing a significant relationship to an area of abnormality. The fissures normally contain two layers of visceral pleura in contact and are seen in the normal chest film only when pleura, x-rayed tangentially, appears as a thin line of density outlined on both sides by lung. The *minor fissure* on the right should be thought of as roughly horizontal, extending forward and laterally from the middle of the major fissure to form the floor of the right upper lobe and the roof of the right middle lobe. On the PA view it is frequently seen as a thin line extending straight laterally from the hilum.

Figure 5-4. Transparent drawing of the right lung, seen from the lateral surface, separated into upper middle and lower lobes (A, B, C) and reassembled (D). The patient faces to your right.

54

Take pencil and paper and make diagrams predicting the block of density you would expect to see on the *lateral* film if each lobe of the five became consolidated. Then try to predict the appearance of the block of density you would see on the *PA view* to go with each lateral. This will be easier if you begin with the right upper lobe, producing a density extending from the horizontal plane of the minor fissure upward to the apex. Work out for yourself these predictable shadow profiles, check them, and you will never forget them. As you reason each one, note which borders of the heart, diaphragm, and mediastinum can be expected to disappear with each block of density.

Remember that a dense sphere within the lung will project as a circular shadow in either PA or lateral view, but that *asymmetrical wedges* of different sorts will project quite differently according to the direction of the ray passing through them. The middle lobe best illustrates this point, since it is a long wedge x-rayed end-on in the PA view and appears as a much smaller shadow than when its full length is seen in the lateral view of the chest. The shadow profile in each instance is to be learned as an exercise in reasoning, independent of anatomic *surface* markings. Decide whether the consolidated middle lobe is going to be more dense-appearing on the PA or lateral chest film. Think sensibly in terms of summation shadowgrams and of the shape and location of the lobe.

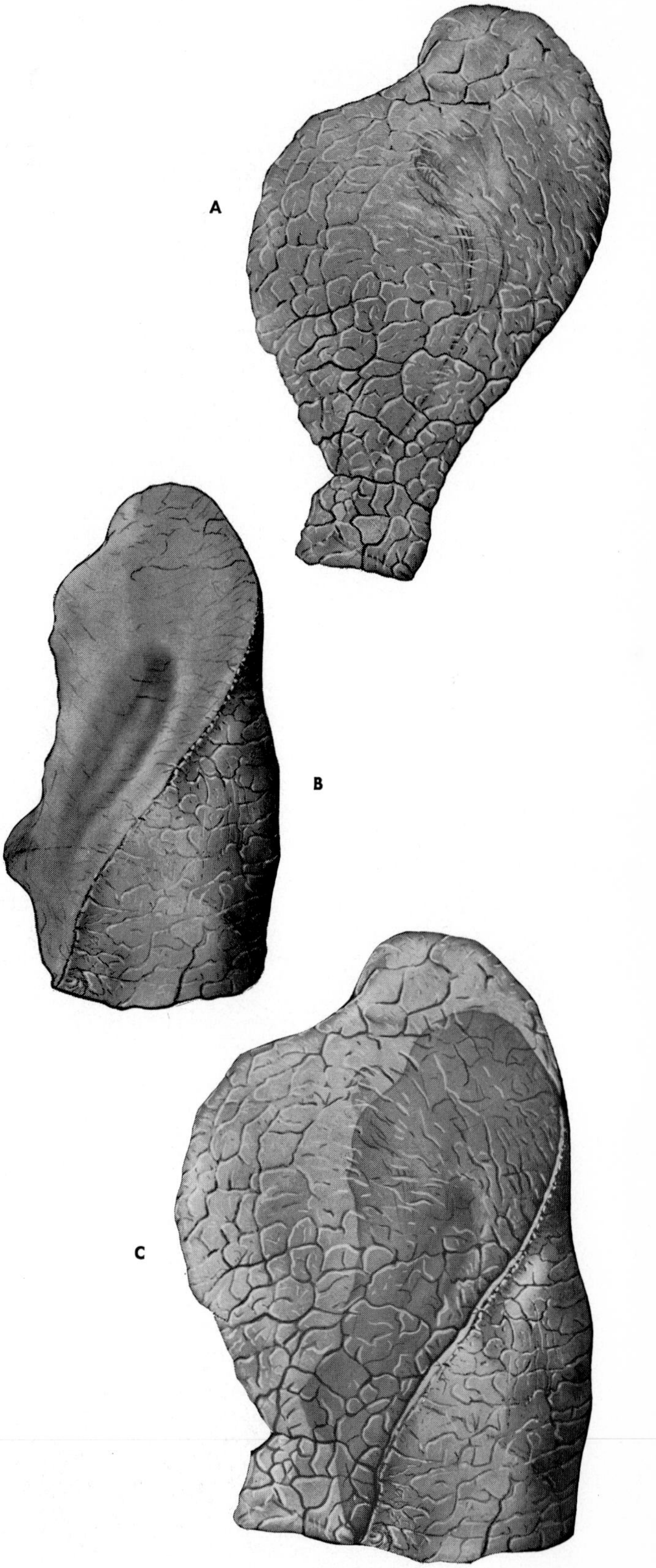

Figure 5-5. Transparent drawings of the left lung, seen from the lateral surface, separated into upper and lower lobes (A, B) and reassembled (C). The patient faces to your left. Note the similarities and differences between the middle lobe on the right and its analogue, the lingular segment of the upper lobe on the left. Density in either will obscure the lower part of the heart profile in the PA view.

The Diagrams You Should Have Drawn
For the Lobes of the Right Lung

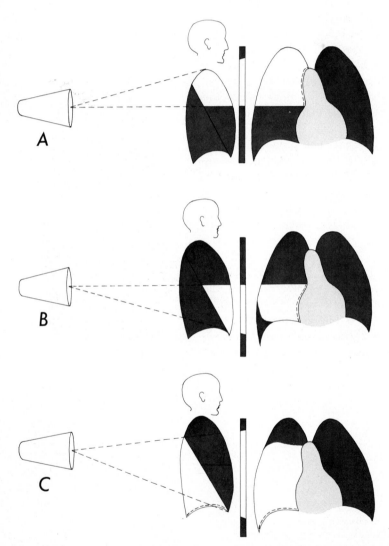

Figure 5-6. Projection shadows of each of the three lobes on the right. In A the right upper lobe is consolidated, its inferior margin outlined by the air-filled middle lobe lying beneath the minor septum. In B the middle lobe alone is dense; note that in the PA view it does not extend into the costophrenic sinus against the lateral insertion of the diaphragm. In C, on the contrary, the lung tissue filling the right costophrenic sinus is seen to be dense because the right lower lobe is dense. The heart shadow has been rendered in gray in these diagrams in order to clarify the shape of the lung mass shadows, but its density would merge with that of the middle lobe in B in an actual radiograph. Disappearing borders are outlined by dotted lines.

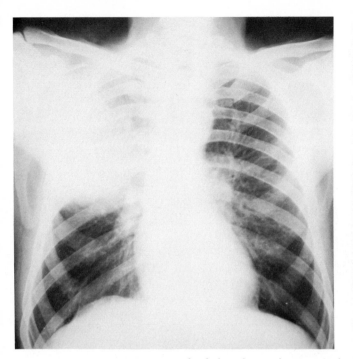
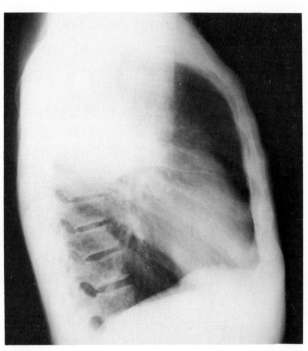

Figure 5-7. PA and right lateral view of a patient with right upper lobe pneumonia. The anterior segment is incompletely consolidated.

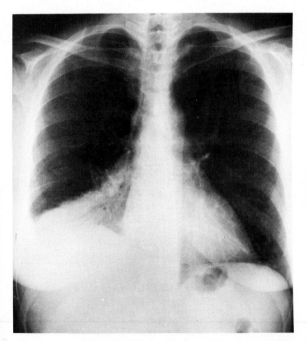
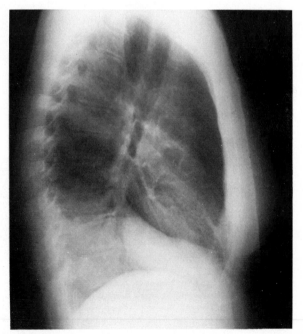

Figure 5-8. PA and right lateral view of a patient with right lower lobe consolidation. Note preservation of the heart profile in the PA and absence of the right diaphragmatic profile in the lateral. Wedge of density in the lateral is due to superimposition of the anterior part of the consolidated lower lobe on the density of the heart. Note air bronchogram. This was chronic inflammation distal to a chicken neck bone in the RLL bronchus.

The Diagrams You Should Have Drawn
For the Lobes of the Left Lung

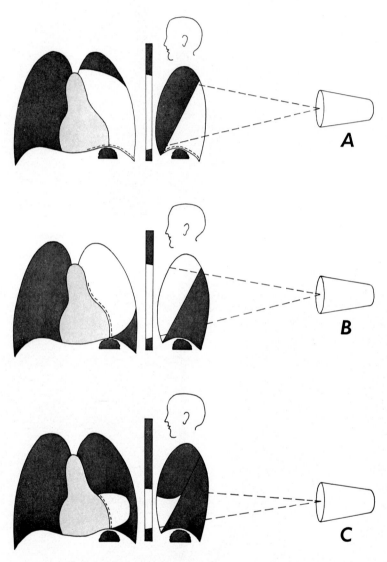

Figure 5-9. Projection shadows of the two lobes on the left. In A the left lower lobe is consolidated; the diaphragmatic shadow disappears (dotted lines), since the roentgen shadows of the lower lobe and spleen are merged into one; the approximate location of the left diaphragm may be indicated by the stomach bubble if one is present; the left heart border does not disappear but is seen through the dense lower lobe because air in the lingula of the left upper lobe anteriorly still throws it into relief. In B the entire left upper lobe is consolidated and the left heart border is lost, but the diaphragm is seen because of lower lobe air above it. In C only the lingular portion of the left upper lobe is solid, erasing the left heart border. Predict the radiographic appearance of the PA and lateral view in a patient with left upper lobe consolidation which *spared* the lingula.

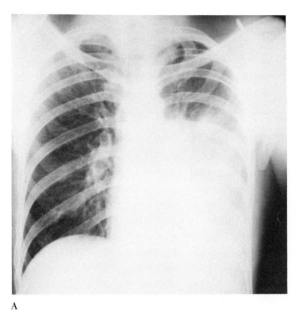

A

Figure 5-10. PA and left lateral views of a patient with left lower lobe consolidation (clinically pneumonia). Note absence of left diaphragm in the lateral view. On original film the left heart border could be faintly seen in the PA view.

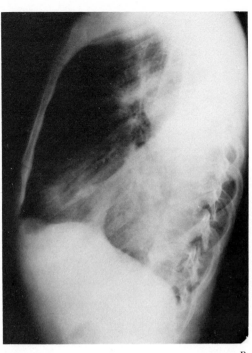

B

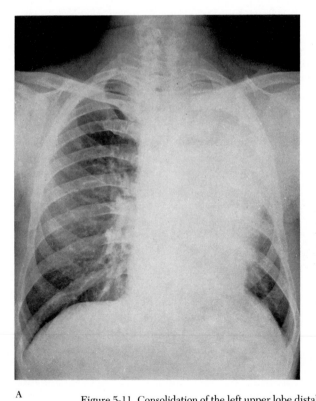

A

B

Figure 5-11. Consolidation of the left upper lobe distal to tumor obstructing the upper lobe bronchus, seen more clearly on the body-section study, B. Note loss of heart profile in A.

Consolidation of Only a Part of One Lobe

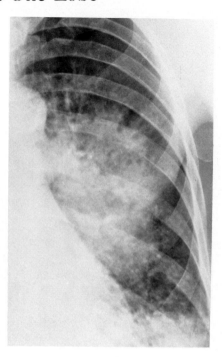

Figure 5-12. Here only a part of the left lower lobe is involved. It is a patch not in juxtaposition to the diaphragm, so the diaphragmatic profile is present. You know the patch of air-space disease is not anterior lying against the heart either, because the heart profile is so well seen. This has been called the "silhouette sign," present when a profile is *preserved*.

When massive densities involve an entire lung or an entire lobe, you have certain clues which tell you how much of the lung is consolidated, and sometimes these same clues help you to determine the location of a patch of consolidation in the lung which does not occupy an entire lobe or bronchopulmonary segment, but only a part of one. Consolidation of all the lung tissue against the diaphragm will cause the outline of the diaphragm to disappear entirely, but a patch of dense lung against the lateral half of the diaphragm will cause the disappearance of only the lateral half of its outline, leaving the medial half visible.

Tomorrow you may see a chest film in which the lower left hemithorax appears dense, but if you can nevertheless see the entire diaphragmatic profile, you will know that there must be air filling the lower lobe. If you cannot see any part of the diaphragm, but still see the left heart border through dense lung, you will know that there must be air in the upper lobe. You will not call either picture consolidation of the entire lung.

Neither will you be prompted to call a patch of partial consolidation like that in Figure 5-12 involvement of a whole lobe, but will think of it as involving most of a bronchopulmonary segment in the posterior part of the chest, since the heart border is so well preserved.

Now that you can recognize and locate anatomically areas of massive consolidation in the lung, as contrasted with the scattered small areas of density you saw in the last chapter, you are probably somewhat impatient to know how one labels them. As I have said, pneumonia and tumor can both produce solid areas in the lung giving the findings outlined above. It is current parlance to speak of "air-space disease" as opposed to "interstitial disease," and to attempt to differentiate them from each other on the PA chest film. It is true that the consolidation of lobar pneumonia *should* be thought of as pure air-space disease. It is also true that other abnormalities of lung in which the entire pathologic change is interstitial *do* produce linear strands of density on the radiograph. However, the student who rigidly attempts to classify all disease as either air-space or interstitial from the roentgen appearance is in for a very disappointing and frustrating experience, because only some diseases pathologically show pure air-space or pure interstitial change. For example, pulmonary edema, interstitial to begin with, often floods alveoli with fluid. Other pulmonary processes (tuberculosis is one) may involve both interstitium and alveoli concurrently.

Lung which is airless because it has collapsed can produce much the same appearance as consolidation except that there will be evidence for change in size and shape of the part of lung involved. Collections of fluid in the pleural space can also produce dense areas in the thoracic cavity, of course, obscuring the otherwise healthy lung it envelops and causing the disappearance of the diaphragmatic outline.

Moreover, in both pneumonia and tumor, some atelectasis and pleural fluid are common in addition to the primary consolidation in the lung itself. One has to remember that these processes go together pathologically and, since they may cast very similar shadows, are often impossible to differentiate from each other from the films alone on the initial study. In the next chapters you will learn how to determine the presence of pleural effusion and how to analyze the particular signals indicating that a lobe has collapsed. Then you will add them to the signs of consolidation we have covered above and interpret chest films systematically on each level.

In Chapter 3 you set up a system for beginning to study a chest film by surveying the bony structures and the soft tissues. In Chapter 4 you added the systematic survey of the hilum and its tapering vessels and the parenchyma of the lung itself. In Chapter 5 you have added a survey to make sure that no large patches of lung appear dense and that the heart borders and both diaphragmatic outlines are present, checking for *disappearance of profiles normally seen.* You are building gradually the sort of careful analysis of a chest film that will help you now in using roentgen data, and serve you all your life in understanding the films on your own patients. Do not be impatient for diagnostic labels.

Did you observe that there was only one breast in Figure 5-2?

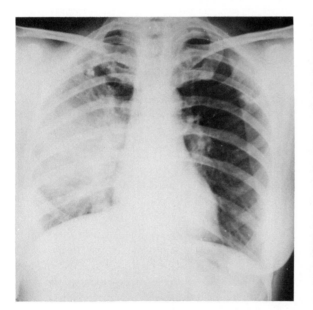
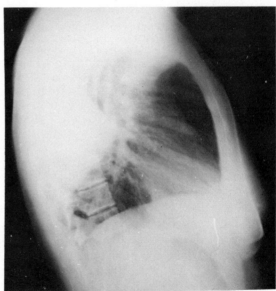

Figure 5-13 (*Unknown 5-1*). Clinically this young woman had pneumonia. Precisely what part of the right lung is consolidated, and where would you hear rales best?

CHAPTER 6 The Diaphragm and the Pleural Space; Pleural Effusion and Pneumothorax; Pulmonary Embolism

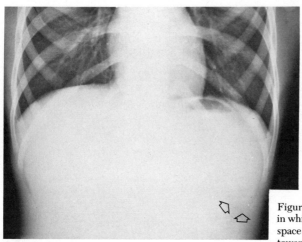

Figure 6-1. Normal diaphragms. Note stomach bubble with fluid level under the left diaphragm. Arrows mark the tip of the spleen. The spleen and the fluid-filled part of the stomach form a continuous shadow.

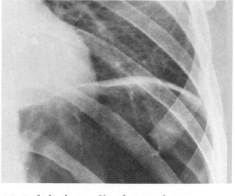

Figure 6-2. Left diaphragm filmed erect after an accident in which large amounts of air were admitted to the peritoneal space. Spleen and stomach are displaced downward and toward the midline. Note the vascular trunks in the lower lobe far posteriorly, extending well below the level of the crown of the diaphragm and, in this patient, superimposed on subdiaphragmatic air. These lower lobe vessels are not seen in Figure 6-1 because they are behind the spleen.

The region of the diaphragm on the chest film affords some fine exercises in the logic of roentgen shadows. Just as you see the profile of the heart, dense between two lucent lungs, so you see the dome of the diaphragm because of a change in the sum of all superimposed densities. The sum of the shadows just below the *level* of the dome of the diaphragm on the radiograph includes a part of the lung posteriorly and the dense liver or spleen solidly applied against its inferior concave surface. Above the level of the dome of the diaphragm the sum of all the densities is dominated by that of the lung, which offers little obstruction to the beam. Hence, on the chest film the diaphragm and its subtended organs are silhouetted, white against the lucency of the lung field above, *even though their shadows are added to that piece of lung which dips into the posterior sulcus.*

Anatomically composed of a thin sheet of muscle attached to xiphoid, lower six costal cartilages, ribs, and upper lumbar vertebrae, the diaphragm itself contributes little to the white shadow on the chest film which we mean when we refer to the "diaphragm." If free air in the peritoneal space interposes between spleen and diaphragm, as it did in the patient in Figure 6-2, the thin sheet of muscle alone is seen with air both above and below it. As usual when a curved, shell-like structure is x-rayed, what you see is that part of the diaphragm which is traversed in tangent by the beam. Although it appears to be linear, you will think in terms of roentgen densities and know it to be a domed shell dividing chest from abdomen. Under the fluoroscope it would be seen to contract downward and flatten with inspiration and to relax upward as the patient breathed out.

62

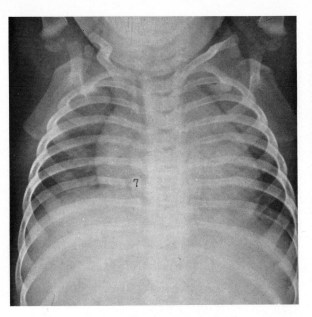 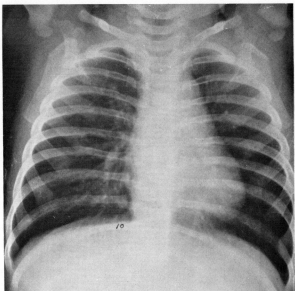

Figure 6-3 (left). The diaphragm at expiration. Figure 6-4 (right). Same patient at inspiration. Note absence of stomach bubble; the patient was lying down.

On most chest films made with the patient standing, the fundus of the stomach will be seen high against the diaphragm, usually containing swallowed air and fluid gastric juice (or lunch). A typical stomach bubble (Figure 6-1) shows a straight line marking the fluid level, above which air provides a radiolucent pocket through which more rays may pass. The same film made with the patient lying down and the beam still directed sagittally will show no level because the beam will strike the fluid level perpendicularly. Notice that in Figure 6-1 you seem to see the thickness of the diaphragm itself because there is air above and below it, but what you are actually looking at is the diaphragm plus the wall of the stomach.

A potentially hollow viscus which is completely filled with fluid and surrounded by dense viscera will not be distinguishable radiologically, but any hollow viscus which contains air will appear on the film as a dark shadow. While you are about it, take time to consider what you can do with air and a fluid level in radiography. Any hollow structure, normal or abnormal, which contains or can safely be made to contain both a gas and a fluid, will show a fluid level provided the beam crosses the plane of that level. Thus, by tilting the patient in several directions and always projecting the beam horizontally across the surface of the air-fluid inter-

face, the entire inside of a cavity can be visualized piece by piece. This can apply to the inside of the stomach, the inside of an abscess cavity, the inside of the ventricles of the brain or of the pleural space when it contains both fluid and air. Air thus becomes a useful *contrast substance*, forming a radiolucent cast of the hollow structure containing it, just as barium sulfate and other safely inert substances form radiopaque casts of the hollow structures into which they are introduced.

Compare a chest film made at expiration (Figure 6-3) and one made when the same patient had taken a deep breath (Figure 6-4). Poorly aerated alveoli and crowded-together vessels naturally decrease the radiolucency of the lung to some extent. Note too that the flexible mediastinum and fluid-filled heart have been compressed upward by the high diaphragms in Figure 6-3, so that they cast an appreciably wider shadow and appear to be enlarged. This will be true of any film made at expiration and is an additional reason why it is important for you to determine the level of the diaphragm in the course of your survey of any chest film. The patient must be cajoled into taking a deep breath if he is at all capable of it, and before you attempt to draw any conclusions from his chest film, you must check the position of his diaphragm and decide whether he has done so.

63

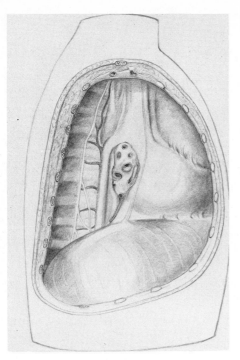

Figure 6-5. Drawing shows diaphragm and costophrenic sinus with lateral chest wall cut away.

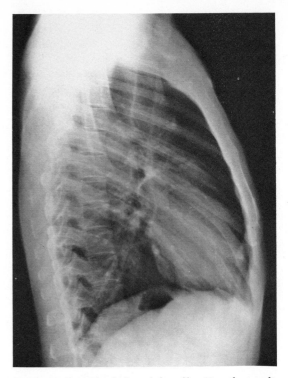

Figure 6-6. Normal right lateral chest film. Note the two diaphragmatic shadows curving down posteriorly. Which is the left diaphragm? Note the vascular trunks in lower lobes extending far down posteriorly, below the level of the crown of the diaphragm.

Because the stomach bubble (present only if there is air in the stomach) normally lies close against the undersurface of the left diaphragm, it should be included in your systematic survey of a chest film. The interposition of anything between diaphragm and fundus of stomach will displace the bubble downward. It may be deformed by the presence of tumor in the stomach. Both its appearance and its location are of importance.

For example, when any massive density in the chest just above the left diaphragm causes the disappearance of the normal diaphragmatic outline, as you have seen in the last chapter, the location of the stomach bubble may tell you where the diaphragm is. In the lateral chest film the presence of the stomach bubble close under one diaphragmatic shadow determines which is the left diaphragm (Figure 6-6).

Although the anatomist thinks of and sees the diaphragm as a single sheet of muscle and tendon, dividing chest from abdomen, the radiologist sees it on the PA chest film and at fluoroscopy as two curved shadows on either side of the heart. He speaks of the "left and right hemi-

diaphragms," in spite of the fact that he knows that usage to be anatomically and semantically not precise. It is convenient to refer to the two halves of the diaphragm in this way because they often respond independently to unilateral disease in the chest above or in the abdomen below.

The two diaphragms, then, as seen on PA adult chest films, normally are smooth curves taking off *from the midline at the origin of the tenth or eleventh ribs.* You should make a practice of counting down the posterior ribs close to the spine to determine the level of the diaphragm. Try it on a few of the chest films you have seen (being sure to identify the first rib by tracing it backward from the sternoclavicular junction). If you determine the level of the diaphragm on a few actual patients' films seen in the course of your clinical day, you will find that hospitalized patients tend to show a considerable variation in the level of their diaphragms. The well person who is having a checkup obeys efficiently the request of the technician to "take a deep breath"; but the anxious, tired, pain-beset hospital patient may fail to do so, even

64

though he has a fractured ankle to be set and nothing at all wrong with his chest or abdomen. The result is of course that the lower part of his lung close to the diaphragm will be poorly inflated with air and consequently more dense on the chest film, giving an appearance of abnormality where, in fact, none exists.

The motion of the diaphragm may be studied under the fluoroscope. When chest films are difficult to interpret and there is some question of abnormality in the lung close to the diaphragm, a fluoroscopic study of the area in question often contributes vital information. A small amount of fluid in the pleural space may not be visible in the PA chest film, for example, but may be seen during various maneuvers under the fluoroscope. The fluoroscopist tilts and turns the patient as he watches the motion of the diaphragm. That motion will be inhibited when there is inflammation near the diaphragm, and the presence of a subdiaphragmatic abscess may first be suspected when the motion is found to be limited at fluoroscopy.

The two diaphragms may be elevated by large collections of fluid in the peritoneal space, as in the patient with heart failure or cirrhosis of the liver. With distension of many loops of large or small bowel in intestinal obstruction, the diaphragms are usually high and may also be limited in their downward motion, responding reflexly to abdominal pain. For the same reason they are normally high and "splinted" in their motion for a few days after abdominal surgery. You would expect them to be high in the third trimester of pregnancy and they are.

On the other hand, the diaphragms may be depressed and flattened in any condition which greatly increases the volume of the structures within the thoracic cage. Thus, in emphysema, with irreversible trapping of air in the lung and gradually increasing overexpansion, the diaphragms are low and flat. They may show serrated margins because then the insertions into the lower ribs become visible. Likewise, with the added volume of large collections of pleural fluid or of tumor masses in the lung, the diaphragm maybe depressed.

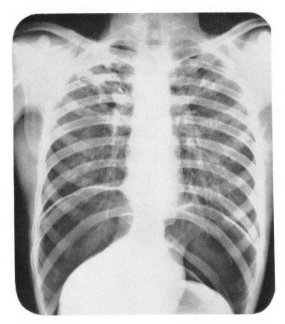

Figure 6-7 (*Unknown 6-1*). Determine the level of the diaphragms in this patient with bilateral upper lobe tuberculosis. Did the patient take a deep breath?

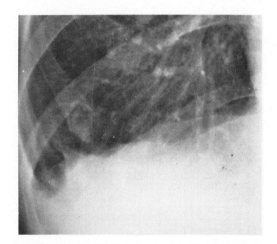

Figure 6-8. A low, flattened, serrated diaphragm is often seen in older patients, most of whom have some degree of emphysema. This diaphragm did not move at fluoroscopy.

65

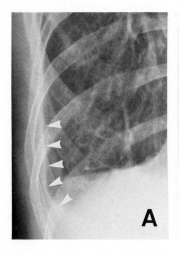
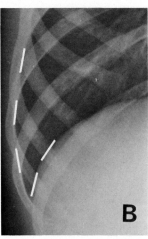

Figure 6-9 (left). A: The old, thickened pleura, caught tangentially by the beam of x-rays here, is actually a cuff of scarred tissue curving away from you and toward you over the surface of the lung and represents parietal and visceral pleura densely adherent to each other. The pleural space in this area is entirely obliterated, and with it the costophrenic sinus. (Compare B, a normal costophrenic sinus.) This is not to be confused with a small pleural effusion: remember that thickened pleura will not change from film to film or with tilting of the patient as free fluid does.

The *pleura* is a closed empty envelope, which on one side invests the surface of the lung, dipping into its fissures, and on the other side is applied against the inner surface of the thoracic cage. Too delicate to be seen radiographically under normal circumstances, it may become visible when it has been thickened by inflammation and catches the beam of x-rays tangentially against the chest wall. The two thicknesses of pleura in the *minor fissure* may frequently be seen as a thin white line extending straight laterally from the right hilum, because the minor fissure is normally horizontal. Both the left and right *major fissures* and the minor fissure on the right may be seen on the lateral chest film whenever they happen to line up with the beam.

The pleural space, although normally empty and collapsed, *may come to contain either fluid or air or both*, any of which will alter the appearance of the chest film. A massive collection of fluid on one side can displace the mediastinum toward the opposite side, depress the diaphragm, partially collapse the lung, and render the entire hemithorax dense and white. Air in large or small amounts may gain access to the pleural space by rupture through the pleural surface of the lung, or after trauma when the lung is punctured by the ends of fractured ribs. Air may be introduced into the pleural space intentionally for diagnostic purposes following a pleural tap. If the amount of pleural air is large, the lung will be seen partially collapsed against the mediastinum. Any amount of air in the pleural space allows you to see some part of the surface of the lung which you do not see in the normal chest film because the lung lies closely in contact with the chest wall. Detection of a small pneumothorax depends on seeing the veil-like pleural margin of the lung beyond which no lung markings extend.

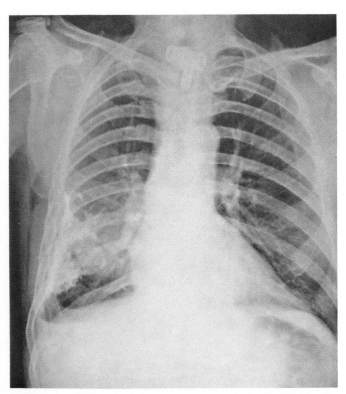

Figure 6-10. Calcification of an extensive plaque of thickened pleura. Note air in soft tissues of the lateral chest wall. There was a draining sinus in this patient with chronic inflammatory pleural disease, which explains the obliterated costophrenic sinus.

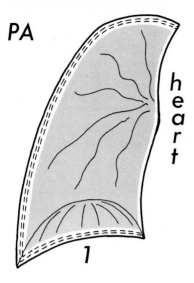

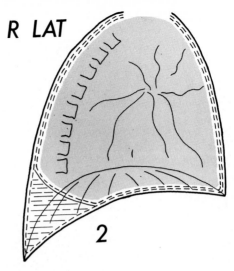

Figure 6-11. Small hydrothorax not seen in the PA view. Short broken lines indicate layers of parietal and visceral pleura between which the fluid lies.

Large amounts of pleural air or fluid are easy to visualize; small amounts are much more difficult. If you will look again at any normal diaphragm shadow in the PA projection, you will see that it dips laterally to form a sharp angle with the chest wall. The base of the lower lobe, cupped convexly over the diaphragm, dips into this recess at the sides and deep posteriorly. The *costophrenic sinus* (or *sulcus*), then, of which only the lateral part appears in the PA chest film, is a continuous ditch formed between the chest wall and the diaphragm at its insertion. The lowest part of this ditch, when the patient sits or stands, is located far posteriorly on either side of the spine, as you have already appreciated from the lateral chest film. Into this ditch extends the base of each lower lobe against the posterior insertion of the diaphragm, and pleural fluid gravitates into it. Thus the first hundred milliliters of pleural fluid which accumulates will not be visible in the lateral costophrenic sinus on the PA chest film but *would* be seen in the lateral chest film obscuring the posterior portion of the diaphragm. It would also be appreciated at fluoroscopy, coming into view as the radiologist turns and tilts the patient.

When enough fluid is present to fill up the posterior sulcus, the lateral part of the sulcus begins to fill, and this will be noted on the PA chest film as a blunting or obliteration of the costophrenic sinus on that side.

(Problem: What happens to the fluid in Figure 6-11 if, in preparing for a diagnostic tap posteriorly, the intern asks the patient to sit on a chair and lean forward?)

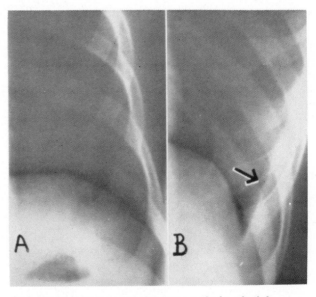

Figure 6-12. A: Patient erect. B: Patient tilted to the left. Fluid which is free in the pleural space can generally be dumped into the lateral costophrenic sinus where it is easy to see. Note that the fluid interface with the lung cannot represent the top of a rib because it is *not in series* with the inclination of the other ribs.

67

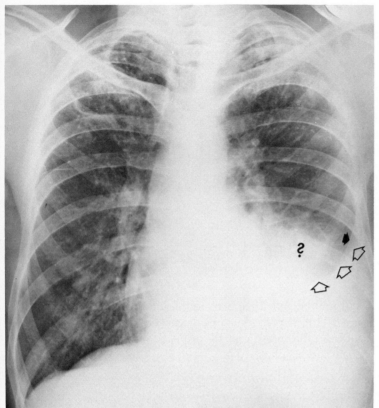

As a greater amount of fluid collects, the density of it obscures the rounded shadow of the diaphragm entirely and will be seen as an upward-curving shadow against the chest wall (Figure 6-13). *It never forms a horizontal fluid level unless there is also air present opening up the pleural space.*

Whenever you see an obscured diaphragm which does not curve downward to the lateral costophrenic sinus, you must wonder whether there is fluid above it and look closely for an upward curve of density against the lateral chest wall or for a fluid level. *Do not call a curved fluid line in simple effusion a "fluid level."* Whenever you do see a fluid level, you must look closely for the margin of lung, which is certainly present with pneumothorax and always visible somewhere. You must not forget to wonder what may be going on in that part of the lung which is concealed by the fluid shadow and to plan its better visualization (Figure 6-13). Massive effusions are more likely to be malignant in origin (Figure 6-14).

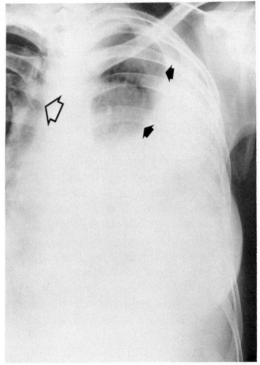

Figure 6-14. Large accumulations of fluid show a crescentic line ascending along the lateral chest wall (black arrows). Note the displacement of the trachea to the opposite side (mediastinal shift).

68

Where small amounts of pleural fluid collect far posteriorly against the diaphragm, small amounts of pleural air collect high over the cupola of the lung apex and against the upper lateral chest wall. They may be very difficult to see there because of the overlapping tangle of bones, and minimal pneumothorax is quite often missed unless you are looking carefully for it. It is more obvious when the lung is less well aerated, so that a film made at full expiration may show clearly the margin of slightly denser lung outlined by darker pleural air against the chest wall. Again, a fluoroscopic study will help, or a film may be made PA with the patient lying on his good side; the air in the pleural space will then collect over the lower ribs where it is easy to see. This is called a "lateral decubitus film" (Figure 6-16).

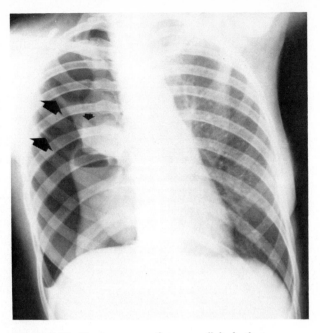

Figure 6-15. Massive pneumothorax; small hydrothorax. The right lung is only partly collapsed because of dense pleural adhesions (larger arrows). The small arrow points to the smaller of two cavities in the diseased lung; the unmarked one has a fluid level in it. You can see the three lobes collapsing separately in the pleural air. Note the horizontal fluid/air interface for the small fluid collection in the right costophrenic sinus.

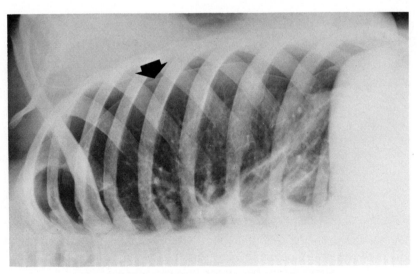

Figure 6-16. Pneumothorax. Margin of the lung outlined by air. PA lateral decubitus film. Patient lying on his side; the weight of the heart pulls the lung away from the chest wall, rendering a small pneumothorax easier to see.

69

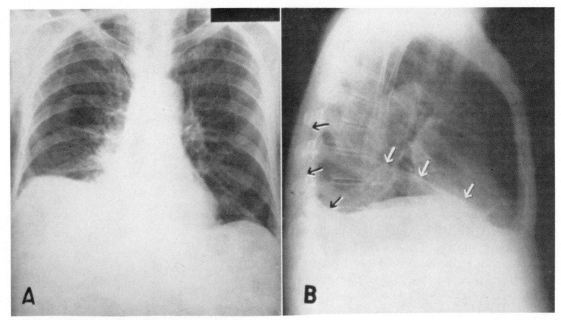

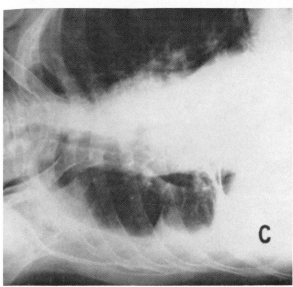

Figure 6-17. A: Subpulmonary collection of pleural fluid imitates a high right diaphragm. B: Lateral film shows fluid curving up along the posterior chest wall (black arrows) and dipping into the major fissure. C: Decubitus film shifts the fluid against the lateral chest wall, where it is seen to dip into the minor fissure.

The lateral decubitus chest film is most useful in determining the presence of subpulmonic fluid. When the patient is placed on his affected side, fluid trapped beneath the base of the lung against the diaphragm can be dumped out into the pleural space against the lateral, now-dependent chest wall as in Figure 6-17C. Without this maneuver the PA film might be interpreted as a "high right diaphragm."

Fluid may also become imprisoned in the fissures and when it does, fluoroscopy and films made at the direction of the radiologist will be able to show that the fluid lies in the known anatomic plane of one or the other of the fissures. Remember that the planes of the two major fissures descend obliquely from high against the posterior chest wall to a point low against the anterior chest wall. Similarly the plane of the minor fissure on the right is normally horizontal, extending forward and laterally from the middle of the major fissure at a level opposite the right hilum. Collections of fluid within these fissures will lie in the same planes, and you can look for them there. Frequently, when enough free fluid has accumulated, you can see it dipping into both major and minor fissures, as you do in Figure 6-17B and C.

70

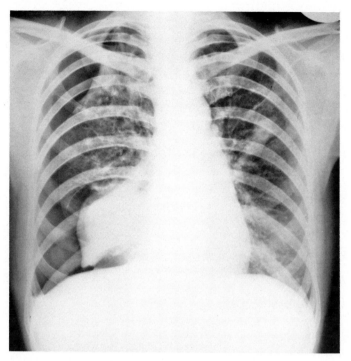

Figure 6-18 (*Unknown 6-2*). Clinically this patient had had fever and cough with hemoptysis for six months but had refused medical attention. Tuberculosis was the working diagnosis. Analyze the film and decide whether it supports the diagnosis.

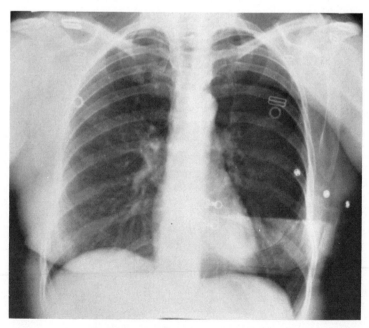

Figure 6-19 (*Unknown 6-3*). Locate this fluid level anatomically.

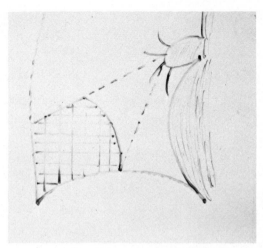

Figure 6-20. Diagram showing the points in the development of the roentgen changes in pulmonary infarction.

Pulmonary Embolism

One cause of pleural effusion often forgotten by students is *pulmonary embolus with infarction*, only now being recognized more regularly because of improvement in diagnosis with the help of isotope scans and angiography.

At first *the chest film is apt to be normal*, but the roentgen changes which develop in lung infarction of any size are now well described and logically related to the pathology.

One could anticipate early evidence of relatively underperfused lung tissue distal to the vessel blocked by the embolus, just as one could predict that the hilar vessel involved would appear to end abruptly and have no branches continuing beyond it. This has been called the *pruned hilum*.

Since infarction is always ischemia of peripheral, pleura-based lung, one could also anticipate that a peripheral density would appear on the chest film when intra-alveolar hemorrhage and, later, organization occur. Remember, though, that there is a good deal of pleura-based lung which abuts the fissures or even the mediastinum, so that infarcts do not *always* appear laterally on the chest film. They *are* more common there, and they often present as rounded densities ("Hampton's hump") near the costophrenic sinus above an elevated diaphragm. This infarcted piece of lung, when it is close to the diaphragm, may have its characteristic shape obscured by the presence of some pleural effusion.

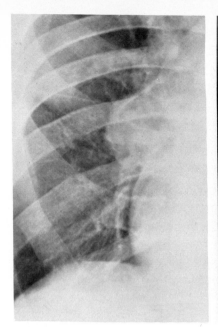 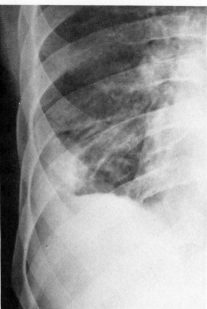 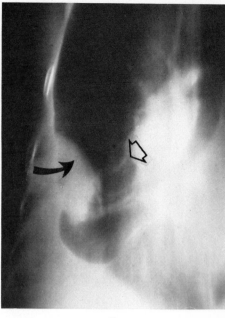

A   B   C

Figure 6-21A and B show the early and late development of characteristic roentgen findings in pulmonary infarction of the right base against the lateral chest wall.

C is a laminagram on the same patient on the same day as B. Dark arrow indicates Hampton's hump and boxed arrow points to pruned hilar vessel.

Nuclear Medicine

The use of isotope studies in pulmonary embolism

Remember that the chest film is frequently normal in pulmonary embolism (PE) even when there are convincing clinical symptoms to suggest that diagnosis. You will look carefully at such a patient's films for an elevated diaphragm and/or some pleural effusion, but today the diagnosis of PE is made as a rule with the help of *isotope studies*, often followed by *pulmonary arteriograms*.

In order to comprehend the field of radiology in the full round, you must be familiar with all of the various imaging procedures by which visual information about the patient's body may be obtained. The field of nuclear medicine is an immensely valuable aid in diagnostic work. It involves the use of *unstable isotopes (radionu-*

clides) which disintegrate, predictably releasing gamma rays. The emission of these rays may be "scanned" to produce an image on a screen and/or recorded photographically with the help of a *gamma camera*.

Lungs, bones, liver, spleen, kidney, heart, thyroid, and brain may all be evaluated with the help of such studies, and you must be prepared to learn their place in the workup of patients with various disease conditions. Currently used procedures will be discussed briefly for each area of the body as we go along. At this point it is the contribution of isotope scans to the diagnosis of pulmonary embolism with which we are concerned.

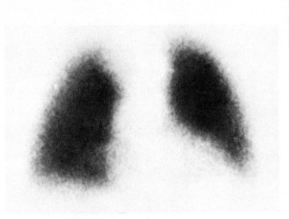

Figure 6-22. Normal perfusion lung scan. Frontal projection.

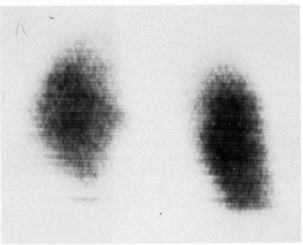

Figure 6-23. Perfusion lung scan in a patient with a large pulmonary embolus at the right base.

In pulmonary nuclear imaging one substance used is a "tagged" (radioactive) human serum albumin. Particles slightly larger than erythrocytes are injected intravenously. As they perfuse the lung, they are trapped in some of the capillary branches throughout the pulmonary arterial tree, where the emission of gamma rays continues until disintegration is complete. The particles become inactive in a matter of hours. Scanning techniques carried out during this interval produce an image of the lung (in terms of its arterial bed) which is photographically recorded. The distribution of the trapped, emitting particles is normally uniform throughout the lung, so the image produced should be that of two blackened lung-shaped shadows with the slightly asymmetrical heart shadow between them—white because it has no trapped particles.

This procedure is useful in the diagnosis of pulmonary embolism because the embolus has blocked a branch artery. The lung tissue peripheral to that block is *not* perfused with the isotope, therefore, so a "defect" (nonblackened area) is produced on the scan. This type of study is called a *perfusion scan.*

If a patient suspected of PE shows no perfusion defect on his scan, he can be presumed not to have an embolism. If the chest film shows no abnormality in a younger patient who clinically suggests embolism, and the perfusion scan shows one or more defects, the diagnosis of embolism is usually presumed to be definite.

Another useful approach to the problem of PE is the *ventilation scan.* This procedure is carried out by the inhalation of a radioactive gas (xenon). In this way the degree of ventilation of all parts of the lung can be imaged.

A number of disease conditions of the lung do cause alterations in ventilation (pneumonia, emphysema, tumors), but uncomplicated pulmonary embolism does not. Thus, a patient clinically suspected of having a pulmonary embolus who has a *perfusion scan defect but a normal ventilation scan* very probably *has* an embolus.

In older patients the presence of chronic obstructive pulmonary disease (COPD), often not apparent on the chest film, creates special problems in the diagnosis of pulmonary embolism. In these patients *matching scans* generally indicate a segment of abnormal lung causing defects on both scans and indicating both underperfusion and underventilation of that segment, probably not an infarct. But even patients with COPD can have pulmonary emboli. In such patients when the clinical suspicion of embolus is high and life threatening, a diagnosis of embolism must be established with the help of angiography. The embolus itself can then be visualized radiographically as a lucent filling defect in a blocked artery.

74

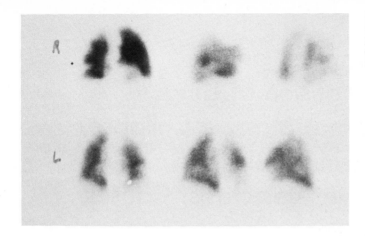

Figure 6-24. Series of *perfusion lung scans* (PA, AP, two laterals and two obliques) on a patient clinically suspected of PE. Note several defects along the right lateral chest wall in first scan.

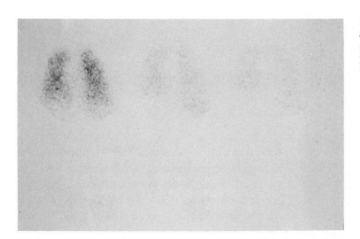

Figure 6-25. Same patient. Six *ventilation scans* show bilaterally symmetrical xenon gas which "washes out" of the lungs completely in three minutes indicating no retention, hence no COPD, and confirms PE.

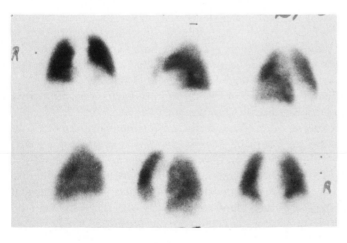

Figure 6-26. Same patient 16 days later. *Perfusion scan* is normal. Emboli have resolved.

CHAPTER **7**   Overexpansion and
Underexpansion of Lung:
Emphysema; Massive Collapse;
Compression Atelectasis;
Obstructive Atelectasis; Causes
of Mediastinal Shift

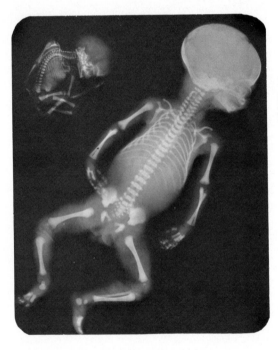

Figure 7-1. Stillborn twins, one dead at 3 months, one born dead at term. Note that lungs, heart, and abdominal structures blend into one uniform shadow.

When lung tissue is inflated with more than its normal content of air, it becomes more radiolucent than usual. No matter how clearly radiolucent the normal tissue on a chest film now looks to you, remember that it is quite logical that a cube of air should be more radiolucent than the same cube of air traversed by blood-filled capillaries. As you would expect, then, the roentgen appearance of overexpanded lung will be an overall *increased radiolucency*, the affected lung appearing too dark with the exposures used for chest work. In addition, the lung markings will be spread apart as the vessels are separated farther and farther by the ballooned alveoli. In ob-

structive emphysema localized to one segment of lung this appearance maybe so exaggerated as to be confused with pneumothorax. The true state of affairs may generally be determined by a careful fluoroscopic study or by inspiration and expiration films.

Atelectasis, on the other hand, causes the lung to appear less radiolucent than usual, and atelectasis of one lobe will be seen first as a difference in density between the two sides of the chest film. Thus you will be looking for an unaccountably dense area in the lung. You have already seen diffusely increased density due to the high position of both diaphragms in a film made at peak expiration, and you realize that that amount of decreased radiolucency at some phase of the respiratory cycle goes with every breath your patient takes.

You see in Figure 7-1 the chest film of a stillborn infant who has never breathed at all. His lungs and bony thorax are collapsed about the heart and mediastinal structures as one uniformly dense shadow within the rib cage, and they blend continuously with the shadows of the dense abdominal structures.

76

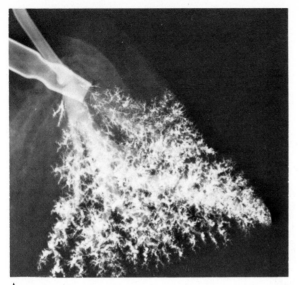
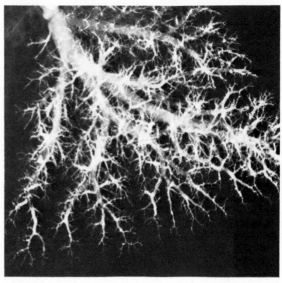

A   Figure 7-2   B

In Figure 7-2 the arterial tree of a dog's lung has been injected with opaque fluid and sealed off, inflation and deflation of the lung being carried out through a tube tied into the bronchus. In Figure 7-2A you see the lung collapsed around its arterial tree in just about the same degree of hypoaeration which would exist near the diaphragm at full expiration. In Figure 7-2B the specimen has been inflated to approximate the lung near the diaphragm at deep inspiration.

Below you see the lungs of a child at expiration and inspiration. (In childhood a range from posterior rib 7 to posterior rib 10 is normal for full respiratory excursion.) In this chapter you will learn the changes in the appearance of the chest film when both lungs are underexpanded (Figures 7-1 and 7-3A) and when both are overexpanded (next page spread). Then we will consider the changes seen when the volume of one hemithorax is altered enough to produce shift of the mediastinum from its midline position.

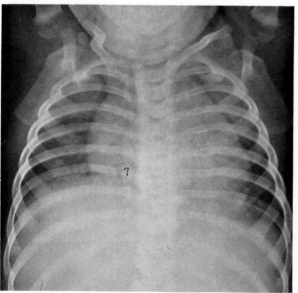
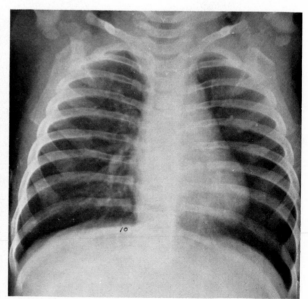

A   Figure 7-3   B

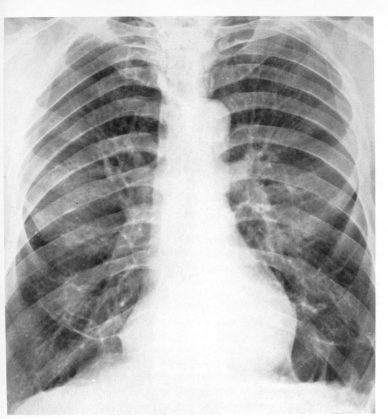

Figure 7-4. Emphysema with bleb formation, both lower lobes. The heart appears normal in size, but remember that right ventricular enlargement (cor pulmonale) is difficult-to-impossible to recognize in the PA view alone. In the lateral view the lower half of the anterior clear space may be obliterated in cor pulmonale because of right ventricular enlargement. The patients with small-looking hearts on this page spread probably have cor pulmonale, the *relatively* large right ventricle being masked in the PA view by its anterior location and the bilateral compression of the heart from the overinflated lungs.

Emphysema

With chronic emphysema the lungs are both generally overexpanded, the diaphragms low, flattened, and often serrated. Many cases will be obvious to you by these tokens, together with the increased radiolucency you will see at the usual roentgen exposures for chest work. Lesser degrees of generalized emphysema may be much less obvious. In those patients the fluoroscopic finding of diaphragms which move down only slightly with inspiration and return only very slowly on forced expiration will help to establish a diagnosis of emphysema. In many patients with emphysema the concomitant development of pulmonary fibrosis adds the shadow of a web of filamentous strands of increased density. These radiate outward from the hilum through the entire lung. Localized emphysematous bullae may be seen anywhere in the lung, like huge air cysts bordered by dense thin walls which enclose them. Rupture of such bullae, producing a spontaneous pneumothorax, is not unusual.

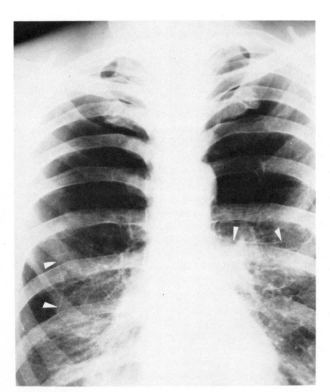

Figure 7-5. Widespread pan-acinar emphysema grade III in a patient with chronic bronchitis. Arrows mark walls of bullae.

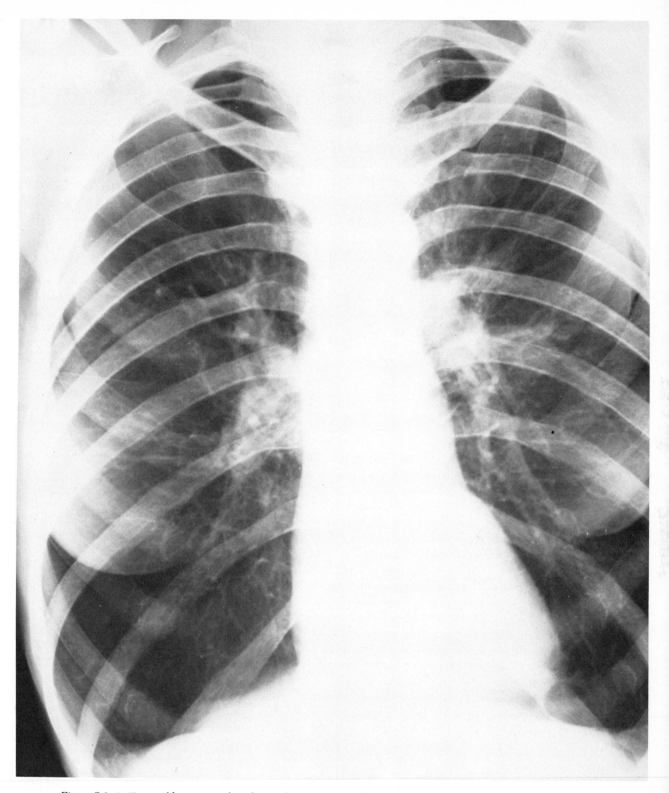

Figure 7-6. A 45-year-old woman with widespread pan-acinar emphysema had severe dyspnea and evidence of airway obstruction but no cough or sputum, no history of asthma, and no wheeze. Note the low position of the diaphragms, the small heart with prominent pulmonary artery and normal hilar vessels which *look* prominent in relation to the actually small peripheral lung vessels. You can use the relatively normal left upper lung field vessels as normal marker vessels to help you observe that the comparable ones on the right are small. In most of this woman's lungs there is really no capillary bed left.

Normal Mediastinal Position

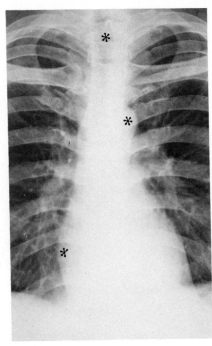

Figure 7-7. Three tag points to be used in checking the midline position of the mediastinum. (See text.)

Anatomists describe the mediastinum as a region. I prefer to think of it as a bundle of structures sandwiched between the two inflated lungs. With the exception of the air-filled trachea, all these structures have the same radiodensity and merge into a homogeneous shadow superimposed upon that of the spine in the PA projection. Thus, the shadows of the mediastinal structures cannot be separated from each other except by a variety of special procedures employing contrast substances or by computerized tomography. On the routine chest film, only the lateral margins of the mediastinum outlined by air in the lungs on either side can be identified.

With important changes in the air content of either lung, or with large accumulations of pleural air or fluid, the mediastinum will bow to one side like an elastic diaphragm. You will need to identify a few anatomic points along the margins of the mediastinal shadow and to know their normal locations if you are to be able to recognize mediastinal displacement. There are three of these signal points which ought to be included in your systematic chest survey.

The first is the column of air in the trachea, visible as a dark vertical shadow on the PA chest film, normally a little to the right of the midline as it approaches the carina. The second is the white knob you see to the left of the spine at about the fifth rib posteriorly. This knob is the shadow margin created by the arch of the aorta as it swings posteriorly and turns downward to become the descending aorta. You see it, of course, only because there is radiolucent lung tissue abutted against it, and it will disappear if that lung tissue becomes airless or if a dense mass lies against the aorta.

Finding the trachea and the aortic arch in their usual locations, then, will tell you that the upper mediastinum is where it ought to be. When there is a marked decrease in the amount of air in the right upper lobe, for example, the trachea will be found shifted toward that side. The arch of the aorta will be pulled with it toward the midline, its shadow disappearing as it becomes superimposed upon that of the spine. In just the same way the trachea and the aortic arch may be displaced to the left when there is a decrease in the air content of the left upper lobe. If you review the anatomic relations of the aortic arch, you will find that normally both upper and lower lobes adjoin it. For this reason, if there is no air at all in the left upper lobe, it will lie, dense and much decreased in size, against the *anterior* mediastinum, and you may actually still see the aorta through it, illumined by the overexpanded lower lobe. Check the position of trachea and aortic arch on some of the chest films you have seen so far.

The third tag point in determining the position of the mediastinum is the shadow of the right heart border. Major changes in the size of either *lower* lobe will swing the heart to one side, and it will look displaced. You may think that since we have not yet discussed the heart and cardiac enlargement, you will not be able to use the right heart border with much sense of security, but be reassured. Up to now I have shown you very few abnormal hearts and a good many normal chest films. Look back over some of them at the right border of the heart as it curves down toward the diaphragm. By the time you have looked at a dozen or so, you should be convinced that the border of the normal right heart shadow is generally about a fingerbreadth beyond the right border of the spine on a full 14-by 17-inch chest film (and proportionately less on these engraved reductions). Of course, this is a very rough working rule, and you will learn how to modify it as you look at more and more films.

Obviously, elevation of the diaphragms compressing the liquid-filled heart from below will exaggerate the lateral projection of both heart borders. Therefore, accuracy about mediastinal position will depend on your having counted down the ribs so that you are sure the diaphragms are drawn down well. Obviously, too, if the right middle lobe lying against the right heart is consolidated, that border will disappear and cannot be used in tagging the position of the lower mediastinum.

If, however, you are satisfied that the diaphragms are well down, that the clavicles and ribs are symmetrical and show no rotation, and that the right heart border appears to be in about its usual position, you can say then that the lower mediastinum is not appreciably displaced.

If the *whole lung* on one side collapses, then all three tag points will show a shift in position, since the whole mediastinum swings to that side. If *only an upper lobe* is involved, you may find that the trachea and aortic arch are shifted, while the right heart border is not. On the other hand, *collapse of only a lower lobe* may cause a definite shift of the position of the heart, although that of the trachea and aorta remains normal. Less massive changes such as collapse of the right middle lobe or of one bronchopulmonary segment will usually not be enough to displace the mediastinum at all and they are readily compensated for by slight overexpansion of adjoining lung tissue.

If you analyzed Figure 7-8 correctly, you realized that the patient was markedly rotated so that the right ribs appear much longer than those on the left. The straight PA film made a few minutes later is seen in Figure 7-9, in which a slightly better inspiration has also been taken. Aortic arch and right heart border are now normal (for an infant with his diaphragms at the middle of the ninth interspace), and the mediastinum is clearly in midposition.

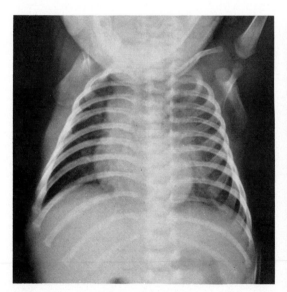

Figure 7-8. Is this mediastinal shift? Before you go on, analyze this film according to every kind of basic information you now possess.

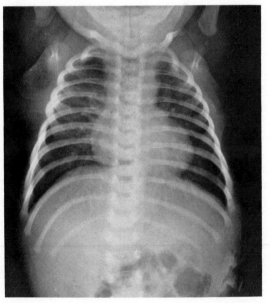

Figure 7-9. (See text.)

Mediastinal Shift

The mediastinum may be displaced *permanently* (for example, by scar tissue in the lung retracting it to one side, or by surgical removal of the whole lung); *temporarily* (as when a major lobe collapses postoperatively); or *transiently* (as when a foreign body in one major bronchus interferes with the inflation or deflation of that part of the lung during each inspiration). Permanent and temporary displacements of the mediastinum will usually be appreciable from the PA chest film, and you will be looking for them every time you check the three tag points in your systematic chest survey.

Transient shifts are often first recognized only at fluoroscopy when the radiologist employs one of the many maneuvers he has developed to demonstrate such findings. One of these is to ask the patient to sniff suddenly, with one border of the mediastinum held in view under the fluoroscope. The sudden inspiratory sniff will cause the mediastinum to jump slightly to one side if inequality of aeration is present.

Because any single chest film only represents the state of affairs in your patient's chest at one particular fraction of a second in time, it is quite possible to expose the film when the mediastinum is in midposition, even though there is a definite mediastinal shift during some other phase of respiration. The single PA film you hold in your hand later that day thus may give no indication at all that there was a transient shift of the mediastinum at expiration. If you suspect there may be one, you ought to ask for *films made at inspiration and expiration,* a commonly used device for recording transient mediastinal shift.

The mediastinum may also be *pushed* to one side by pressure from an overexpanded lung, as in obstructive emphysema when air is drawn into that part of the lung with every breath but incompletely expelled. A check-valve foreign body may do this. The same dynamics exist when faulty bronchi with inadequate cartilaginous support collapse with each attempted expiration.

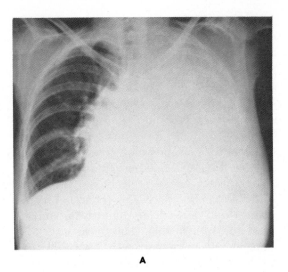

A

Figure 7-10A. Temporary mediastinal shift due to a massive pleural effusion. The trachea and heart are displaced to the right by the accumulation of fluid in the left pleural space. B shows the patient after recovery. Note sharp, clear costophrenic sinuses.

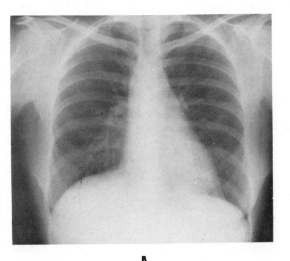

B

Obstructive emphysema probably also exists at some point in the natural history of any endobronchial tumor, although soon the obstruction is completed as the tumor grows, and the lung beyond it collapses as its air is absorbed or escapes to other segments. On serial films one would be able to observe the mediastinum at first displaced *away* from the side of the lesion by the overexpanded lung and a week or so later displaced *toward* the side of the lesion as the affected lobe collapses, another illustration of the value of serial films and the proper evaluation of changing roentgen signs.

If you make a practice of thinking of the mediastinum as a flexible disc held in the midline *whenever the volumes of the two hemithoraces are equal*, you will not find it difficult to understand and remember how mediastinal shift occurs. The mediastinum *must* shift whenever there is an important change in the volume on one side. Massive pleural effusion shifts the mediastinum to the opposite side, as you have seen in Figure 7-10A. It would be pushed to the opposite side by the overexpansion of the remaining lung in congenital absence of one lung, or after pneumonectomy, or in massive collapse of one whole lung. Unilateral bullous emphysema may shift the mediastinum, compressing the good lung as in Figure 7-12.

The mediastinum may *not* shift, on the other hand, if the various additions and subtractions in volume on one side cancel each other out, so that the volume of the abnormal hemithorax remains equal to that on the normal side. For example, in Figure 7-11 you see a patient with a large pneumothorax. Air trapped in the pleural space has added to the volume of the left hemithorax, but at the same time the left lung has collapsed to one-third its normal volume. Note that the mediastinum remains in the midline.

The mediastinum *may* not shift because it has become fixed as a result of adhesions subsequent to inflammation, or from tumor invasion. It may also be checked in its displacement by pleural adhesions which prevent the full collapse of one lung.

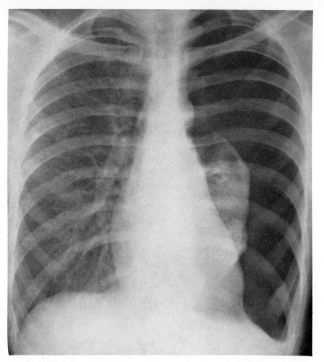

Figure 7-11. Pneumothorax with the mediastinum in the midline. The volume of pleural air is compensated for here by the degree of collapse of the left lung.

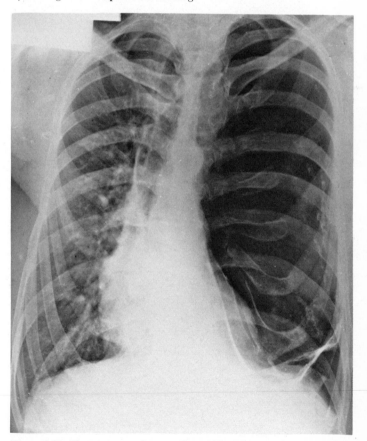

Figure 7-12. Obstructive emphysema of part of the left lung, causing shift of the mediastinum to the right. No pneumothorax was present.

Mediastinal Shift due to Abnormality of One Lung

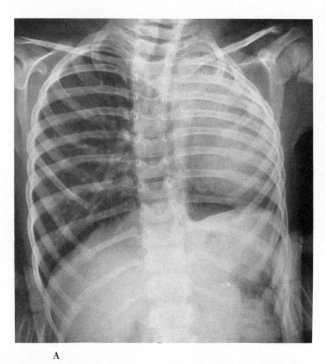

A

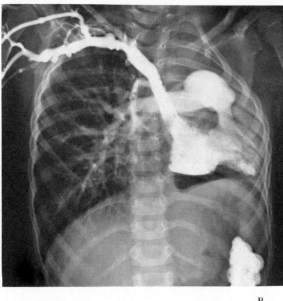

B

Figure 7-13A. Permanently displaced mediastinum in a 4-year-old who had agenesis of the left lung and compensatory overexpansion of the right lung coming across the midline. The dense mass in the left hemithorax is the heart, as proved by angiography, B. Note absence of left pulmonary artery.

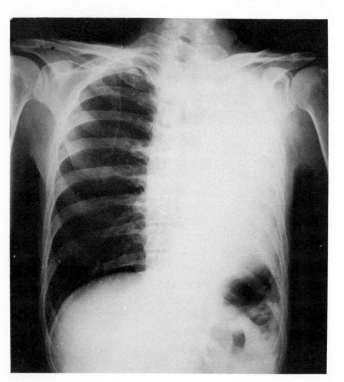

Figure 7-14. Massive collapse of the left lung. Note pronounced mediastinal shift and high diaphragm. A late postpneumonectomy film would look the same.

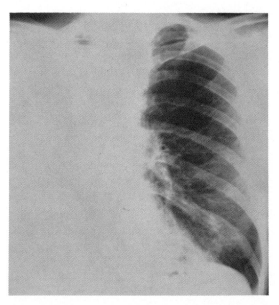

Figure 7-15. Have you evidence here for mediastinal shift? (Answered in the text.)

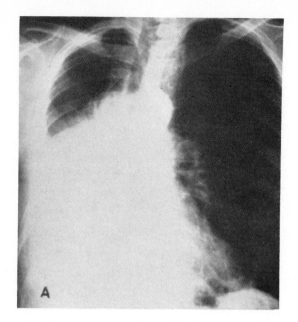

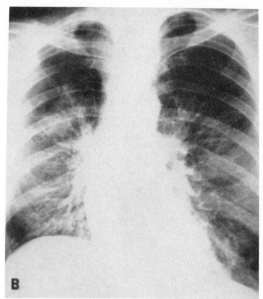

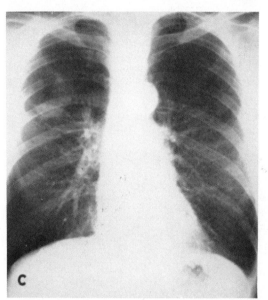

Figure 7-16. (See text.)

The patient in Figure 7-15 has a massive collapse of the right lung. The heart shadow is shifted to the right and merged with that of the atelectatic right lung. The trachea is not seen on this film, but there is no aortic arch visible to the left of the spine. The right heart border can be of no use to you here because of the increased density of the lung against it.

The presence of lung carcinoma with atelectasis was established by bronchoscopy and aspiration of malignant cells, and the patient in Figure 7-15 received a course of radiation therapy. The three parts of Figure 7-16 are a series of subsequent studies made during that treatment and at three months after it had been completed. In A, part of the right upper lobe has reexpanded but not enough to allow the trachea, now clearly seen, to return to midline. However, the aortic arch is now well seen. The right heart border and diaphragmatic profile are still absent. In B, they have reappeared with the reexpansion of the entire lung. The primary lung tumor mass may now be seen in the mid-lung field overlying the right seventh rib, and both hila are seen enlarged with tumor-invaded nodes. In C, made three months after the completion of treatment, there is further regression and the mediastinum is clearly in normal position, although the primary tumor in the right lung is still seen. Collapse of the right lung was doubtless the result of compression of the right main bronchus by the hilar mass of secondary nodes (no obstruction of the airway due to endobronchial tumor could be considered here, since the tumor mass is seen peripherally). In lung cancer this type of massive early bilateral hilar and mediastinal metastases is fairly common.

Mediastinal Shift due to
Collapse of One Lobe on the Right

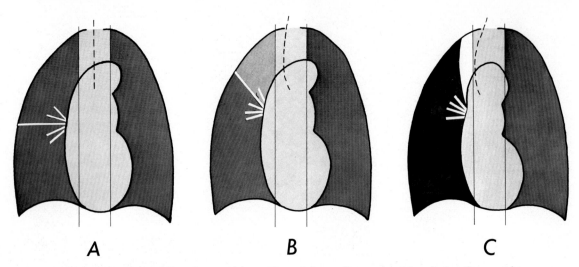

A   B   C

Figure 7-17. Collapse of the right upper lobe. A: Normal chest with normal position of minor fissure, right hilum, trachea, aortic knob, and right heart border, and equal aeration of all lobes. B: Right upper lobe collapsed 50 percent. Minor fissure deflected upward, trachea pulled slightly to the right. No change in right heart border. Changes in aortic knob and hilum equivocal. C: Major collapse of the right upper lobe, which is now a flat wedge of density against the superior mediastinum. Trachea and aortic knob deflected to the right. Right hilum drawn upward. Overaeration (hyperradiance) of lower and middle lobes. No change in right heart border. (Hilar displacement upward or downward is sometimes the first evidence of a collapsed lobe to be noticed.)

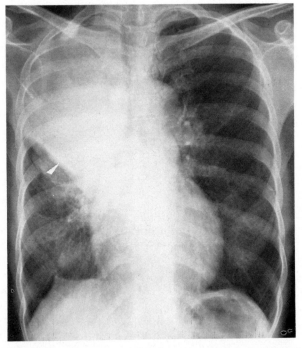

Figure 7-18. Patient with right upper lobe atelectasis distal to a bronchogenic carcinoma. Arrow indicates elevated minor fissure.

A collapsing lobe tends to fold up fanwise against the mediastinum in a characteristic manner, and a dynamic concept of these collapse patterns and the roentgen signs by which they are to be recognized is, again, nothing more than an exercise in the logic of radiodensities applied anatomically. You would anticipate, for example, that with atelectasis of the *right upper lobe* the location of the minor horizontal fissure dividing it from the middle lobe could be seen increasingly well as the contrast increased between the poorly aerated lung tissue above it and the well-aerated lung tissue below it. Moreover, since the fissure is fixed at the hilum, it is natural that it would be seen to tilt upward from that fixed point as the upper lobe collapsed. When completely collapsed, the pancake-flat upper lobe would apply itself against the upper mediastinum and merge its shadow with that of other mediastinal structures. The shadow of the trachea would be drawn to the right, and the aortic knob would be drawn with it. The right hilum would appear to be drawn upward slightly.

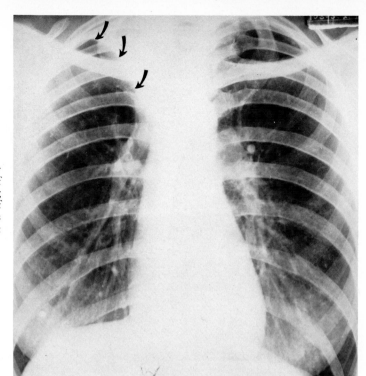

Figure 7-19. Nearly complete collapse of the right upper lobe in a patient with a ten-year history of symptoms of cough and occasional hemoptysis. Arrows indicate curving margin of elevated minor fissure. At surgery obstruction of the right upper lobe bronchus by a bronchial adenoma was discovered and lobectomy performed. Note high right hilum and stretched lower lobe vessels.

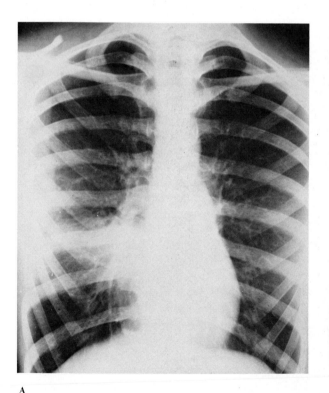

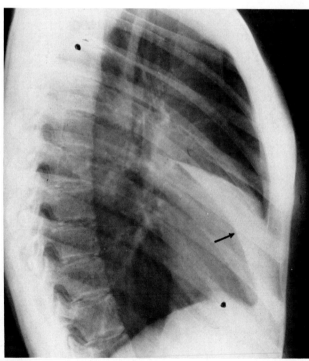

A

B

Figure 7-20. Collapse of the right middle lobe. A line drawn between the two black dots in the lateral view (B) would indicate the normal location of the major (oblique) fissure. Hence its lower part must be bowed forward (arrow).

87

Mediastinal Shift due to
Collapse of One Lobe on the Left

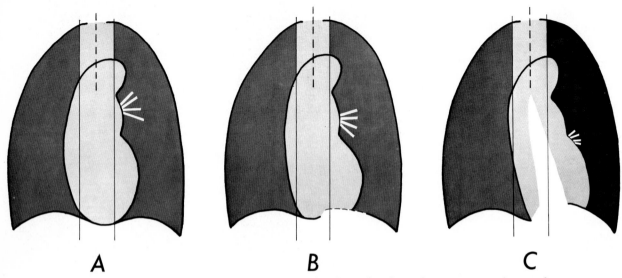

Figure 7-21. Collapse of the left lower lobe. A: Normal profiles and mediastinal tag points. B: Early signs of left lower lobe collapse. Less of the heart is seen to the right of the spine. Vague decrease in lucency of lower left lung field with preservation of the diaphragmatic profile, which becomes slightly elevated and less sharp medially. C: Massive collapse of the left lower lobe. Little or no heart profile seen to the right of the spine. Medial half of the left diaphragm profile missing. Left lower lobe seen as a wedge of density through the heart shadow. Left hilum depressed. Increased radiolucency of the left upper lobe.

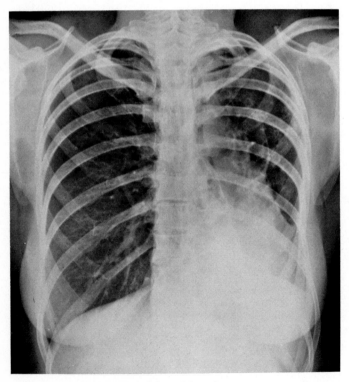

Figure 7-22. Left lower lobe collapse in a woman postappendectomy with inhalation anesthesia.

Now put together the signs of *left lower lobe* collapse in just the same deliberately logical way. Since the major fissure on the left lines up with the beam of x-rays only in the lateral view and is always quite oblique to the ray in the PA view, no clear-cut margin between the normal and atelectatic lung tissue is to be seen in the PA film as the left lower lobe begins to collapse. However, the heart gradually shifts toward the left, so that you see less and less of the heart border to the right of the spine. You watch the left diaphragm become slightly more elevated and less and less clearly seen medially as the left lower lobe collapses, although the *lateral* half of the shadow profile of the diaphragm remains clear because of the compensatory expansion of the lingula of the left upper lobe, now touching it. The left hilum is depressed, gradually disappearing behind the left border of the heart, an important and often missed roentgen sign of left

88

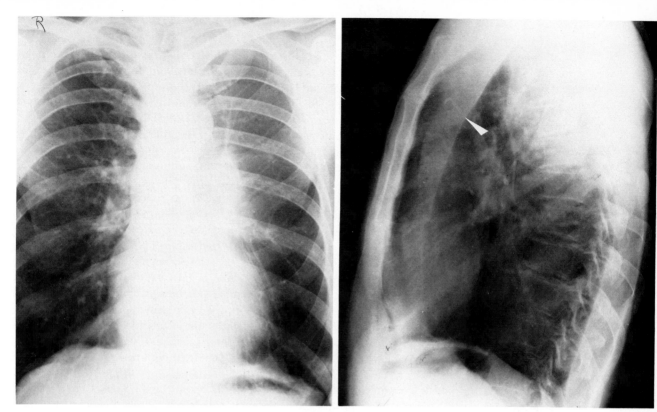

A

B

Figure 7-23. Collapsing left upper lobe due to obstructing carcinoma. Note veil-like density of left upper lung field and obscured left heart profile. The trachea is pulled to the midline and the aorta is too prominent, implying upper mediastinal shift. Lateral view (B): arrow indicates main fissure bowed forward as left upper lobe collapses. It is seen here as a slender wedge of density.

lower lobe collapse. The lung markings of the left upper lobe appear spread apart and the lung tissue more lucent than that in comparable interspaces on the right. The totally collapsed lower lobe appears, finally, as a wedge-shaped shadow against the mediastinum posteriorly. Its outer margin is visible through the heart shadow, thrown into contrast by air in the normal lung tissue against it laterally, that is, in the overexpanded upper lobe (Figure 7-22).

No matter how subtle the findings may be radiologically, if you are making a practice of going over each chest film in a systematic fashion, one day soon you will discover suddenly that the mediastinum you are looking at is shifted or that the medial half of one diaphragmatic shadow is missing. Any such finding must be accounted for, and it is then that you will begin to look more closely at the relative position of the two hila, compare the radiolucency of

the lung tissue on the two sides, and check for the presence of slim wedges of density against the mediastinum. In the next patient in whom you suspect atelectasis of a lobe, you ought to arrange to be present when the radiologist carries out the indicated fluoroscopy. There you will watch the mediastinum shift conspicuously and observe inequality of aeration to be exaggerated at some phase of respiration.

Although collapse of any of the four major lobes will generally result in the findings outlined for you above, collapse of the smaller *right middle lobe* or of a *single bronchopulmonary segment* will be too minor a change in volume to cause mediastinal displacement, hilar shift, or much variation in lung markings. Collapse of these smaller structures must be diagnosed from their appearance and anatomic location, with heavy reliance on the history and change from film to film.

Roentgen observations which imply the presence of extensive emphysema or massive atelectasis will serve to remind you of distortions in architecture and aberrations of function which you might otherwise forget to consider in a particular patient. The old man with chronic emphysema is most concerned with his respiratory difficulties, but you will not be able to look at those overexpanded lungs and fibrous traceries of shadow without thinking of the increased work being done by the right side of his heart. In the same way, the signs of a collapsed lung must remind you that its vessels are crowded together, that the pulmonary circulation of blood is greatly decreased, and that the functioning of the heart must be embarrassed.

Finally, you must not forget, in looking at such films, that changes in volume within the thorax may compensate for other changes and obscure them. If the mediastinum seems in its normal midline position in spite of the fact that one entire lung field is dense, you can know only that the volumes of the two hemithoraces *are* equal. Underneath that white density there may be just enough collapse to compensate for the added volume of tumor or pleural effusion.

Remember that the radiograph is a shadowgram. Although you know that inflammation and tumor both render the lung dense, you must anticipate, for example, that in either condition some atelectasis is likely to be present as well, adding to the density of the already involved lung. Tumor or inflammation may cause collapse of a lobe even though the entire lobe is not actually involved in the primary process.

The consolidated pneumonic lobe often remains normal in size, as you saw it in Chapter 5, but equally often such a lobe will be distinctly decreased in size. In a good many patients with the clinical signs of pneumonia, therefore, you must expect to find some additional roentgen indications of atelectasis. As you expand your knowledge of medicine, you will learn to evaluate the roentgen signs of lobar collapse according to whether, for example, your patient was admitted with clear-cut pneumonia or has only a minor degree of fever and cough the day following surgery. In the former you must think in terms of pneumonia-plus-atelectasis and treat accordingly. In the latter you must think in terms of atelectasis primarily, and of the possibility of inflammation developing in the collapsed lobe. That they may look the same, or very nearly so, on the films should not disturb you, since you are using the radiographic findings as part of the entire clinical analysis rather than as oracular information.

In just the same way, bronchogenic carcinoma quite often presents itself initially as atelectasis, that is, as a lobe which is gradually collapsed beyond the invisible obstructing bronchial tumor. Indeed, all three explanations for increased density may be present together in a patient who develops pneumonia in a partly collapsed lobe behind a tumor of the bronchus. A respectable percentage of lung cancers are at first thought to be pneumonia with atelectasis, and only the unaccountable failure of the atelectasis to resolve and the lungs to reexpand fully with proper treatment eventually raises the question of tumor.

Up to this point in the book I have avoided giving you diagnostic labels. It is immensely important for you to realize that the type of analysis of roentgen findings you have been learning offers you an improved understanding of the dynamic pathologic changes within the thoracic cage of your patient. As such it is much more useful to you than any collection of diagnostic tags and labels. When you see mediastinal shift on a chest film or appreciate exaggerated radiolucency or the disappearance of normal profiles, you are recognizing roentgen findings rather than diagnoses. Such findings are heavy with implication as to what is going on inside your patient. Their presence will often go a long way toward confirming, expanding, or exploding an original working diagnosis based on the history and physical examination. The trained radiologist's daily experience with roentgen shadows increases his capacity for similar but more sophisticated deductions, and some of these permit him to conclude beyond all reasonable doubt that a specific condition must be present. Be satisfied yourself with recognizing roentgen signs a bit longer.

90

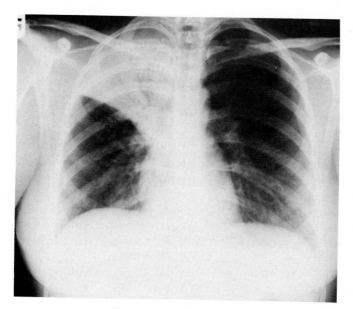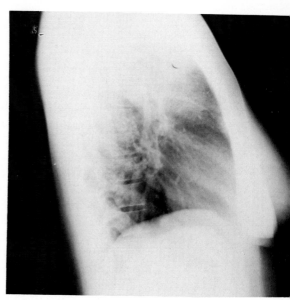

Figure 7-24 (*Unknown 7-1*). Young woman with fever and cough for one week; well before. Analyze film, make a provisional diagnosis, and plan workup and management.

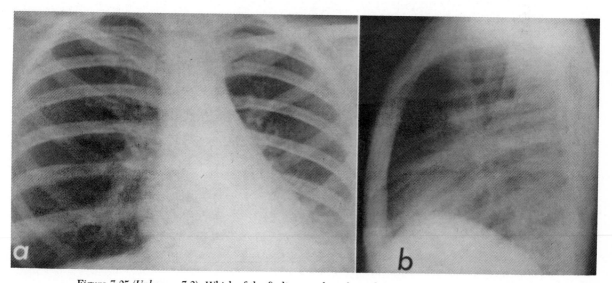

Figure 7-25 (*Unknown 7-2*). Which of the findings we have been discussing are present in this patient?

The heart is the largest of the mediastinal structures, and all of the profiles which bulge beyond the shadow of the spine on both sides represent parts of the heart or of its great vessels. You can think of these profiles as nine intersecting arcs. Justify their identity on the basis of the angiocardiograms on the opposite page. Remember that some of the structures producing these shadows are more posterior in the chest (8,9) and others far anterior (2,7). Remember, too, that when an opaque substance mixed with

blood fills a particular chamber of the heart, its shadow may seem to you quite different in shape from what you have learned about that chamber based on a gross examination of the heart and its surface markings. Where a chamber is thickest its shadow will be most dense in the angiogram, and where it tapers off and becomes very thin a much less dense shadow is produced. Look at the shadow of the right ventricle, for example, in Figure 8-3. The slender, flattened part of the chamber which extends far

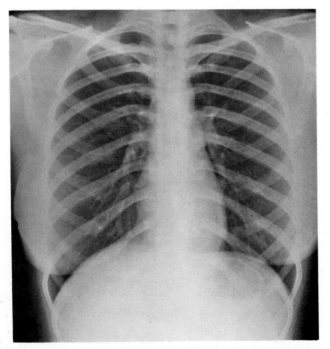
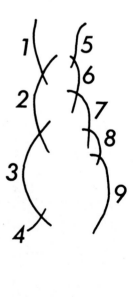

Figure 8-1 (left). The normal mediastinal profiles are all vascular and resolve into a series of nine intersecting arcs, as shown in Figure 8-2 (right): (1) superior vena cava; (2) ascending aorta; (3) right atrium; (4) inferior vena cava and cardiac fat pad; (5) left subclavian vein and artery, left common carotid artery; (6) aortic arch; (7) pulmonary artery; (8) left atrium; (9) left ventricle.

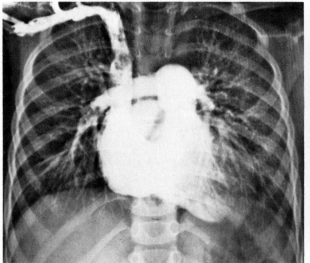

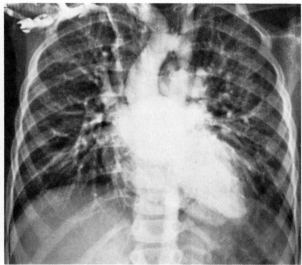

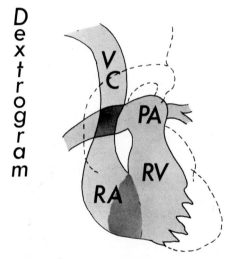

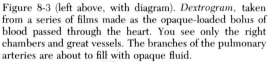

Figure 8-3 (left above, with diagram). *Dextrogram*, taken from a series of films made as the opaque-loaded bolus of blood passed through the heart. You see only the right chambers and great vessels. The branches of the pulmonary arteries are about to fill with opaque fluid.

Figure 8-4 (right above, with diagram). *Levogram*, taken three seconds later when the right side of the heart had been cleared of opaque-containing blood. You see only the shadows of the left chambers and great vessels. This child had coarctation of the aorta (indentation below the arch of the aorta).

to the left against the interventricular septum in the PA view hardly seems to belong to the dense massive shadow of the rest of the ventricle. Note also that you appreciate only vaguely the location of the tricuspid valve in this view, because the right atrium and right ventricle are partly superimposed. In the levogram notice that you see the dense upper margin of the crab-shaped left atrium through the shadow of the ascending aorta, in spite of the fact that you know the left atrium is on the posterior surface of the heart and that the ascending aorta arises anteriorly. Their opaque-filled cavities have cast separate shadows outlining them for you, and the two shadows overlap in this view.

The plain film of the chest made PA, then, shows you a number of mediastinal bulges seen in profile against the radiolucent lung on either side of the spine, all of them vascular shadows. In addition, you can usually see air in the trachea, but all other mediastinal organs merge with one another and their shadows are superimposed upon those of the spine and the heart. You cannot account for the shadow of the esophagus or distinguish lymph nodes, thymus, or nerves; the thoracic duct merges with the shadows of other soft tissues and fluid-carrying vessels. Except for their marginal profiles and their branches entering the lucent lungs, even the great vessels are merged with other shadows.

Fortunately most of the mediastinal structures can be visualized safely in one way or another by the use of specialized techniques. The vascular structures, of course, have been studied in the past decades in an impressive variety of ways. In Figure 8-5 the aortic arch and its branches in the superior mediastinum are seen studied in two projections after a radiopaque contrast material has been injected via a catheter inserted into the right brachial artery. The chambers of the heart are studied by injecting an opaque substance through a catheter placed in the antecubital vein and observing the bolus of radiodense blood as it passes through the heart. Angiocardiograms will be discussed further in a subsequent chapter.

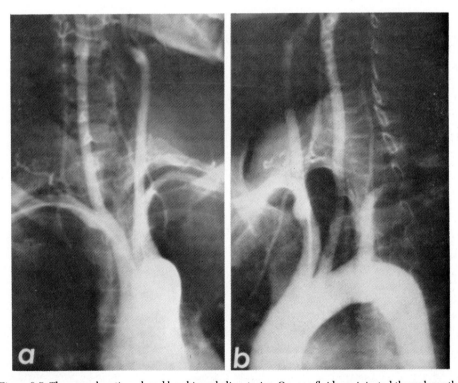

Figure 8-5. The normal aortic arch and brachiocephalic arteries. Opaque fluid was injected through a catheter in the brachial artery. The patient in *a* is almost PA (very slightly rotated to the left). In *b* he has been sharply rotated to his right, unrolling the aortic arch so that its branches no longer overlap. Remember that both venous and arterial shadows account for arcs 1 and 5 in Figure 8-1.

Much information may be obtained by study of the radiolucent column of air in the trachea. The compression or displacement of the trachea or major bronchi is often not apparent on the plain PA chest film, but is well seen on Bucky films, on films made with supervoltage techniques, or in body-section studies.

On this page you are employing as a contrast medium the normally present air within the bronchial tree. While it is perfectly feasible also to instill opaque fluid into the trachea, coating the inner surface of the structures to be studied (as in bronchography), films which depend on air alone for contrast may be very informative. The air column will be seen well in Bucky films. It is visualized in even better detail in body-section studies, such as the one in Figure 8-6A. Body-section studies give you more precise details because the confusing superimposed shadows of structures in front of or behind the tracheobronchial tree have been eliminated.

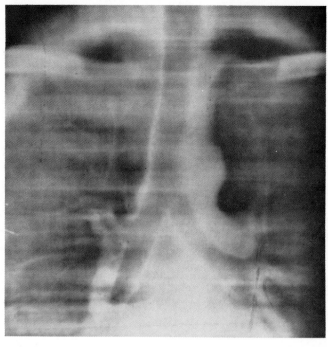

A

Figure 8-6. Coronal body-section study of the normal tracheobronchial tree.

(1) Clavicle
(2) Normal opacity of great vessels and tracheal wall
(3) Azygos vein
(4) Right main stem bronchus
(5) Right upper lobe bronchus
(6) Site of origin of right middle lobe bronchus
(7) Right lower lobe bronchus
(8) Normal opacity of vessels and tracheal wall
(9) Trachea
(10) Aortic arch
(11) Concave profile between aortic knob and left pulmonary pedicle
(12) Left pulmonary pedicle
(13) Left main stem bronchus
(14) Left upper lobe bronchus
(15) Left lower lobe bronchus
(16) Carina

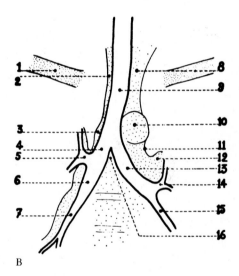

B

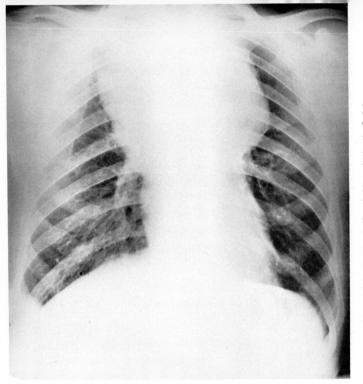

Here you can study the abnormal soft tissue profiles produced by mediastinal masses and compare them with the normal arc profiles identified in Figure 8-2. In all such patients the initial plain film of the chest shows a mediastinal bulge or fullness. In some of them the radiologist would be able to weight his interpretation very heavily in favor of a particular type of pathologic condition (as in the patient with mediastinal lymphoma in Figure 8-7) because of the smooth bilateral bulges. In other types of soft tissue mediastinal bulges the list of differential possibilities may be very long indeed, and from the plain films one can only note the presence of a mass and describe it.

Figure 8-7. Abnormal profiles due to a large mediastinal mass projecting to both sides. With this type of malignant mass, most commonly produced by lymphoma, there is tracheal compression and dyspnea.

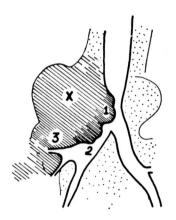

Figure 8-8. Coronal midthoracic body-section study of a man, 65, with dyspnea and weight loss. Note irregular narrowing of the trachea (1) and right main stem bronchus (2). The mass (x) would appear on the regular chest film as an abnormal bulge on the right, opposite the aortic arch. Note downward deflection of a branch of the upper lobe bronchus (3). Final diagnosis: bronchogenic carcinoma with spread to mediastinal lymph nodes.

96

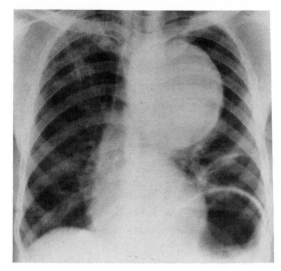

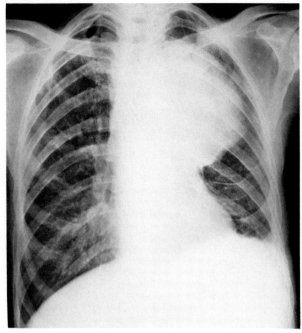

Figures 8-9 (above) and 8-10 (right). Similar chest films; different conditions. (See text.)

You will find that some abnormal mediastinal profiles seem to you to be quite clearly neither cardiac nor pulmonary. Unfortunately, with others it will not be so easy to make this decision. Look, for example, at Figures 8-9 and 8-10. In many ways they are quite similar. Each has a dense rounded mass in the left upper chest, which seems to protrude from the upper mediastinum. Both men were dyspneic, had chest pain and cough. Yet one was found to have a large left upper lobe bronchogenic carcinoma, which obscured his normal left mediastinal profile, and the other had a large aortic aneurysm. Either mass could have resulted in enough phrenic nerve pressure to paralyze the left diaphragm. Note the position of the diaphragm in each. Either mass could have involved the vertebrae, destroying bone and causing back pain. Of course, supplementary procedures would have given the important additional information needed to make a diagnosis in each case. The aneurysm could have been seen to be clearly a part of the aorta at fluoroscopy or angiographically, while the lung tumor might have shown an abnormal air bronchogram on a Bucky film and would probably have been diagnosed at bronchoscopy. *The inconclusiveness of initial chest films should not discourage you, for they are not very often diagnostic.*

Today the differentiation of mediastinal masses is frequently aided by the use of *computerized tomography*. By providing a cross section of the living patient, CT enables the radiologist to identify all normal structures and to decide whether they are in a normal location or displaced. He can identify any abnormal masses, then, even ones which on the chest film merged their shadows with those of normal structures. In the two patients above, the CT scan would have informed us that one mass was solid and the other blood filled. The attenuation coefficients would have been quite different for blood and tumor. Vascular structures can have their attenuation *enhanced* (exaggerated) by angiography, the blood stream being rendered more opaque by the injection of a soluble contrast substance. By CT the vascular structures would then be shown to be much denser than nonvascular structures next to them. Similarly, well-vascularized parts of an organ or mass will show a different density from avascular parts by such enhancement.

The CT scan is of particular importance in the identification of tumor-invaded and enlarged lymph nodes in the mediastinum which are not visible on the chest film. You can imagine how different the prognosis and management would be for a patient with a malignant solitary nodule in his lung if it could be shown that he already had metastases to his mediastinum.

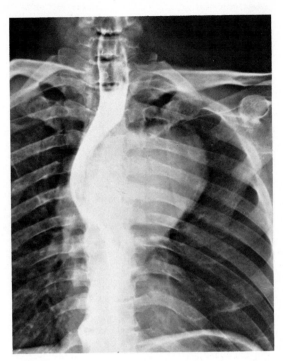

Figure 8-11. Another patient with an aortic aneurysm shows you the deflection of the barium-filled esophagus.

Deflection to one side of either the trachea or the esophagus can be appreciated readily in the PA view and may indicate significant mediastinal abnormality. Such deflections are very common, and you will probably see one in the near future. When you do, be sure to note whether you are looking at a whole mediastinal shift or at the deflection of only certain of its structures, as in Figure 8-11. You can see the trachea on most conventional and all Bucky PA films of the chest. Barium paste, often given to a patient to swallow during chest fluoroscopy, leaves a streak of barium caught in the mucosal folds of the esophagus for a few minutes after the main bolus has passed into the stomach. The first chance you have, notice that the normal esophagus deviates slightly to the right at the level of the arch of the aorta.

When you see the barium-filled esophagus in the lateral view, on the other hand, notice that it bisects the chest cavity, reaching the diaphragm at about its midpoint (Figure 8-13). It lies close against the posterior surface of the heart. One could anticipate from this relationship that the esophagus would be displaced backward by enlargement of the left atrium.

The lateral chest film offers you an excellent view of the *anterior mediastinum*. Note the radiolucent area in front of the heart shadow (Figure 8-12A). Many types of tumor masses occur here. The thyroid gland may extend downward into the anterior mediastinum. Thymic masses as well as certain teratomas may be found there. When such anterior mediastinal masses are viewed laterally, they *fill in the normal anterior clear space* and merge their shadows with that of the heart.

Masses of many kinds occur in the *posterior mediastinum*, those of neurogenic origin being found there commonly. Such masses will fill in the normally radiolucent area behind the heart in the lateral view (Figure 8-12A) and may obscure part of the diaphragmatic profile. In looking at the lateral film you should make a practice of always checking the anterior and posterior clear spaces.

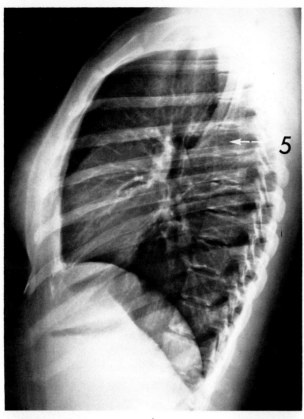

A

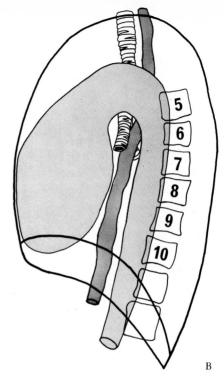

B

Figure 8-12. A is a left lateral radiograph of the normal chest; B is a tracing of the outline of the chest from A. The heart outline and vertebrae have also been traced. Arrow indicates T5. Outlines of the approximate positions of trachea, esophagus, and aorta have been added.

Note that on the radiograph you locate the hilum precisely by the white spot representing the density of the left pulmonary artery coming toward you and x-rayed end-on. The vascular branches radiating in all directions also help pinpoint the location of the hilum. Two vertical crenulated white lines bound the dark column of the trachea and represent its cartilaginous walls. Note the two dark areas where the lungs come close together, one in front of and above the heart and one behind and below the heart. These are the anterior and posterior clear spaces and may sometimes be seen to contain soft tissue masses.

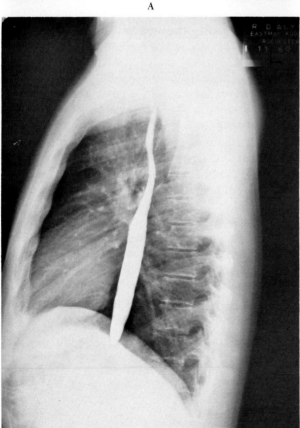

Figure 8-13 (left). Another patient with the esophagus full of barium. Note that although it lies close to the spine, it could be said to bisect the chest in this view.

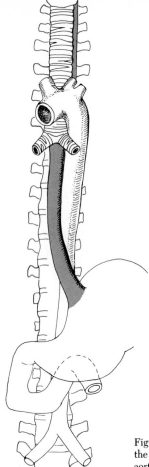

Figure 8-14. Relationships of the trachea, esophagus, and aorta.

The normal relationships of trachea, aorta, and esophagus to each other and to the vertebral column behind them may be reviewed from the diagram in Figure 8-14. Deflections of any of these structures as seen on the chest film become more comprehensible, and the origins of abnormal masses more easily remembered, if you can readily recall the normal relationships.

In the computerized tomogram in Figure 8-15 you are looking up from the patient's feet at the undersurface of a cross section of the patient's chest taken at the level of the arch of the aorta. The patient is lying on his back, so of course the vetebral body is below. The vertebra has been recognized by the computer as a cluster of *dense* cubes in the mosaic, arranged so that it at once strikes you as having a characteristic cross-sectional shape, and it is therefore a *white* vertebra-shaped shadow on the screen-photograph. In fact, it looks precisely as it would if we had been able to radiograph a cross-sectional slice of the patient!

Note that the computer has also recognized the relative radiolucency of the contents of the spinal canal. The arch of the aorta curves from right anterior in the body to left posterior. Remember that you are looking up at it from below, and justify its appearance. Find the superior vena cava and the trachea. Note calcification in the wall of the aorta.

In Figure 8-17 on the opposite page, you see a computerized tomogram of a patient who had had a diagnosis of bronchogenic carcinoma made from cell washings taken during bronchoscopy although the primary lesion was small, located in a branch bronchus far peripherally. It was 1 centimeter in size on the routine chest film, an excellent candidate for resection and a hopeful prognosis. However, the computerized tomograms showed mediastinal nodes not seen at all by plain radiography, which completely altered the prognosis and plan of treatment for this patient, who was then referred to the radiation therapist rather than to the surgeon.

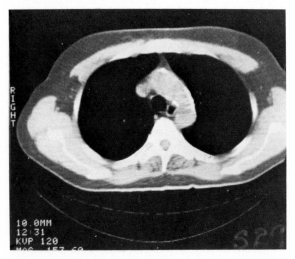

Figure 8-15. Computerized tomogram at the level of the aortic arch.

100

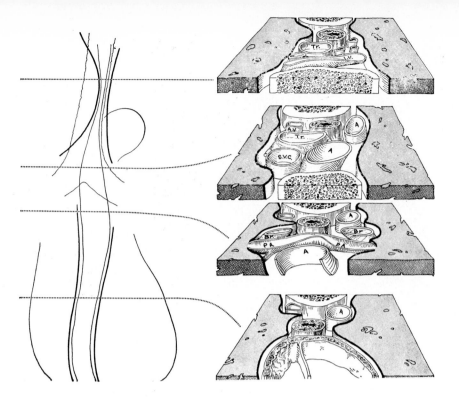

Figure 8-16. Mediastinal relationships in cross section. *Tr*, trachea; *IV*, innominate vein; *AV*, azygos vein; *A*, aorta; *SVC*, superior vena cava; *Br*, bronchus; *PA*, pulmonary artery; heavy lines, pleural reflections.

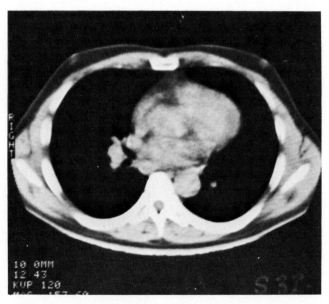

Figure 8-17. Computerized tomogram at the level of the carina in a patient with one peripheral metastasis in the left lung.

Patients with Anterior Mediastinal Masses

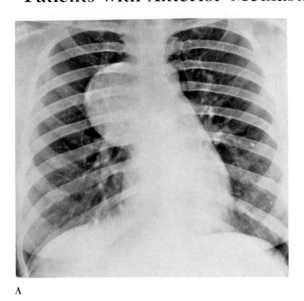
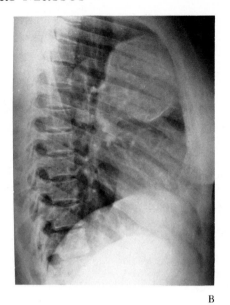

A

B

Figure 8-18. A large spherical, anterior, mediastinal mass protrudes to the right and shows a shell of calcification. Note high anterior location in the lateral view (B), filling in the anterior clear space.

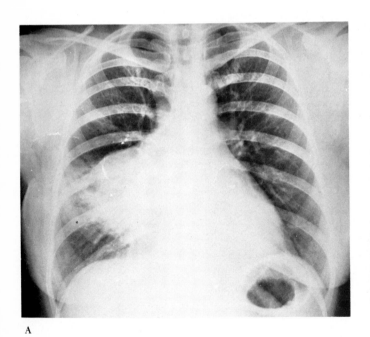
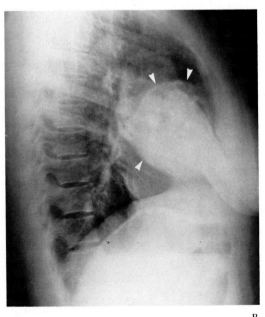

A

B

Figure 8-19. Patient who proved to have a mediastinal teratoma, probably arising anteriorly but projecting far to the right. In the lateral view (B) it is seen as a dense shadow superimposed on the heart.

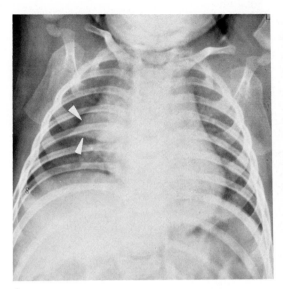
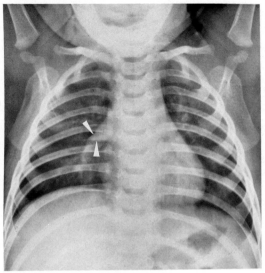

A   B

Figure 8-20. The normally enlarged thymus of an infant, seen as a triangular, sail-shaped shadow overlapping the hilum as it projects laterally from the anterior mediastinum. It will be better visualized at expiration (A) than at inspiration (B).

The Infant Thymus

Few mediastinal masses have anything distinctive about their outline. One which does is the normally enlarged infant thymus, which will be seen to project from the mediastinal margin like a triangular sail, often bilateral but usually more prominent on the right. The projection will be exaggerated at full expiration, as in Figure 8-20A. Note the diminution in the size of the mass in Figure 8-20B, a film made on the same patient at inspiration. The mediastinum is much more difficult to appraise in the infant and young child than it is in the adult, since the proportionately greater flexibility of the structures involved tends to produce buckling, folding, and compression, which give an appearance of widening when no abnormality exists.

Hilar Adenopathy

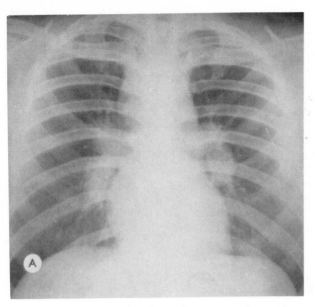
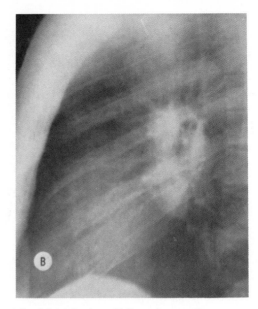

Figure 8-21. Hilar adenopathy. Patient with sarcoidosis, stage 1, has bilateral enlarged hilar nodes as well as a mass of paratracheal nodes, more prominent on the right but present on both sides and widening the mediastinum. Note that the lowest node in each hilum is clearly a spherical density superimposed on the tapering densities of vessels.

Unknowns

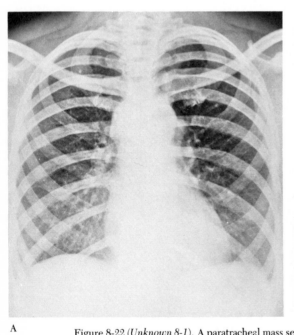
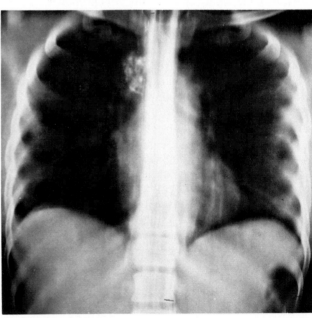

A

B

Figure 8-22 (*Unknown 8-1*). A paratracheal mass seen on the chest film is shown by plain coronal tomography, B, to contain granules of calcium. Figure out how it would have appeared on a CT transaxial scan.

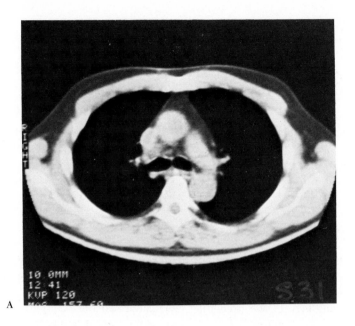

Figure 8-23 (*Unknown 8-2*). A man, 44, had a carcinoma of the colon resected ten days ago. At surgery the liver looked normal and no local involved nodes were found. The patient is demanding a prognosis. One radiologist feels the plain chest film shows questionable metastases, but others do not agree. Computerized tomography is carried out. A shows the scan just at the level of the carina, and B has been made lower through the heart, with the technique varied for soft tissues. What does it show?

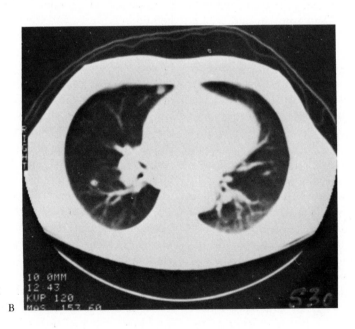

CHAPTER 9 How To Gather and Use Radiologic and Other Imaging Data

You already know that this book is not at all intended to be a reference book in radiology but rather an instruction in how to study films, how to recognize important roentgen changes, and how to confer intelligently with the radiologist in the whole-patient study. The importance for all graduating physicians of knowing some radiology has been increasing steadily, and no medical student should allow himself a defeatist attitude about his chances of learning a good deal about radiology while he is in school. You have learned some basic radiology in the preceding chapters, perhaps more than you realize.

On the other hand, the field of diagnostic roentgenology has expanded so much and in so many detailed ways that you should not expect to learn to interpret films regularly and with confidence in a four- or five-year period of initiation in medical training. You can and should learn to study the films on your own patients, using them to check your clinical impressions, and to appreciate the magnitude of any changes which may be present.

The preceding chapters will have given you some idea of how to go about analyzing chest films, but I am sure you feel less self-confidence about approaching actual films than you would like. How to proceed to build your own store of roentgen knowledge on this admittedly sketchy beginning should be your next concern. Almost everyone does this after a fashion; some build at random and without much sense of organization or direction; some do it systematically and deliberately. The latter usually find that radiologic facts are considerably easier to remember when gathered together in clumps and groups.

Now suppose you say to yourself, "I have learned how to look at the bony thorax, the lungs, diaphragm, pleural space, and mediastinum . . . but I don't feel that I know anything about diagnosing tuberculosis, for example. Of what use is it just to be able to recognize a pleural effusion?" There, indeed, you can begin.

Stop and list for yourself the ways you know tuberculosis *can* manifest itself on the chest film, and you will see that you already have some idea about the radiologic spectrum of the disease. Tuberculosis can, of course, be manifest initially as a simple pleural effusion (the organism being recoverable from the tapped fluid), even when there are no visible abnormalities in the lung by x-ray. It can be discovered on a routine chest film in an asymptomatic patient as a shadowy infiltration in the infraclavicular area of one lung, visible to you when you compare the interspaces carefully. It can show itself as a more extensive infiltration with or without cavitation, all of which you have seen in the preceding chapters and would be able to recognize. You have seen enlarged hilar and paratracheal lymph nodes, which occur in childhood tuberculosis, and you know that clusters of calcifications in these areas remain in adult chest films to indicate where such nodes have healed.

Tuberculosis can cause pneumothorax, with or without pleural effusion, and you know where to look for small amounts of air or fluid in the pleural space. Miliary tuberculosis will result in the appearance of innumerable tiny densities scattered throughout the interstitium of both parenchymal lung fields, as you would expect. Endobronchial tuberculosis may cause scarring, bronchial obstruction, and atelectasis.

In more advanced chronic cases tuberculosis produces extensive scar tissue formation and cavitation in the lung, distorting its structure and altering the position of the hilum or of the mediastinum. You need not be told that Bucky films, body-section studies, or special lordotic apical views may be needed in order to discover an open cavity in a mass of scar tissue behind a heavy overlap of bony rib cage and clavicle. Solitary tuberculous granulomas in the lung may closely resemble solitary tumor nodules. You are certainly anticipating my reminder that serial studies made at intervals will afford information as to the progress or control of the disease which cannot be obtained in any other way. In sum, you already *have* a good deal of knowledge about the roentgen shadows which this single disease might be expected to produce in the lung.

Remember, however, that both for you and for the radiologist, *these are roentgen findings and not diagnoses.* In the new patient being studied medically for the first time, the finding of a fluffy, infiltrative shadow in the lung does not make a diagnosis of tuberculosis. *In fact, the diagnosis of tuberculosis is never a matter for the radiologist to settle.* If he phrases his report rather positively in the direction of that disease as a most probable explanation for the shadows he sees, he does so with the certainty that you, the clinician, will not consider the diagnosis established *without bacteriologic confirmation.*

Thus, certain diseases ought never to be "diagnosed" in written roentgen reports. Others show an almost pathognomonic roentgen appearance, and then time is saved for everyone if the radiologist simply states that the findings *are* those of such and such a condition. Remember that the more expert and knowledgeable the radiologist becomes, the more confidently he will undertake to help direct your thinking, and the more reliance you may place on his diagnostic suggestions. Furthermore, he can do your patient as much service by ruling out as "very unlikely from the roentgen appearance" some items included in your differential slate as he can by making diagnostic suggestions of his own.

The roentgen literature is full of well-researched and well-written articles reporting the statistical incidence of this or that roentgen finding in this or that disease condition. Familiarity with such studies helps the radiologist in advising you. He knows, for example, that patients with bacterial pneumonias of the lobar type usually show beginning density in the lung by x-ray between 5 and 10 hours after the onset of symptoms, while those with viral or atypical pneumonias frequently show no changes for 24 to 48 hours. Patients with pulmonary tuberculosis may not show any demonstrable roentgen shadow for 4 or 5 months after exposure. The radiologist must always interpret the shadows he

sees in the light of such considerations.

Never forget, however, that *your patient is not a statistic.* The radiologist may interpret his findings in the light of statistical probabilities, but you are treating one specific human being. No matter how well-informed and experienced a radiologist may be, he is not an oracle, and his advice and interpretations of shadows must always be fitted into the clinical picture and weighed against conflicting evidence. A good many radiologists prefer to study the films at first with no knowledge of the clinical story, purely as an exercise in roentgen interpretation, and then to reconsider their own ideas about the shadows in light of the clinical findings. Their report to you often does not include, therefore, all the possibilites they considered on first looking at the film, and it is a shortcut in the press of work to suggest in writing only those disease entities which are still believed possible at the time the first film studies are being reported. Subsequent film studies and subsequent clinical findings will narrow the list of possibilities until a diagnosis is made.

Some disease conditions, of course, produce no roentgen changes whatever. For example, the usual course of typhoid fever is not accompanied by any useful radiologic findings; but when the organism invades bone, an osteomyelitis differing somewhat roentgenologically from more common forms of bone inflammation will be visible in the films. In the course of your training in medical school you will learn in which of the common disease conditions you can or cannot expect radiologic help.

A negative roentgen examination in the patient with a compelling story and clinical findings in whom radiologic changes *are* to be expected, on the other hand, is one of the most constant and disturbing problems the radiologist has to face. He has to be familiar with, and remind you constantly about, the *occasional fallibility of the roentgen method* and also about the point in any disease at which roentgen changes may be expected to be present. The patient with miliary tuberculosis, for example, febrile and very ill, may show minute miliary densities in the parenchyma of the lung in the chest film relatively late in the illness, several weeks after a presumptive clinical diagnosis has been made and therapy begun. The patient with a history suggestive of gallbladder disease may have negative x-ray studies for years before he finally shows positive imaging evidence for chronic cholecystitis and stones. In the patient with enough scarring from duodenal ulcer it may be impossible to demonstrate a newly recurrent crater by barium study, and much more reliance must be placed on this patient's own evaluation of his worsening condition than on the fact that the roentgen study reports no change.

You have, thus, two types of roentgen data to accumulate and clump together. You must have a clear visual image of the various sorts of informative roentgen changes a particular disease *may* produce. At the same time, in another compartment of your mind, you must gradually accumulate information as to the fallibilities of the roentgen method *in that same disease.* You must be prepared for the negative examination and wise enough to discount it in the patient about whom you are justly worried. In general, positive roentgen findings are helpful, but a negative study is not a clear slate.

Your procedure, then, from this point on in extending your knowledge of radiologic diagnosis should be to become a collector. Reasoning always from your increasing knowledge of pathophysiology, you will add, day by day, to each group of visual images representing the roentgen changes which may be produced by a disease entity. You will discover that as you collect visual images, each one serves as a review of the pathophysiology involved. It is unquestionably in this way that you will find them most useful in medical school, since they provide a visual device for remembering data which seem much more complex when learned first from the printed page.

Gradually building in your own mind a familiarity with the varied roentgen appearances of a particular disease is somewhat the same procedure most radiologists carry out when they build what is affectionately referred to as "The Teaching Collection," a tangible accumulation of film cases, arranged and catagorized for reference use. Few such collections are really complete, any more than your mental collection will be, but they are added to and reworked and improved constantly, just as your own set of intellectual images will be. If you approach in a deliberate way the collection of grouped roentgen images representing gross pathologic changes, I believe you will find that when you are ready to assume postdoctorate responsibilities, you will indeed have a fair grasp of diagnostic radiology. It will not stop there, of course, because you will have developed the habit of adding to the catalog of images from daily experience.

You will also be making a practice of filing away learned instances in which the roentgen examination was negative in the face of clinical evidence *for* a disease process. To be sure, this is a more sophisticated procedure, but just as important and just as much a question of collecting. Remember that candor between you and the radiologist is to be recommended strongly. You must be able to say to him, "How sure are you?" and he must be able to reply, "I am not sure at all, but I believe it is the most probable explanation." At other times he must be able to say to you, "I can't, of course, guarantee what the microscopic study will show, but I personally have no doubts whatsoever." Occasionally he must say to you, "I have little experience with this disease. The literature describes the changes we have here, but let's get another opinion." In time you must be accomplished enough to say, on receiving a negative report, "That's all very well, but I feel strongly that my patient *has* the disease. How soon might a repeat study show changes?"

You must also *listen* to the radiologist when he feels strongly about a diagnosis and insists that no other should be entertained. Argue with him if you like, but listen; and explore with him the possible additional information that might be obtained from other imaging studies such as computerized tomography, sonography, or isotope scans.

Start Your Image Collection with the Following Cases of Proven Pulmonary Tuberculosis

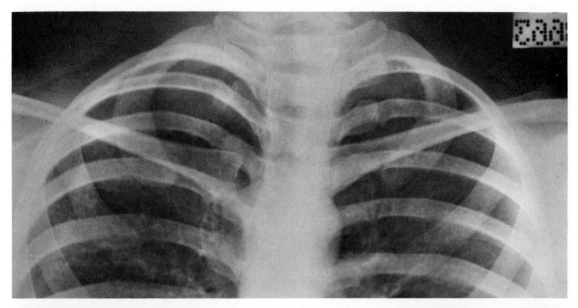

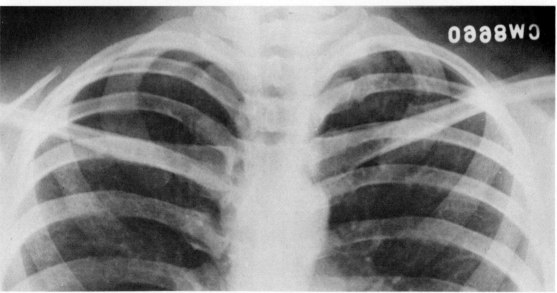

Figures 9-1 and 9-2. An example of *minimal apical tuberculosis* in details from two chest films made on the same patient. Figure 9-1 (above), a routine film made in September, is normal. Figure 9-2 (below), made five months later, shows numerous small, fluffy shadows in the lung tissue at the left apex, in the second and third interspaces, and superimposed on the first three ribs. Compare the interspaces. Up to this point in the book you have seen a number of instances of the roentgen shadows which may be produced in the chest film by tuberculosis. Add to them now the cases of tuberculosis which follow, and you will have a nucleus of images to start your collection.

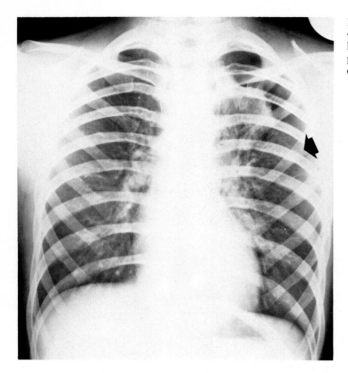

Figure 9-3. *More extensive tuberculosis*, left upper lobe, with small pneumothorax (arrow indicates visible margin of lung). Strands of shadow extending to the chest wall are pleural adhesions over the apex, restricting the degree of collapse.

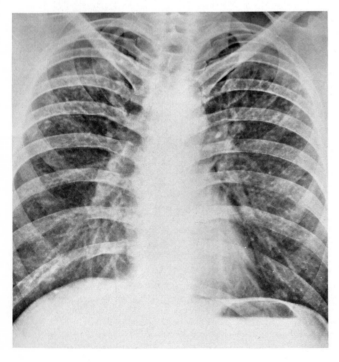

Figure 9-4. Silicosis in a miner with sputum positive for acid-fast bacilli. Most of these myriad lesions must be silicotic nodules, but at least a few represent infiltrative granulomas. No diagnosis of "tuberculosis" is to be made from this film, of course.

Figure 9-5. *Bilateral chronic upper lobe tuberculosis.* Note that in addition to the obvious infiltrative parenchymal streaks in both upper lobes, there are ring-like cavities present. The one on the right can be seen rising above the medial end of the right clavicle, and the one on the left overlies the fourth rib near the lateral chest wall. Note also the very characteristic vascular lung markings extending down into the lower lung fields from the hila. These are longer, straighter, and more vertical than the normal lower lung markings and may be likened to the taut guy ropes of a tent. Their appearance is easy to remember when you realize that in this type of upper lobe tuberculosis there is so much scarring and retraction that the upper lobes are markedly reduced in size and both hila are drawn upward, stretching the vessels to the lower lobes.

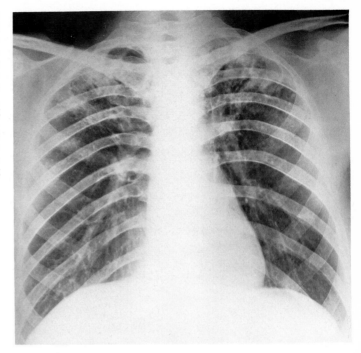

Figure 9-6. *Cavitation in a relatively new tuberculous lesion.* Considering the size of the cavity here, there is less extensive parenchymal density than might be expected in chronic involvement. When you compare carefully the lung seen in the seventh, eighth, and ninth interspaces on the two sides, those on the left appear normal, while those on the right show scattered soft shadows.

Think now of the pathologic process which is going on, rather than of the roentgen shadows. Consider that the balance between the resistance of the patient and the virulence of the disease must determine the rate of tissue breakdown. This being so, it must follow that the relation of the size of the cavity to the type of inflammatory density in the involved lung around it, as you see them in the x-ray, provides an index to the state of the host-disease balance. In a portion of lung showing many soft, fluffy shadows, the sudden appearance of a large, thin-walled cavity probably means rapid tissue breakdown in poorly resisting lung. A similar cavity in a segment of lung known to have been diseased for a long time, and showing instead the dense, discrete, and stringy shadows of healing fibrotic lesions, would not carry the same implications. Just so, the progress of changes in a series of films made at intervals provides a useful index to the patient-disease relationship and all the factors which may influence it.

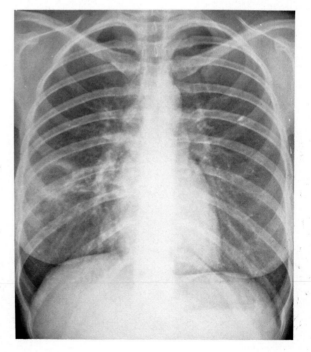

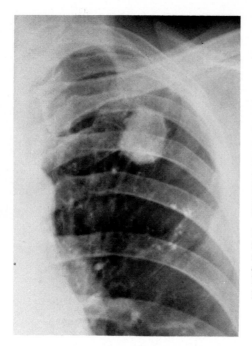

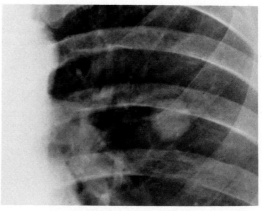

Figures 9-7 (left) and 9-8 (above). *Tuberculous granulomas* in the lung may closely simulate solitary tumors, either primary or metastatic. Some granulomas contain no calcium, others calcify centrally (or expand around and engulf an earlier calcific focus). Still others calcify peripherally and appear to have a shell.

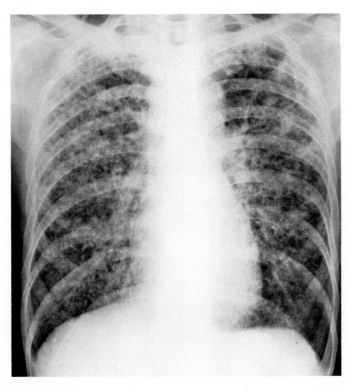

Figure 9-9. *Miliary tuberculosis.* The innumerable lesions scattered throughout the parenchyma here, and probably resulting from hematogenous spread, have been engrafted upon a lung field in which there was already some tuberculous infiltration in the upper lobes. *In looking at any film, you have to consider that the shadows you see may represent acute changes superimposed on chronic ones.*

112

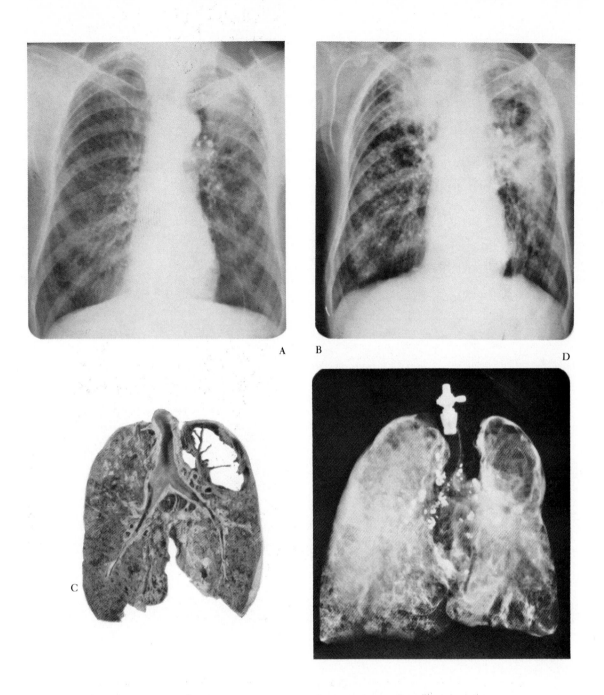

Figure 9-10. *Silicotuberculosis.* A stonemason, 61, admitted with a productive cough (A), showed extensive calcification in both hila and an infiltrative density in the left upper lobe. Sputum was positive for tubercle bacilli. Patient was discharged after two and a half years of hospital care, went back to work for four months, and was readmitted (B) with extension of involvement and cavitation. He died two months later. Lung specimen shown in C, photograph, and D, radiograph.

113

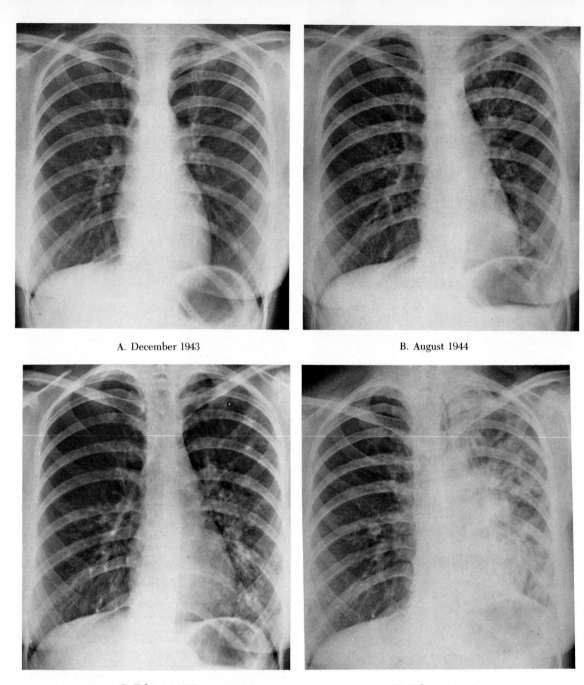

A. December 1943

B. August 1944

C. February 1945

D. February 1946

Figure 9-11. *Serial films over a period of three years in a patient with tuberculosis.* In A she has a soft infiltrative lesion extending upward from the left hilum to the apex. In B, made eight months later, there is progressive involvement of the left upper lobe and new areas of density extending downward toward the left diaphragm, which may be either in the lingular segment of the upper lobe or in the lower lobe. In C, made six months later, there is involvement throughout the left lung, but with the development of scar tissue the patches of shadow have taken on a harder, denser, and more discrete appearance. D, a year later, gives you radiographic indications that there is much more scar tissue retraction than on the earlier films. Note that the trachea and the heart have been drawn over to the left. Cavitation is obvious in the upper lobe. You see the profile of the diaphragm still. In E, there appears to be an immense cavitation replacing the upper lobe (absence of lung markings). The left diaphragmatic profile and that of the left heart border have disappeared, indicating consolidation, and there is new spread of the disease to the right lung. Some pleural effusion on the left cannot be excluded. F is a radiograph of the postmortem specimen of the two air-inflated lungs, the vessels of which have been injected with an opaque substance.

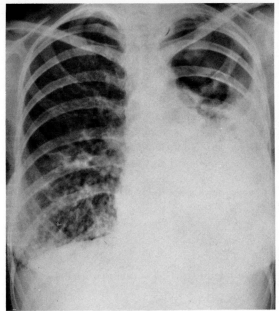

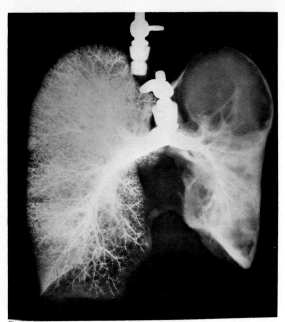

E. August 1946

F. October 1946

You can understand now why I have deferred so long giving you illustrations clearly labeled as a particular disease entity. To do so, without first showing you how to make roentgen findings serve you, would have been to invite the card-sorting approach to radiologic diagnosis. From this point on you will become a collector of all the roentgen images which can be produced by a particular disease, but I hope you will always do so by relating the shadows to the pathologic condition.

Unknowns

As an unknown for this chapter try listing all the roentgen changes which could be produced by bronchogenic carcinoma. You have already seen a number of them in the course of the preceding chapters, but you will be able to imagine others. As an embellishment for this exercise, think of each one as belonging to a patient who presents himself in your office for the first time today—so that, in addition to going over all the types of shadows caused by lung cancer, you will also be preparing yourself for the modes in which patients with the disease may first be encountered. If you make the effort of writing down your list, you will able to tick it off against the answer in Appendix A (which is admittedly incomplete).

115

Evaluation of cardiac disease is firmly based upon the clinical findings from auscultation and electrocardiograms. Confirmatory and sometimes helpful findings may be obtained from radiology in the cardiac patient, but you will find that the chest films are often not very helpful in the commoner types of heart disease. For example, the patient with myocardial infarction seldom has any helpful x-ray findings either during the attack or later, and congestive failure is usually no more apparent on chest films than from careful clinical appraisal. To be sure, the routine chest films made on most hospitalized patients will need to be reviewed by you personally, and therefore you must learn how to examine them and when to avail yourself of the more complex methods of study. Those methods include fluoroscopy expertly carried out by the radiologist, cardiac catheterization with cardioangiography using serial films or cineangiography to document the progress of the radiopaque bolus passing through the heart and lungs, coronary arteriography, echocardiography, computerized tomography, and procedures using radioisotopes.

Measurement of Heart Size

We are a race of measurers, partly perhaps because it is easier to measure than to think. Before angiocardiography was developed, making possible the study of the individual cardiac chambers, the overall size of the heart was measured in its every dimension and some of these measurements proved useful. Since heart catheterization and angiocardiography have come into wide use, however, much less reliance is placed on plain film measurements in a cardiac patient and the attention of clinicians is directed toward a variety of more precisely meaningful procedures.

Nevertheless, in the day-to-day routine patient problems, evaluation of the shadow of the heart on the plain film of the chest will prove useful to you. Detailed studies in cardiac evaluation you will relegate to experts, of course, but you can develop for your own daily use a *rough* estimate of the size of the heart, using only the measurement you make on a 6-foot PA film (which enlarges the heart by projection less than 5 percent). If you know one easy-to-carry-out measuring system and employ it on every PA chest film you study, you will soon develop an ability to *estimate* heart size. A left lateral film, now a routine part of the chest film study, will enhance the accuracy of plain-film assay of heart size.

You must add to this mode of assaying the status of the heart an awareness of *the ways in which cardiac enlargement may be (1) simulated or (2) masked.* Even more important, you must have some familiarity with changes in the *shape* of the heart due to specific chamber enlargements, since a change in shape either with or without enlargement may sometimes indicate the type of heart disease which is present more clearly than any other single clinical sign.

In sum, then, you must be able to estimate overall cardiac size while accepting the important limitations of that estimate, to discount conditions which may simulate enlargement, and to be aware of the changes produced in the shape of the cardiac profile by various disease processes. These things every physician ought to know comfortably.

The simplest method of measuring the heart is to determine its relation to the width of the chest at its widest part near the level of the diaphragms. This is called the *cardiothoracic ratio,* and is carried out on the 6-foot PA chest film only. Measure between two vertical lines drawn tangential to the most prominent point on the right and left cardiac profiles. The prominence of the bulge on the right is usually a little higher than the apex of the left profile. *In adults the width of the heart should be less than half the widest thoracic diameter, measured from inside the rib cage at its widest point.*

No ruler is necessary for this measurement, nor do you need to remember anything more than the 50-percent figure. Using any handy piece of paper with a straight edge (the handiest will often be the margin of the patient's own film envelope), determine the width of the heart. Then decide whether this width exceeds the distance from the midpoint (spine) to the inside of the rib cage (half the transthoracic diameter). Still more simply, you can measure from the midline to the *right* heart border and see whether that distance will fit into the piece of lung field to the *left* of the heart, something you can do from the back row at ward rounds! For example in Figure 10-1, is the distance A to midline less or greater than B to D?

The left lateral film is an excellent check on the PA appearance of the heart. When apparent enlargement to the left in the PA view is checked on the left lateral chest film, increase in the *mass* of the left ventricle will extend the border of the heart posteriorly and low against the diaphragm. Conversely, increase in the mass of the right ventricle will be seen to fill in the lower part of the anterior clear space behind the sternum but will not extend the heart posteriorly.

No doubt you measured the heart in Figure 10-1 and found it normal in size, but compare it now with almost any of the chest films in the preceding chapters and you will certainly be struck by the flat, almost absent, aortic arch. This young patient had been discovered to have sustained hypertension. Someone finally felt for his femoral pulses, found them absent, and measured his blood pressure in both arms and legs. The possibility of coarctation of the aorta was suggested in view of unobtainable pressure in his legs. Reinspection of his chest film revealed the saucered erosions of the undersurface of his ribs, where the dilated intercostal arteries had developed as collateral pathways. His coarctation was successfully revised surgically, restoring him to normal health and life expectancy. It is nothing short of criminal neglect for a physician to fail to measure leg pressures in any young hypertensive. Figure 10-3 (next page) is a detail on the chest film in Figure 10-1. The radiologic manifestations of coarctation are seldom

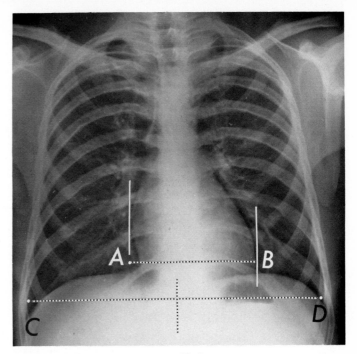

Figure 10-1. This young man was told after an insurance examination that he had a heart murmur. Is his heart enlarged?

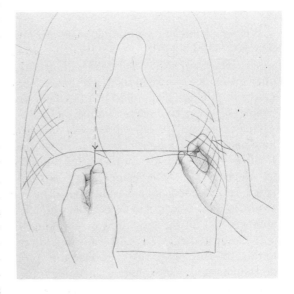

Figure 10-2

present as yet in children under 10. You must remember too that a number of other conditions can cause rib notching. Neurofibromatosis is one.

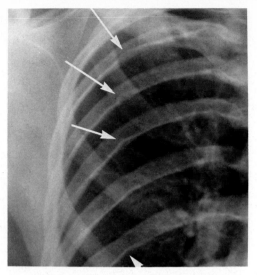

Figure 10-3. Detail from Figure 10-1.

Factors Limiting the Information Obtained by Measurement

It is a good thing to realize that heart shadows may be abnormal in shape even though normal in size. They may also be enlarged with or without a distinctive change in shape, for *tone* is necessary to produce shape, and hearts which decompensate may be enlarged and shapeless.

Hearts may also be only *apparently enlarged* for a variety of reasons which you must be able to discount. You already know some of the ways in which cardiac enlargement may be simulated. You have seen it in chest films made at *expiration*, and it is logical to expect that a high diaphragm will tilt the heart upward bringing its apex closer to the lateral chest wall. In addition to this, the flare of the ribs is greater at inspiration and decreases at expiration, further altering the apparent cardiothoracic ratio. In any patient in whom you would have reason to expect the diaphragm to be high, you will be anticipating an apparently enlarged heart shadow. In the presence of *any kind of abdominal distension* (late pregnancy, ascites, intestinal obstruction) you may not be able to estimate heart size for this reason.

Remember too that portable bedside chest films are usually made AP and result in an appreciable enlargement of the heart shadow by projection, since the heart is farther away from the film. *The factor of projection* may be further exaggerated if, because of awkward arrangements of furniture in crowded hospital rooms, the technician must make the film at a distance much less than 6 feet. Important and valuable data may be obtained from bedside films on the very sick patient, but an estimate of heart size is not among them.

The next point to be checked, after you have counted down the ribs to determine the level of the diaphragms and made sure you are looking at a 6-foot PA film, is that there is *no rotation off the sagittal plane*. You have already seen in an earlier chapter the degree to which rotation may produce an appearance of widening of the heart and mediastinal shadows, and you know that symmetry of the clavicles and ribs gives you assurance that no rotation is present. We will be discussing the intentionally rotated oblique films in more detail, and there you will be able to study more closely the precise effect of rotation on the cardiac shadow.

Deformity of the thoracic cage will, of course, often render impossible any attempt to measure the size of the heart, and you would not expect to be able to do so in severe scoliosis, for example. The solitary (but symmetrical) deformity of a depressed sternum usually displaces the heart to the left, and your suspicions will be aroused when you find no right heart border from which to measure. A lateral film will settle the matter. In severe cases the posterior surface of the sternum is only a few centimeters from the anterior margins of the vertebral bodies, so that mediastinal shift and cardiac displacement simulating enlargement are inevitable.

You might wonder whether the size of the heart shadow would be increased if the film happened to be taken at full diastole, and decreased if it were made at the end of systole. The shadow *is* slightly different at the extremes of the cardiac cycle, but the difference is not usually enough to matter in using a rough estimate like the cardiathoracic ratio, at least in adults.

118

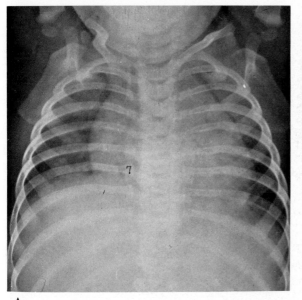
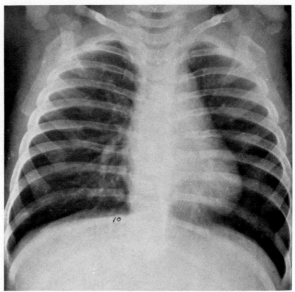

A

B

Figure 10-4. Seven-month-old infant, examined because of cough and upper respiratory infection, appears to have cardiac enlargement until high diaphragms and hazy lung fields are noted (A). When a second film is made at full inspiration (B), the heart is not enlarged to measurement.

It is important for you to develop an immense degree of caution with regard to making pronouncements about apparent enlargement of the *infant* heart as you see it on chest films. This is particularly true in the infant under 1 year of age. Because of the greater flexibility of all the structures and because of the basic difference in proportion of abdominal size to thoracic size, the normal diaphragmatic level in the infant is higher than in the adult. He is usually filmed AP and supine (although at a distance proportionate to 6 feet in the adult). He wiggles and is hard to immobilize, which produces rotation. He has not yet developed the proportion of lung size to heart size characteristic of the adult and present already in the older child. Beware of x-ray appearances suggesting cardiac enlargment under 1 year, therefore, without supporting clinical evidence.

On the other hand, always remember that *overdistension of the lungs* for any reason compresses the heart and mediastinal structures from both sides and narrows their PA shadow. Therefore, in the dyspneic patient with low diaphragms and in the emphysematous patient, the heart size as measured on the PA chest film may be *deceptively small*, not informing you reliably about the cardiac status at all. In patients with chronic emphysema the heart is often found at autopsy to be enlarged by weight as a result of right ventricular hypertrophy (cor pulmonale), although no cardiac enlargement had ever been noted radiologically (see Figure 10-6).

Noncardiac disease may mask true cardiac enlargement. If you think back through the earlier chapters, you will have no difficulty in appreciating the degree to which mediastinal or pulmonary disease may render the dimensions of the heart unobtainable. Any density which obscures one cardiac profile makes it futile to try to estimate heart size. Thus, neither the size nor the shape of the heart can be studied from plain films in the patient who has a massive pleural effusion, consolidation in the anterior part of either lung, or a large anterior mediastinal mass.

True mediastinal shift is usually the result of some important change in intrathoracic dynamics and may so alter the position of the heart that measurements are meaningless.

119

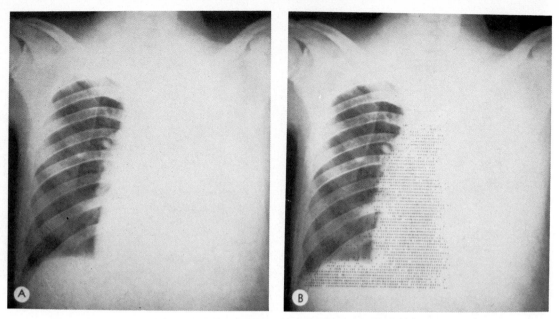

Figure 10-5. A: Patient with massive pleural effusion on the left. Chest film affords no information whatever about the heart, which might be very much enlarged. B: Visualization of the heart is effected by scintillation scanner technique, the blood contained in the heart having been rendered radioactive by an intravenous injection of radioiodinated serum albumin. Heart is small and displaced slightly to the right by the effusion.

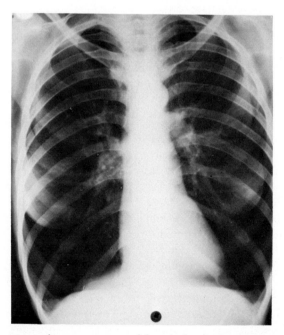

Figure 10-6. The heart in emphysema, compressed from both sides by the overexpanded lungs, looks deceptively small although the right ventricle was enlarged (later postmortem).

Interpretation of the Measurably Enlarged Heart Shadow

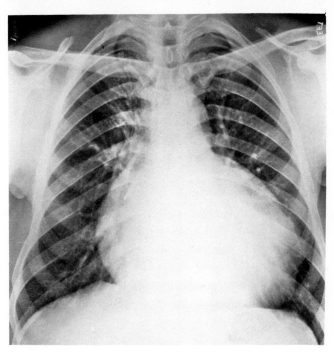

Figure 10-7. (See text.)

Consider now a chest film in which, after checking out all potentially misleading factors, you find that the measured heart shadow exceeds its allowed 50 percent of the transthoracic diameter. How can you distinguish between cardiac hypertrophy, cardiac dilatation, and the shadow cast by a pericardial effusion around the heart?

This problem is a very real one. The heart muscle, the blood contained within the cardiac chambers, and any fluid encasing it in the pericardial sac all have about the same roentgen density and will be quite indistinguishable on a chest film.

Figure 10-7 gives you an example. A patient with acute rheumatic fever and pancarditis shows obvious enlargement of the heart shadow. From similar cases which you have seen at autopsy, you know as you look at this film that there may well be valvular involvement, myocardial damage, and pericarditis with effusion. The heart disease is properly termed "pancarditis," and dilatation of the chambers due to poorly functioning valves and an inflamed, inefficient myocardium, as well as the pericardial fluid, all could contribute to the production of a large shadow. The obvious advantage to you of thinking in terms of gross pathology as you look at the film can scarcely be overemphasized.

There are some roentgen details which will help you in distinguishing between hypertrophy and dilatation. The well-compensated, hypertrophied heart tends to have sharply outlined, firmly rounded contours for its measurably enlarged heart shadow, just as you would expect with good myocardial tone. Left ventricular hypertrophy, when it predominates as it so commonly does in the hypertensive or older patient, produces relatively more enlargement to the left and a moderate alteration in *shape* without much measurable enlargement. When the heart goes into failure, decompensates, and dilates, it will lose to some extent its well-rounded contours, the shadow increasing in width by projection to both left and right.

Ventricular hypertrophy without dilatation is very difficult to recognize, and you will not be able to say that cardiac enlargement is present in patients with hypertension or aortic or pulmonic stenosis, for example, until the hypertrophied ventricular wall decompensates and the ventricle dilates. In clinical practice a *review of the patient's old films* is probably the best way to assay the development of cardiac enlargement.

121

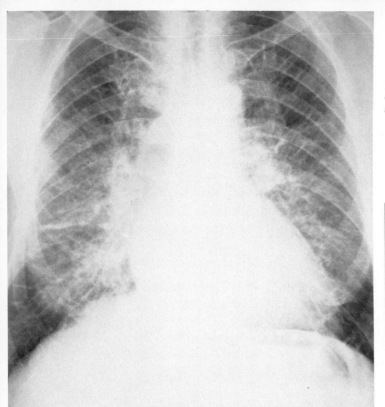

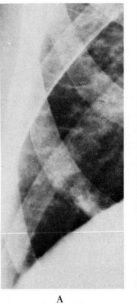

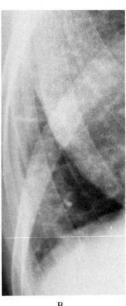

Figure 10-8. Moderate congestive failure. Note general increase in vascular markings, engorged hila, Kerley's B-lines, and fluid in the horizontal fissure.

A   B

Figure 10-9. Kerley's B-lines represent thickened interlobular septa. One of these patients had mitral stenosis with a history of repeated bouts of failure. The other had lymphatic spread of carcinoma.

The Heart in Congestive Failure and Pulmonary Edema

Additional important indications of the physiologic state of the failing heart will be found on studying the hilar shadows and lung fields carefully (Figures 10-8 and 10-9). In acute left ventricular failure which develops very rapidly, fluffly increased densities about both hila may indicate pulmonary edema. In failure developing more gradually, the hilar vessels (pulmonary veins) will appear enlarged and tortuous and will be seen to extend farther out into the lung fields than they do normally. With long-standing failure, very informative changes appear in the lung fields. The lungs as a whole appear hazy and less radiolucent than usual. Short parallel horizontal lines of increased density at the lung base close to the costophrenic angle, which have been identified as distended lymphatics of the interlobular septa, become visible as interstitial edema increases. These are called "Kerley's B-lines." (The "A-lines" and "C-lines" extending upward and downward from the hilum are hard to distinguish from vascular shadows and have not proved very useful.) Ker-

ley's B-lines are *not* associated with cardiac failure only, but may be present in any condition in which there are distended lymphatics in the interlobular septa, as you see in Figure 10-9. A subpleural accumulation of fluid seen tangentially just inside the rib cage close to the costrophrenic sinus should also be looked for and will generally precede the appearance of frank pleural effusion.

The patient in Figure 10-10 has the peculiar densities about both hila which the radiologist would unhesitatingly label pulmonary edema. It looks much the same whether resulting from sudden left ventricular failure, as after a myocardial infarction, or accompanying uremia and kidney failure.

You may have some difficulty in distinguish-

122

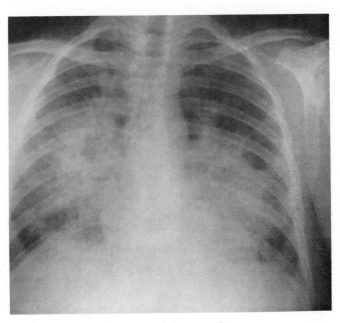

Figure 10-10. Pulmonary edema.

ing between the lung fields of failure and those of acute pulmonary edema. In general, the perihilar densities of edema are whiter and more homogeneous, and often extend about halfway out toward the chest wall. You are struck by the density and fluffiness of the bilateral shadows, whereas in failure you can usually see the lung root well enough to say that the vessels are engorged; the density provided by interstitial fluid is less impressive. Of course, the differences are due to the quantities of interstitial fluid present in frank pulmonary edema engulfing the shadows of engorged vessels. Sudden left ventricular failure may produce the picture of pulmonary edema in a previously normal lung, or may superimpose it on that of chronic failure.

In advanced cardiac failure you will be seeing bilateral pleural effusions commonly, and many instances of heart failure in which the fluid is seen only on the right. Fluid occurring only on the left side, with a clear costophrenic angle on the right, is so rarely due to cardiac failure that you should think of other possible explanations when you see it.

Thus the diagnosis of cardiac failure is made from the enlargement of the heart shadow together with its tendency toward shapelessness, plus the confirmation provided by secondary signs in the hila and lung fields. The tendency of the heart shadow to lose its former distinctive shape is not easy to assay if you are seeing the patient for the first time when he is in pronounced failure. It may be impossible at times to determine anything at all about the probable shape of the heart before it decompensated. In other patients (like the one in Figure 10-8) the degree of failure, although pronounced as indicated by the hila, has not as yet altered the preexisting shape of the heart with its relatively greater left ventricular predominance.

After response to treatment and with improvement of the physiologic state of the heart, the signs of failure which are reflected in the lungs, pleurae, and hila are seen to gradually diminish as the tone of the heart improves and its size decreases. Serial chest films provide an excellent means of following the progress of a cardiac patient through an episode of failure, and you will find that they tally well with other clinical signs available to you.

123

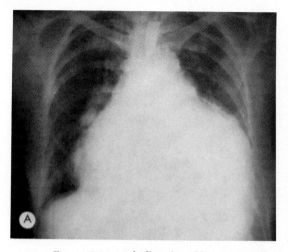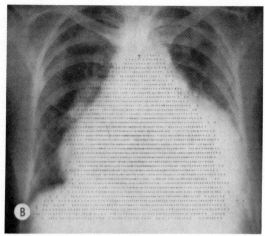

Figure 10-11. Markedly enlarged heart. Clinically there is some question whether this shapeless shadow represents a massive pericardial effusion or cardiomegaly. Radiologically either diagnosis is tenable. The heart is so large that it partly conceals the hila, although the one on the right is definitely engorged. The diminution of pulsations remarked at fluoroscopy would still be compatible with either diagnosis. In B a cardioscan establishes the presence of a very large heart. (The discrepancy along the left border is technical and cannot be taken here as an indication of the presence of pericardial fluid.)

Pericardial Effusion

Distinguishing between cardiac dilatation and an enlargement due to pericardial effusion can be impossible from the chest films. If clear-cut signs of failure are present in the hila and lungs, dilatation is the more probable explanation statistically, but the presence of *some* pericardial fluid as well certainly cannot be excluded.

Pure pericardial effusion without failure tends to show a cardiac shadow resembling a bag of water set down upon the diaphragm with marked and equal enlargement to left and to right and normal hila. So large and formless a shadow as the one you see in Figure 10-11 might well be due either to a much enlarged heart or to a pericardial effusion.

Much has been written about the damping of cardiac pulsations as visible under the fluoroscope in pericardial effusion, but a diagnosis is seldom quite as simple as that. It is true that with massive collections of fluid in the pericardium the cardiac pulsations are strikingly diminished in amplitude, but they are also diminished in myocardial failure severe enough to produce the same large heart shadow.

Sudden increase in heart size to both sides without evidence of failure is probably the most reliable signal that pericardial fluid may be present. The presence of small amounts of pericardial fluid is usually unsuspected radiologically. It is important to remember that a smaller pericardial effusion may not convincingly enlarge the heart shadow but still cause cardiac tamponade.

Of the various methods applied to the diagnostic problem posed by pericardial effusion the newest, least invasive, and most reliable is *sonography*. With this technique different echograms are obtained when the pericardium is applied normally close against the surface of the heart, and when it is separated from that surface by a layer of pericardial fluid. In Figure 10-12B you see the layer of pericardial fluid (which is said to be *anechoic*) interposed between the recorded sound waves reflected from the posterior wall of the heart and from the pericardium.

124

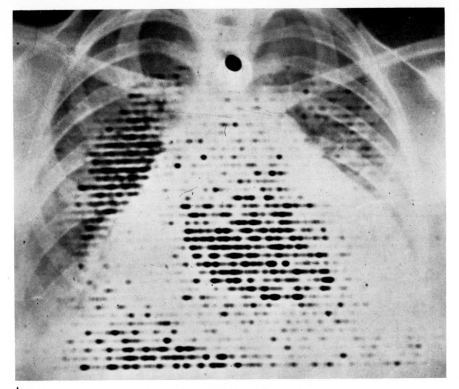

A

Figure 10-12. A: Isotope scan superimposed on the chest film of a patient with pronounced enlargement of the cardiac shadow to both sides, suggesting pericardial effusion. The intracardiac blood pool containing the circulating isotope produces a small cluster of dots and leaves a wide "cold" area enveloping the heart. This is the thick layer of pericardial fluid, which of course contains none of the blood pool isotope. B: Echocardiogram in a patient with pericardial effusion.

B

—ANT. WALL

—RV

—SEPTUM

—LV

—POST. WALL

—PERICARDIAL FLUID

—PERICARDIUM

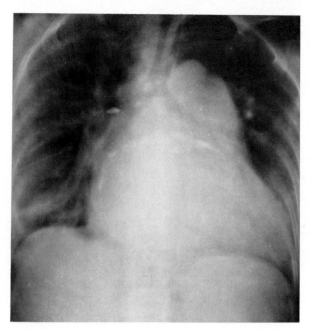

Figure 10-13. Body-section radiograph shows extensive calcification of the right lateral and superior walls of the left atrium in a patient with mitral insufficiency.

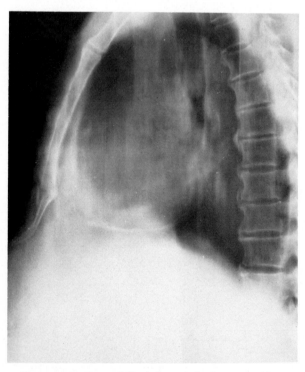

Figure 10-14. Pericardial calcification clearly seen in a lateral midsagittal body-section study. Patient had constrictive pericarditis.

Intracardiac Calcification

Constrictive pericarditis is particularly interesting radiologically because clinical signs of *right* heart failure may be manifest even though the heart is not enlarged and the lungs and hila remain clear. The "small, still heart" of constrictive pericarditis was described by early fluoroscopic observers and is seen in patients with advanced and uniform constriction. Most patients with early obliterative or partially constricting pericarditis do not have such dramatic findings. For example, the heart *may* be enlarged, especially if it was already enlarged before the episode of pericarditis. Pulsations *may* be diminished on the right or at the base of the heart, while those at the apex on the left remain normal or are even exaggerated. This probably occurs because the base of the heart moves least and the apex most during normal cardiac pulsation, so that it would be logical to expect early obliteration at the base while the apex behaved like a tambour at the end of a rigid cylinder.

When the process is long-standing, *pericardial calcification* may be present. Such calcification is only one of several types which can be detected best by fluoroscopy. Calcification of the valves in both rheumatic and arteriosclerotic heart disease has been studied at fluroscopy for many years. The location of the valves in all conventional projections has been carefully studied and is well-known. When only one valve is calcified and there is any question as to which one it is, fluoroscopy usually determines its identity.

Calcification of the coronary arteries may also be seen at fluoroscopy and identified on cinefluorograms. *Calcification of the aorta* is commonly seen in arteriosclerosis, and the calcified intima of the arch in many persons past middle life may be seen as a shell just inside the margin of the aortic knob. Calcification of the ascending aorta is often syphilitic in origin, and the walls of aneurysms, etiologically either arteriosclerotic or luetic, may show calcium. *Calcification of the wall of the distended left atrium* in mitral valvular disease with insufficiency may often be seen on Bucky films or on body-section studies (Figure 10-13).

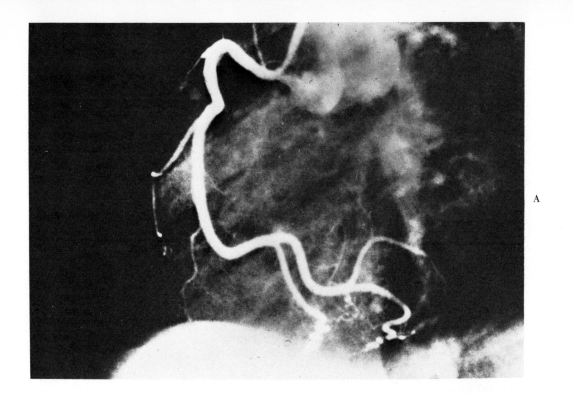

A

Figure 10-15. *Normal coronary arteriograms.* Familiarity with the location of the coronary artery branches makes it easy to identify certain kinds of intracardiac calcifications as being within the walls of those vessels. A: Normal *right* coronary injection with opaque fluid through a catheter hooked into the coronary ostium at fluoroscopy. B: Normal *left* coronary arteriogram. (*In both these cuts you are looking from the patient's left anterior axillary line* in the plane of the interventricular septum. Arteriograms are illustrated here; coronary calcification is difficult to see on films because of the motion of the heart.)

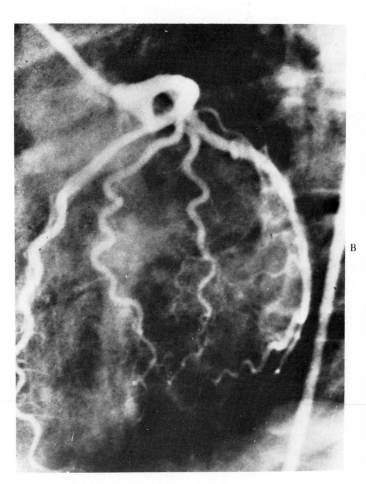

B

127

The Anatomy of the Heart

Left and right anterior obliques

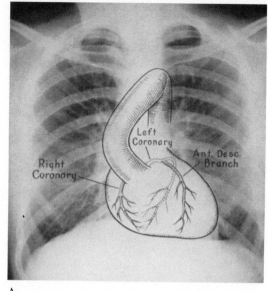

A

Figure 10-16A. In learning to recognize the two commonly used oblique views, you can help orient yourself on the degree of rotation if you review the position of the branches of the coronary arteries. The heart pictured here, although not enlarged to measurement, shows left ventricular prominence and a rather wide-swinging ascending aorta.

Figure 10-16B (opposite page, above left). *The right anterior oblique view.* Made technically as pictured below, with the right anterior axillary line against the cassette holder. This view roughly superimposes the two ventricles upon each other. Note that the right coronary artery bisects the heart shadow in this projection. The posterior surface of the normal heart looks flat and parallel to the spine. Note the resulting triangular shape of the heart shadow.

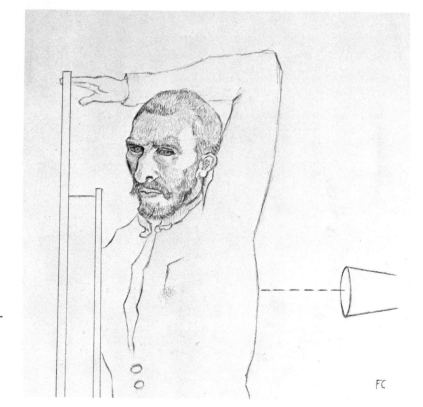

Figure 10-17

Figure 10-18

128

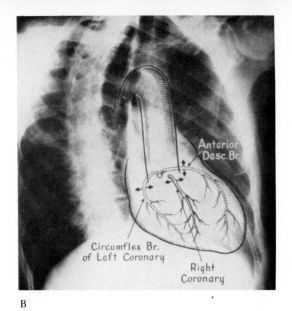

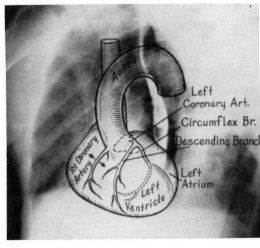

B   C

Figure 10-16C (above right). *The left anterior oblique view.* Made technically as pictured below, with the left anterior axillary line against the cassette holder. This view separates the two ventricles, the left ventricle lying posterior to the descending branch of the left coronary, which bisects the shadow of the heart and marks the position of the interventricular septum. Anterior to this point lies the mass of the right ventricle, on the anterior and inferior surface of the heart. Note that this view also unrolls the aorta, and its ascending and descending limbs are seen enclosing the "aortic window." This produces a quite different shape of the heart shadow roentgenologically, which can be likened to a goosenecked flask. Note that as the mass of the left ventricle enlarges, the characteristic shape in this projection will be exaggerated because the left ventricle will project farther back, overlapping the vertebrae. Note also the position of the left atrium on the posterior surface of the heart. Enlargement of the left atrium could be expected to fill in the aortic window and elevate the bronchi (particularly the left), producing a splaying of the carina, as you will see in the next few pages.

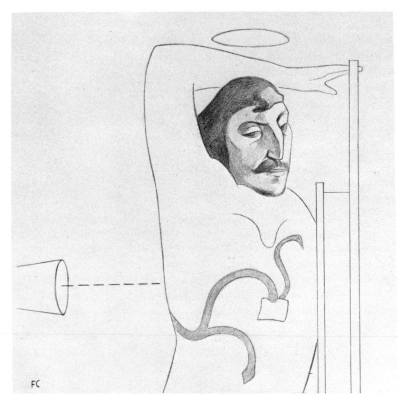

Figure 10-19

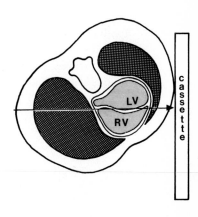

Figure 10-20

129

*Identifying the chambers composing
the profiles in PA and right and left
obliques*

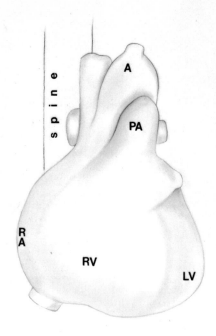

Figure 10-21A. Anterior surface of the heart.

Your initial difficulty in distinguishing the right from the left oblique radiographs may be solved if you learn to study the shape of the heart rather than the various confusing labels on the films. Take any two oblique films in your hands, reversing each until you have a *right oblique in which the heart is to the right of the spine (your right) and looks triangular with a flat posterior surface, and a left oblique in which the heart lies to the left of the spine and is much more bulbous in shape with a rounded posterior surface.* You will then be looking through the two films in the correct way (that is, with the patient facing you but turned a little to each side). Notice that when you reverse a left anterior oblique film and look through it the wrong way, it will *look* wrong to you. This is because it presents the mass of the heart to the right of the spine (as you expect to see it in the right oblique), but its posterior surface is not flat, as you know it ought to be in a right oblique. Watch out for oblique films placed on the view boxes reversed in this fashion, thereby becoming, of course, unreadable paradoxes.

It is easy to learn to identify the portions of the profile of the heart shadow for which each chamber is responsible, and you can do this in the PA and in the two obliques. On the next page spread you have AP angiocardiograms made at the peak of filling of the right chambers and then at the peak of filling of the left chambers after the opaque-loaded bolus of blood has returned from the lungs. Compare them with these diagrams.

Remember that during the angiocardiographic study the patient is filmed AP, but that of course similar studies *could* be made at any degree of obliquity if needed in researching a particular patient's cardiac problem. Later in the chapter you will see a study made by retrograde injection of opaque through the aortic valve and filmed in the lateral projection.

130

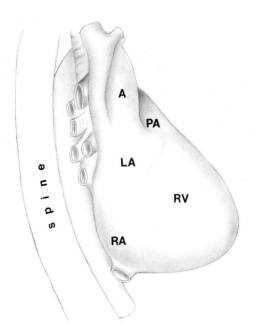

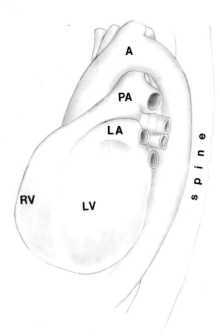

Figure 10-21B. Right anterior oblique surface of the heart. Figure 10-21C. Left anterior oblique surface of the heart.

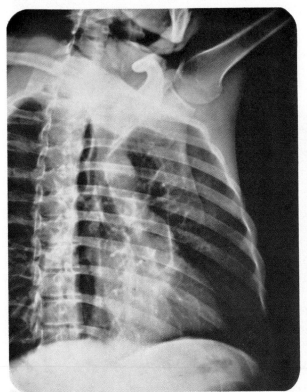

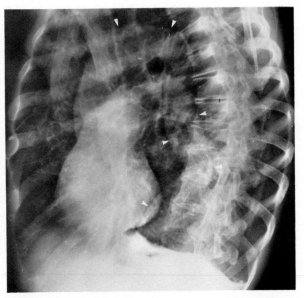

Figure 10-22. Right oblique radiograph of a patient with a normal heart. Note the generally triangular shape of the heart shadow and its flat posterior surface, which will help you to distinguish this view from the left oblique.

Figure 10-23. Left oblique radiograph, with the somewhat elongated and tortuous aorta well unrolled. Note the rounded posterior surface of the heart and shape, differing markedly from that seen in the right oblique.

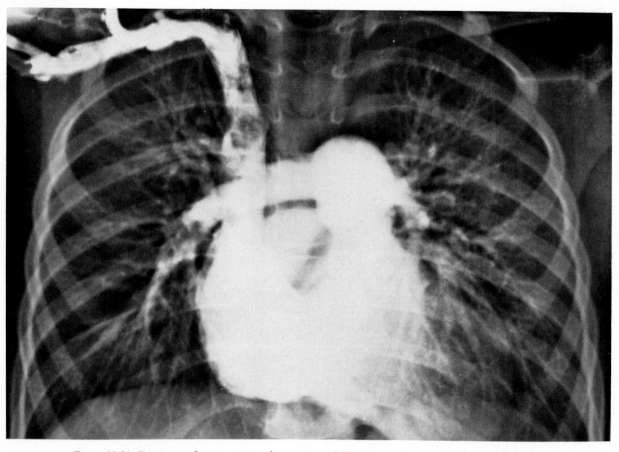

Figure 10-24. Dextrogram from an angiocardiogram on a child with coarctation. Identify: superior vena cava, right atrium (estimate location of tricuspid valve and decide why it is not visible), right ventricle, pulmonary outflow tract, location of pulmonary valve, main pulmonary artery and its branches.

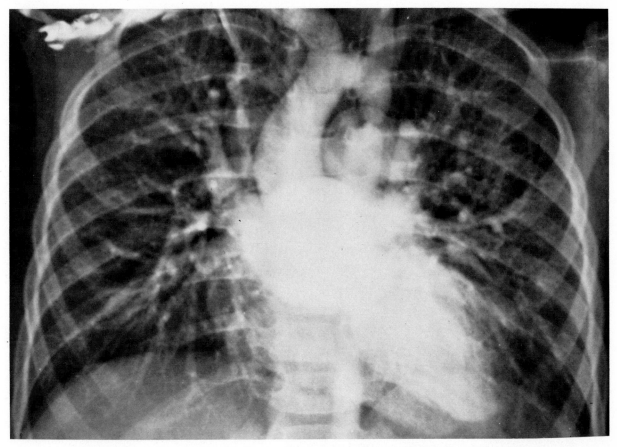

Figure 10-25. Levogram from an angiocardiogram on a child with coarctation. Identify: pulmonary veins approaching the left atrium (is there still any opaque material at all in the arteries?), left atrium high on the back of the heart, location of mitral valve (and why is *it* not seen?), left ventricle, aorta and its branches, and, finally, site of the coarctation.

Changes in the Shape of the Heart due to Enlargement of a Specific Chamber

As you look at the size and shape of the projected shadow of opaque material filling the *left ventricle* in Figure 10-25, try to predict what you might expect to happen to the shape of that ventricle (and consequently to heart shadow itself) with increasing degrees of left ventricular hypertrophy and subsequent dilatation. Imagine that this child's heart responds to years of undiagnosed coarctation and predict its change in shape and the change in the angiocardiogram which could be anticipated. As you do this, you will comprehend better the shape of the adult hearts with left ventricular hypertrophy and failure which you saw several pages back. You will also understand that in a plain film made in the left oblique projection (and even the left lateral which you see more often), the lower posterior surface of the heart becomes increasingly round in cardiovascular disease involving left ventricular enlargement and projects farther and farther posteriorly and to the left. Its surface in the left oblique should normally clear the anterior margin of the spine, but in decompensated hypertensive cardiovascular disease the left ventricle commonly overlaps the spine and is seen superimposed upon it.

Now imagine as you look at the shadow of the *left atrium* in Figure 10-25 that *it* gradually dilates, as it would in a patient with mitral valvular disease with insufficiency. What would you expect that to do to the heart shadow on the PA plain film? You would anticipate an increase in the width of the heart through the base in the PA, and in both the other views you would expect to see the result of crowding upon the structures which are in close relation posteriorly with the enlarging left atrium. Thus the left main bronchus would be elevated and the carina splayed. The esophagus may be displaced to either side and is generally bowed backward. In the left oblique the aortic window may disappear, filled in by the fluid-filled atrium of about the same radiodensity as the aorta itself. In the next few pages you will be able to study examples and to confirm these predictions.

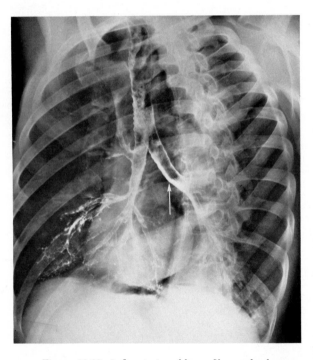

Figure 10-26. Left anterior oblique film made during a bronchogram. The carina sits atop the left atrium normally. When the LA dilates, the left main bronchus (arrow) will be lifted.

134

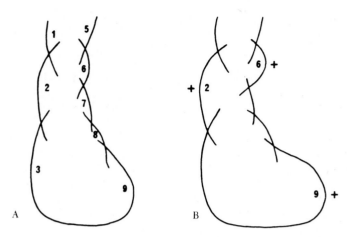

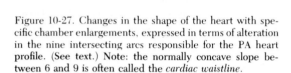

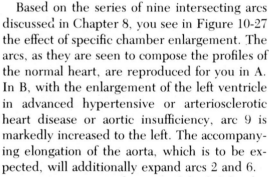

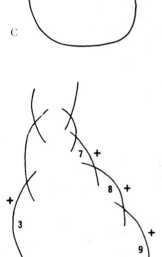

Figure 10-27. Changes in the shape of the heart with specific chamber enlargements, expressed in terms of alteration in the nine intersecting arcs responsible for the PA heart profile. (See text.) Note: the normally concave slope between 6 and 9 is often called the *cardiac waistline*.

Based on the series of nine intersecting arcs discussed in Chapter 8, you see in Figure 10-27 the effect of specific chamber enlargement. The arcs, as they are seen to compose the profiles of the normal heart, are reproduced for you in A. In B, with the enlargement of the left ventricle in advanced hypertensive or arteriosclerotic heart disease or aortic insufficiency, arc 9 is markedly increased to the left. The accompanying elongation of the aorta, which is to be expected, will additionally expand arcs 2 and 6.

In C you see straightening of the left border of the heart so that its normal waistline becomes convex rather than concave, a change to be expected in minimal-to-moderate mitral valvular disease in which there is still only moderate enlargement of the left atrium. This straightening of the left heart border in early mitral disease can be shown to be due to the shadow of the dilated auricular appendage.

In D you see the cardiac shape you might expect in advanced mitral valvular disease with marked insufficiency, often resulting in so much enlargement of the left atrium that it even projects beyond the shadow of the right atrium

on the right border of the heart at arc 3. In addition, there is fullness of arc 7, the pulmonary outflow tract, because of chronic obstruction to the lesser circulation. There is left ventricular enlargement as well, expanding arc 9. Left ventricular enlargement in the patient with a long history of mitral insufficiency may be the result of overload and resultant hypertrophy and dilatation, or of combined aortic and mitral valvular lesions.

In combined mitral and aortic valvular lesions, the cardiac shape which evolves will depend on the lesion which effectively dominates, arc 9 becoming more prominent in hearts in which there is relatively more aortic valve involvement, and fullness of arcs 7 and 8 prevailing when the degree of mitral insufficiency is relatively greater than the aortic valvular disease.

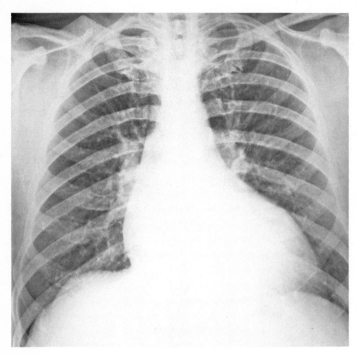

Figure 10-28. *Aortic insufficiency.* Measurable enlargement with dominance of the left ventricle. Note concave waistline and flat aortic arch.

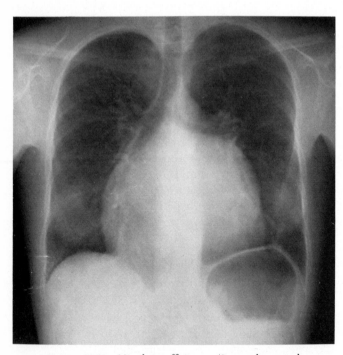

Figure 10-29. *Mitral insufficiency.* (Supervoltage technique). Note elevation of the left main bronchus and splaying of the subcarinal angle.

Try Analyzing the Four Hearts on These Pages Before Reading the Text.

You begin now to have a feeling for the basic differences in shape between the heart shadow with predominantly left ventricular enlargement and the heart in which the left atrium is dilated. They are the most important specific chamber enlargements for you to be able to recognize. Whenever you suspect either, you will try to confirm your impression by examining the obliques.

With left ventricular enlargement, the left oblique will be helpful, showing you rounding and extension of the left ventricle posteriorly overlapping the spine, and possibly some elongation of the aorta if the basic disease is arteriosclerotic. With left atrial dilatation, the left oblique may show you filling in of the aortic window, and the right oblique, posterior displacement of the barium-filled esophagus. Both obliques will show you the same thickening of the heart shadow through the base which you are beginning to recognize as the "mitral heart" in the PA chest film.

Change in the shape of the heart resulting from enlargement of the right chambers is more difficult to recognize, even for the radiologist. The right atrium is to be found immensely dilated, of course, in tricuspid atresia, which is so rare you may never see a case of it—and if you do you will have the impression, more than likely, that you are looking at something you have not seen before. Right ventricular hypertrophy and eventual dilatation are not at all uncommon, but because the right ventricle lies against the diaphragm and the anterior chest wall, juxtaposed to structures of equal density, enlargement of this chamber may be very difficult to recognize, even for the experts. There are one or two points to be remembered about it, however.

Hypertrophy of the right ventricle often displaces a normal-sized left ventricle to the left, so that such a heart shadow may occasionally suggest left ventricular hypertrophy on first glance at the PA. Examination of the two obliques, however, will show the right ventricle (along the anterior profile of the heart shadow) to be rounded and full, and careful correlation with the clinical finding will usually prevent misinterpretation. Remember that in judging the heart x-ray, the PA view is only a beginning and has limitations which must be kept in mind. You will expect to find right ventricular enlargement (cor pulmonale) in many types of chronic lung disease. The right ventricle is hypertrophied in pulmonic stenosis and in several other types of congenital heart disease. Few of these are analyzed from their plain-film studies alone, inasmuch as surgical correction can be planned only after a meticulous and precise delineation of the abnormalities which are present. Though one may expect such changes from the shape of the heart, this type of cardiac patient is invariably studied by specialists, in the cardiopulmonary laboratory, and by either serial angiocardiograms or cineangiocardiography.

One more point to remember: in young girls the left border is often straight without any demonstrable evidence of clinical heart disease. This may be because in young women the left ventricle has not yet assumed its normal slight dominance. The two patients in Figures 10-30 and 10-31 will have puzzled you in this regard. Both show slightly convex left borders. Only the patient in 10-30 has measurable cardiac enlargement, and she had the classic murmurs of mitral stenosis with minimal insufficiency. Her left bronchus is slightly elevated, to confirm our impression from this film alone that a slightly dilated left atrium acounts for the fullness of the left border. The girl in Figure 10-31 has no cardiac enlargement, nor had she any cardiac symptoms. Her dyspnea was due to an incipient attack of asthma. She had a history of one or two attacks a month for several years, and on fluoroscopy her straightening of the left border was easily shown to be caused by slight fullness of the pulmonary outflow tract, or, in other words, arc 7. In the original PA chest film her left main bronchus could be seen to form a perfectly normal angle at the carina, and there was nothing in the oblique views to suggest atrial abnormality. Thus the straightened left border in 10-30 is due to posterior fullness, while that in 10-31 is due to fullness of an entirely different structure located anteriorly.

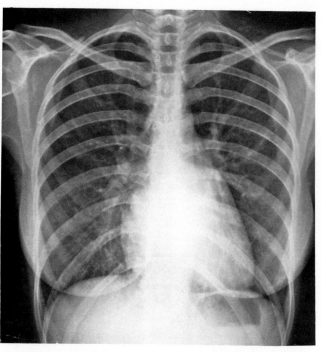

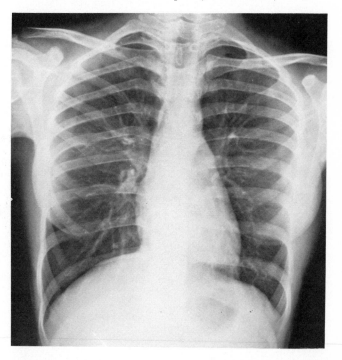

Figures 10-30 (above) and 10-31 (below). Analyze the heart contour in these two young women. Both were short of breath on admission to the hospital. (Answers in text.)

137

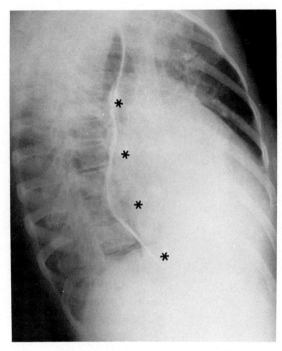

Figure 10-32. Right oblique in a patient with mitral valvular disease and insufficiency, showing posterior displacement of the barium-filled esophagus by the dilated left atrium. Asterisks indicate normal course of the esophagus.

By the time you have studied the films of 50 heart patients in addition to the introductory grounding I have tried to give you in this chapter, you ought to feel fairly secure about the following decisions: (1) you ought to be able to evaluate heart shadows on 6-foot PA chest films, checking the factors which might be producing spurious changes and deciding whether there is true enlargement; (2) you ought to be able to recognize alteration in shape referable to left ventricular dilatation or left atrial dilatation and to check your PA impression on the two obliques and lateral films; (3) you should be able to place the obliques on the viewing boxes correctly most of the time; (4) you will be beginning to know where to look for fullness in the profiles with any particular chamber or great-vessel enlargement; (5) you ought to be able to decide whether a shapeless enlarged heart is in failure, from inspection of the hilar and pulmonary vasculature; and (6) you ought to have some idea as to what help you can expect from the roentgen examination and the radiologist in various sorts of cardiac disease. Try your hand at the following unknowns before you go on to the abdomen.

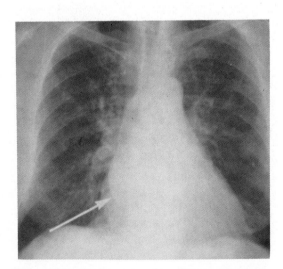

Figure 10-33. Mitral stenosis and insufficiency. The shadow of the dilated left atrium projects to the right, producing a "double shadow" above that of the right atrium.

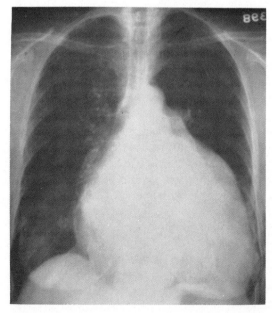

Figure 10-34. Patient, 65, with advanced mitral valvular disease and mitral insufficiency. Note elevation of left main bronchus and shadow of large left atrium seen through the heart shadow.

Unknowns

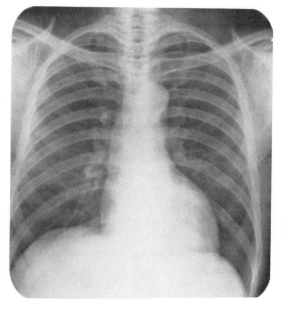

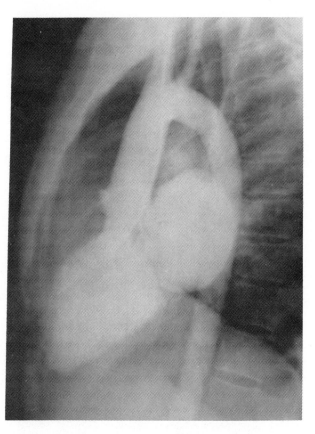

Figure 10-35 (*Unknown 10-1*). Evaluate this heart in view of the fact that it belongs to a young man of 28.

Figure 10-36 (*Unknown 10-2*). Identify the projection and the special procedure being carried out. What do the findings prove?

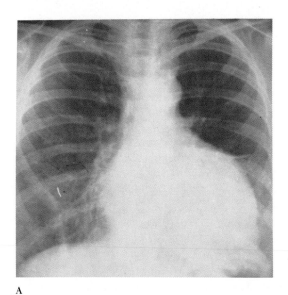

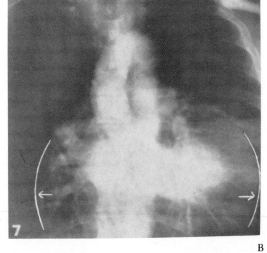

A

B

Figure 10-37 (*Unknown 10-3*). Decide whether the heart on the plain film (A) is measurably enlarged, what its shape suggests, what special procedure is being carried out in B, and what the findings prove.

CHAPTER 11 The Abdomen: Study of the Plain Film I

logic of its appearance is much more easily retained because it can be reasoned out again if it is forgotten. Roentgen study of the abdomen is largely reasoning.

The wide differences in radiodensity of the chest structures provide profiles and margins which are easy to see and to interpret as you first begin to look at x-ray films. In the abdomen, however, organ masses and great vessels merge into a confluent gray shadow so that their borders and profiles vanish. *Only when some structure of differing density lies against one you wish to know about can you see its boundary*—often only a small segment of that boundary—from which you may be able to construe something about the size and shape of the organ in question.

The striking radiolucency of air within the gut will occur to you at once as providing the sort of boundaries and outline segments you need. You will use this kind of information constantly in assaying from plain films the size and shape of organs and masses within the abdomen.

Thus, for example, all air-containing gut may be swept into the left side of the abdomen by a grossly enlarged liver whose mass is seen as a large gray shadow, but whose margin is often only visible to you outlined by air in the colon (Figure 11-3). The stomach, when filled with fluid, lies against the spleen and blends with its shadow invisibly, giving no information as to its size; but if the stomach is inflated with air, it may be seen to be clearly indented from the left and displaced medially by an enlarged spleen. All air-containing structures may be displaced upward out of the pelvis by a large ovarian cyst, and individual large and small bowel loops, like a circle of dark beads, will outline the cyst's upper surface.

Variable as the actual content of air in the gut certainly is, it will prove extremely useful to you in tagging abnormalities in the size and shape of other organs, and you will soon form a visual baseline with regard to the amount and location of air-in-gut which you can expect to see. There is normally at least a little air in the stomach and a fair amount distributed throughout the colon. In the healthy, ambulatory adult the small bowel usually contains little or no air, but normal infants and bedridden adults often show

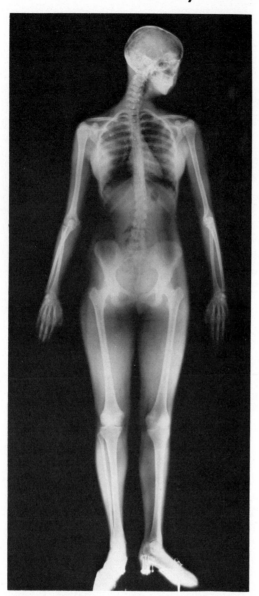

Figure 11-1. Radiograph of an entire (female) human model is helpful in demonstrating the basic differences between chest and abdomen in regard to radiodensities.

Radiographic study of the region of the abdomen is, in its way, perhaps a little more difficult and a little more subtle than that of the chest, but it is equally interesting from the standpoint of the opportunity it affords you to discover how much of roentgen data can be learned through reasoning. Material learned by appreciating the considerable amounts of small-bowel air without any abdominal pathology to account for it.

By definition a "plain film" is a film made without any artificially introduced contrast substance. For this reason you should call it a *plain film* rather than a "flat plate," a meaningless term. The so-called KUB is a plain film. Although we must in this chapter discuss first the plain film of the abdomen, you will find that you will anticipate better the location and appearance of the air-outlined gut *after* you have seen all parts of the gastrointestinal tract filled with barium. *In barium studies the entire gastrointestinal tract is rendered visible, but in the plain film you will be depending on transient air content alone for information,* and you will realize that many parts of the gut are ordinarily invisible because they contain fluid feces or are collapsed. Sometimes parts of the colon will be outlined by their content of semisolid feces with which bubbles of air have been mixed. This casts a distinctive speckled shadow and may be just as useful as air-filled gut in indicating the position of neighboring structures or in locating parts of the colon itself. Such speckled fecal shadows always identify colon and are not seen in the small bowel.

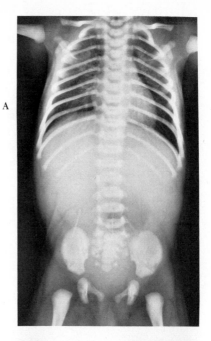

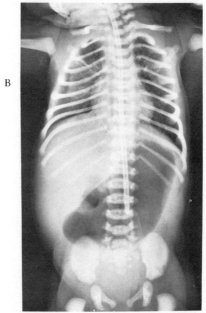

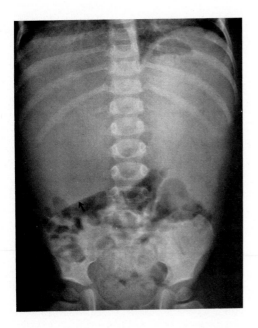

Figure 11-2. A: Airless abdomen in a 4-day-old girl who had been vomiting since birth. All organs blend together as one confluent gray shadow. B: Same patient, stomach inflated with air. Note density of catheter. Upper margin of the antrum of the stomach lies against the margin of the liver.

Figure 11-3 (left). The margin of the liver outlined by air in the gut. You know the film to have been made with the patient standing because of the fluid level in the fundal stomach bubble. The liver in this small boy was immensely enlarged by tumor.

Identifying Parts of the Gastrointestinal Tract from Barium Casts and then from Air Content

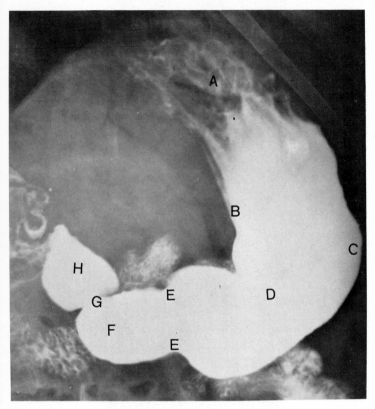

Figure 11-4. The stomach is visible here because it is filled with barium sulfate. (A) the fundus, (B) the lesser curvature, (C) the greater curvature, (D) the body, (E-E) the indentation of a peristaltic wave, (F) the antrum, (G) the pyloric canal, and (H) the duodenal cap or bulb.

Barium casts of various parts of the gut produce white shadows on the film, the margins of which distinctly reproduce the character of the mucosal pattern. The rugae of the stomach are quite different from the plicae of the small intestine and from the smoother, more widely spaced haustra of the colon with their serosal indentations. To distinguish their barium casts is to anticipate differences in their dark air shadows on the plain film.

The distribution through the abdomen of air in the gut is determined to some extent by the degree of fixation of the various structures. The stomach may alter widely in size, but it *is* fixed at the diaphragm and to the retroperitoneal part of the duodenum. The small bowel enjoys the liberty of its ample mesentery, folded into the midabdomen. The transverse colon varies widely in position too, but the ascending and descending portions of the large bowel are normally tethered in the lateral gutters by their shorter mesocolons. Within this degree of latitude you will learn to identify different parts of the air-filled gut by their locations as well as by their distinctive mucosal patterns. Remember which are the fixed points in the gut, and that the stomach, cecum, and rectum are very distensible.

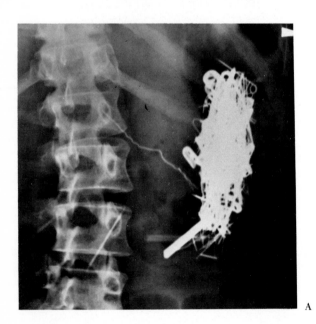

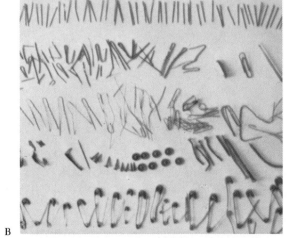

Figure 11-5A (left). The position of the stomach indicated by its accidental content of hardware. A mental patient complained of abdominal distress. At gastrotomy 287 metal and glass objects were removed (B, above.)

142

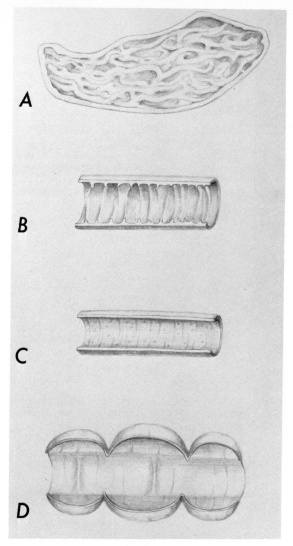

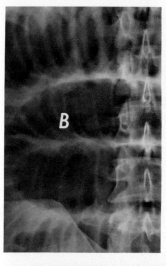

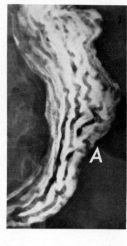

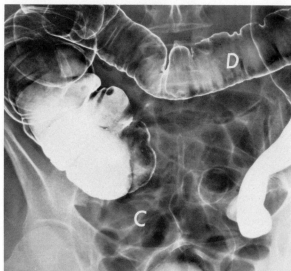

Figure 11-6. The mucosal linings of stomach (A), jejunum (B), ileum (C), and colon (D) differ anatomically enough to be identified from the appearance of their respective air shadows. Remember that hollow organs *full of barium* (as in Figure 11-4) look quite different from the same organs *filled with air* or lightly coated inside with a smear of barium.

Figure 11-7 (above). Examples to help you. A: The rugae of the stomach are seen as black wavy shadows. These radiolucent soft-tissue ridges are visible because opaque barium lies in the valleys between them. The reverse is often seen when the stomach contains only air, that is, soft-tissue ridges with more radiolucent air in the valleys between them (Figure 11-8). B: The distinctive plical folds inside the jejunum appear as transverse, denser ridges with air between (here seen in distended small bowel of intestinal obstruction). C: Air-filled loops of ileum, filled from the colon during a barium enema, overlap their shadows in the pelvis and lower abdomen. D: The colon with its characteristic serosal indentations, or haustra, filled with barium and air. Reason out why the transverse colon appears to be outlined in white, whereas the descending colon is uniformly opaque.

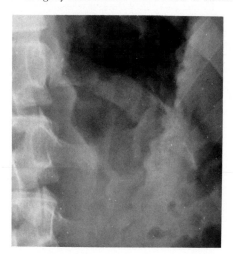

Figure 11-8 (left). The rugae thrown into relief by air in the stomach as the only contrast substance.

143

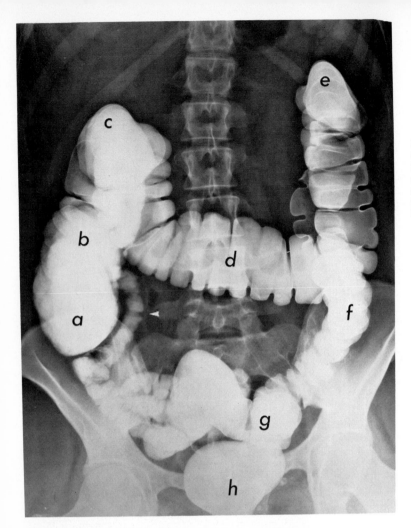

Figure 11-9. Normal distribution of the colon. (a) cecum, (b) ascending colon, (c) hepatic flexure, (d) transverse colon, (e) splenic flexure, (f) descending colon, (g) sigmoid, and (h) rectum. Note overlap at flexures. Small white arrow points to the terminal ileum, which often fills during the barium enema.

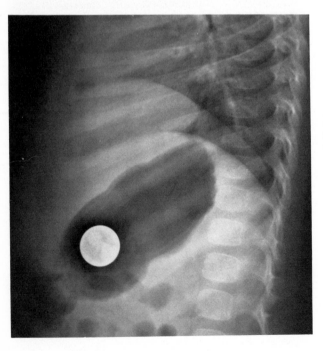

Figure 11-10. Lateral view of the air-filled stomach containing a Lincoln-head penny. Would you be likely to be able to identify the coin if the stomach were filled with (1) barium, (2) lunch?

Identifying Fat Planes, Tangentially Viewed, as Normal Markers

Fat distributions within the abdomen also help you to make certain decisions about the structures they invest. The wide apron of the omentum will not help you because it is distributed across the abdomen and never seen in tangent. The perirenal envelope of fat, however, provides a tangential radiolucent layer outlining the kidney mass with a dark line where more x-rays reach the film to blacken it.

In the same way precisely, the fatty layer next to the peritoneum in the abdominal wall is not seen where the sagittally directed ray of a supine plain film strikes it en face anteriorly in the midline. At each side, however, where the fat layer turns posteriorly toward the patient's back, the beam catches it tangentially and the dark line produced on the film is called the "flank stripe"*.

The flank stripe disappears when the flank itself becomes edematous. This is perfectly logical: fluid infiltrating the fat renders it as dense to the x-ray beam as the largely fluid muscle which adjoins it. With inflammation near the flank (as in appendiceal abscess, for example) the flank stripe on that side may disappear, while the opposite one remains normal. In exactly the same fashion, perirenal inflammation erases the perirenal fat line.

The subcutaneous fat of a fetus near term may be traversed tangentially by the ray, outlining a leg or an arm or the buttocks against the inside of the uterine wall. Concentrated accumulations of fat, such as may be present within a dermoid cyst, produce localized round radiolucent shadows on the film, appreciable to the eye because of their juxtaposition with surrounding structures of greater density.

As you will see in the next chapter, it is their surrounding radiolucent fat that renders abdominal organs and masses so clearly identifiable in cross section by computerized tomography. Obese patients are harder to examine clinically and often have confusing plain films, but they will be easy to examine by CT.

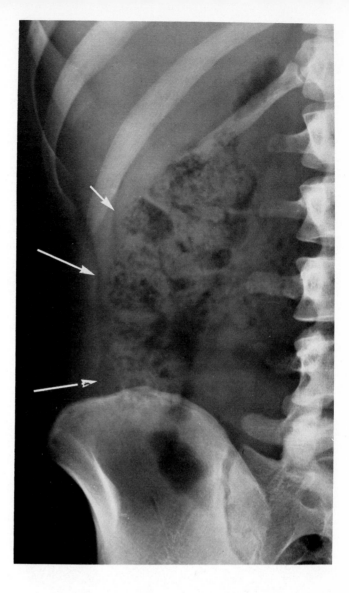

Figure 11-11. Right flank stripe, close against which lies the ascending colon, indicated, as it so often is on the plain film, by the characteristic speckled shadow of feces mixed with air. Note margin of liver above. Dark shadow overlying the wing of the ilium is air in cecum or terminal ileum.

* You will also hear it referred to as the "preperitoneal" or even "properitoneal" fat line, both of which seem to me semantically poor terms. I advise you to stick to "flank stripe," which is short and direct and does not involve abused word root derivations.

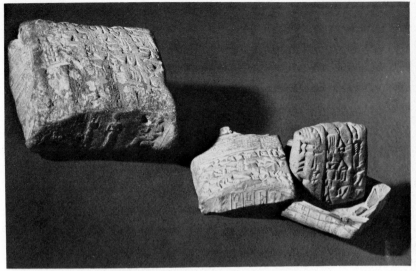
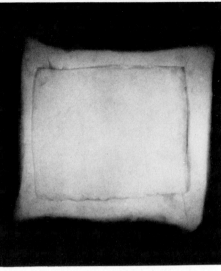

A   B

Figure 11-12. A: Clay tablets from the ancient Sumerian city of Ur. Records of business transactions were recorded in this way, and because the tablets were fragile and the records precious, an outer envelope of clay was added bearing the same information in duplicate. B: The envelope of air between the inner and outer layers of clay is well shown in this radiograph of the intact clay tablet. The parallel between this and any fat- or gas-encased anatomic structure of greater density is obvious.

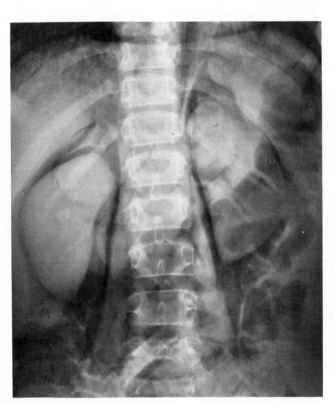
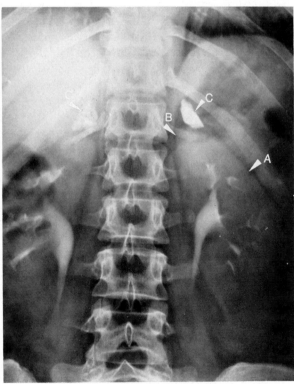

Figure 11-13 (left). A gas injected into the retroperitoneal space has outlined the kidneys even more dramatically than does the fatty envelope you usually depend upon to locate them on a plain film. Compare this with Figure 11-14 (right) where A is the margin of the parenchyma, B the upper pole, and C the calcified adrenal gland. (This patient had Addison's disease.)

146

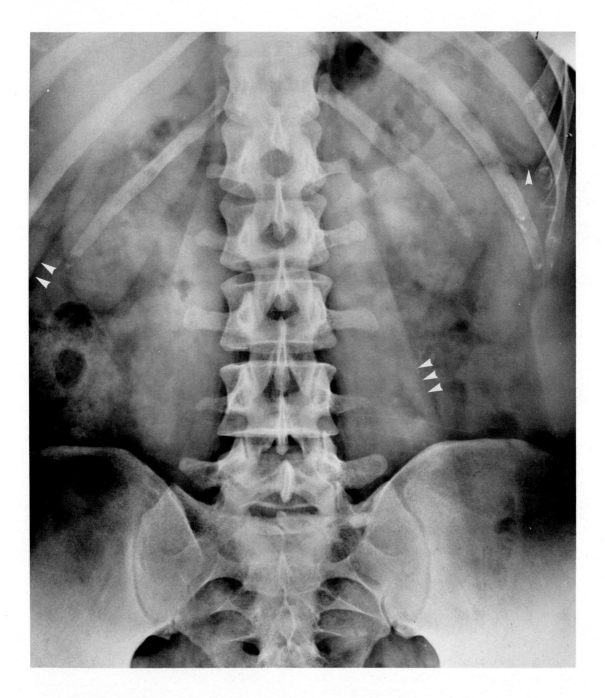

Figure 11-15. Soft tissue unusually well seen on the abdominal plain film. Single arrow indicates the tip of the spleen. Double arrow marks the lower margin of the liver, which you can follow obliquely upward across the shadow of the kidney. Triple arrow indicates the left psoas margin. The psoas shadows are generally symmetrical. Here the lower part of the right psoas is obscured by something of equal density lying against it. Note dark air in the stomach overlying the upper tip of the left kidney and haustrated, air-filled shadows representing the distal transverse colon lying across the middle of the left kidney. The entire outline of the right kidney is seen but not that of the left. The left kidney is a little larger than the right. Note speckled fecal shadows in the right colon and excellent flank stripe on the left.

147

Identifying Various Kinds
of Abnormal Densities
in the Abdomen

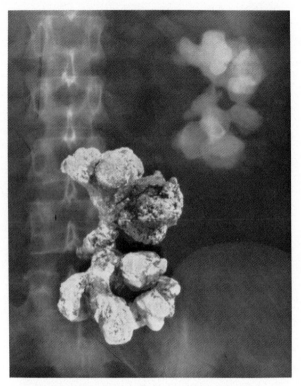

Figure 11-16. Stag-horn calculus in the left kidney. The photograph of the surgical specimen has been superimposed on the radiograph (plain film) for comparison.

and calyces, closely resembling the shadow of opaque fluid you see on a pyelogram (Figure 11-16).

Calcification within the capsule of any organ will resemble the radiograph of an egg shell, more dense peripherally where it is caught tangentially by the ray (Figure 11-19). Calcification in the wall of a hollow organ will look very similar, and you will often see this type of calcification in the aorta in older patients. Sometimes it will bound an aneurysm of that great vessel (Figure 11-21). Plaques of calcium scattered throughout the wall and caught by the ray in tangent will provide an interrupted white outline, as you would expect. A vessel of smaller caliber, when its wall becomes calcified, will show linear white margins like the rose stem in the first chapter and they will be serpiginous and parallel if the vessel describes a tortuous course (Figure 11-20). You will recognize them as characteristic for a hollow cylinder of dense material about a more radiolucent core, x-rayed from the side.

Abnormal radiodensities can be provided by any area of calcification sufficiently large to absorb some of the beam. Calcified thrombi will be seen as dense white nuggets. Gallstones calcify much less commonly than kidney stones, but kidney stones and gallstones will both have a characteristic location and may often show a distinctive radiographic structure in their shadows as well; calcified gallstones are frequently laminated and faceted. If you stop to think for a moment, both the lamination and the faceting are to be expected. Gallstones, more often than kidney stones, form over a long period of time in a pool of fluid of slowly changing metabolic composition; hence the lamination seen in the radiograph. They are also more often multiple and are made to rub against each other with the contractions of the gallbladder—hence the faceting. Kidney calculi are not very often laminated and rarely develop facets. The very characteristic stag-horn renal calculi fill up the entire pelvis

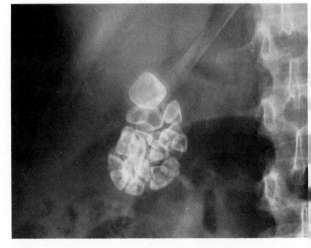

Figure 11-17. Cluster of faceted calculi in the gallbladder. Note that these have formed in such a way that their outer surfaces seem to contain more calcium. Now look closely. The large, square, uppermost calculus shows a distinct new layer of *lesser* density. This illustrates the process of the development of lamination.

148

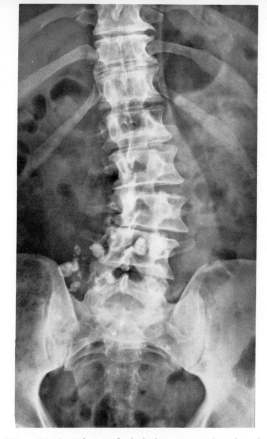

Figure 11-18. A cluster of calcified mesenteric lymph nodes overlie the course of the right ureter near the upper border of the sacroiliac joint. This patient was positioned as straight as possible in the supine position. Note the obliquity produced in the midlumbar spine by his degree of scoliosis. The psoas shadows are asymmetrical, as you would expect.

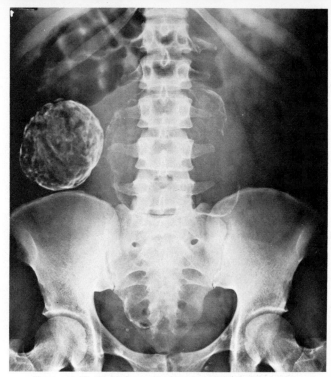

Figure 11-19. Multiple uterine leiomyomata in a 42-year-old woman complaining of constipation and dysuria. The patient had lived all her life in a remote rural area and had never consulted a physician before. There had been a large, painless, lower abdominal mass present for ten years, the top of which was palpable 28 centimeters above the pubic symphysis. The specimen removed at surgery showed many intramural, pedunculated, and submucous fibroids, with varying degrees of calcification. Note displacement of gut.

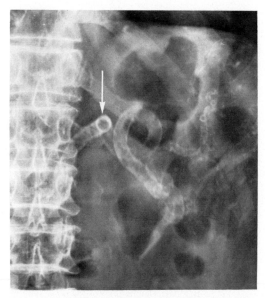

Figure 11-20. Calcified, tortuous splenic artery. Note parallel winding white lines. Arrow indicates segment passing sagittally and hence filmed end-on, appearing as a white ring.

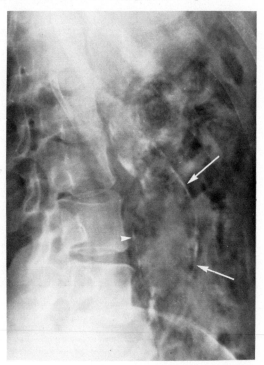

Figure 11-21. Lateral abdominal plain film showing plaques of calcium in the wall of an abdominal aortic aneurysm.

149

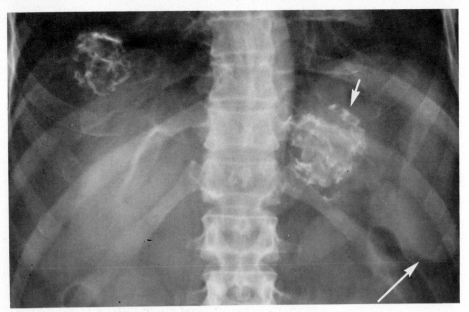

Figure 11-22. Calcifications in the liver, probably representing healed abscesses in a patient with amebic dysentery. Long arrow indicates the tip of the spleen, which is not enlarged. Short arrow points to abscess in the left lobe of the liver.

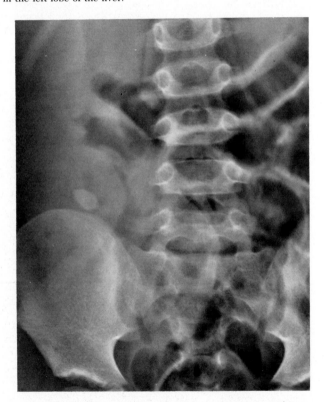

Figure 11-23. Abdomen of a 5½-year-old boy. Air-filled gut is seen displaced to the left away from the right flank where a soft-tissue mass can be seen, in the middle of which there is an oval dense shadow suggesting calcium. This proved to be a fecalith within a large appendiceal abscess.

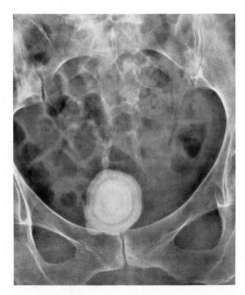

Figure 11-24. Bladder calculus present for some time was finally removed via the suprapubic route. Note lamination.

150

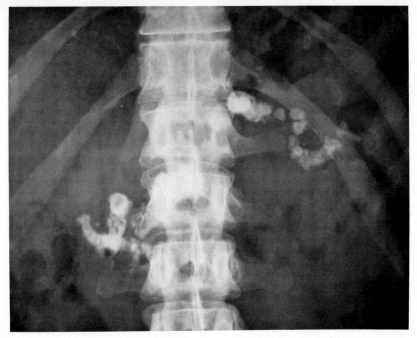

Figure 11-25. Plain film of the upper midabdomen, showing many calcium-containing concretions in the pancreas that outline its entire ductal structure. This occurs in some cases of chronic pancreatitis and is frequently associated with alcoholism.

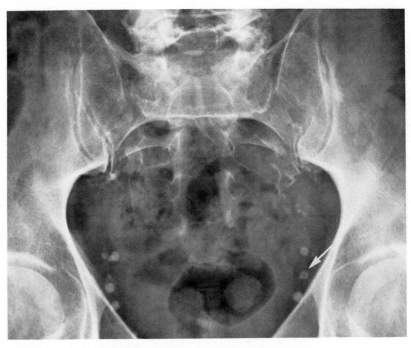

Figure 11-26. Plain film of the bowl of the pelvis, showing clusters of phleboliths on both sides. The one indicated by the arrow shows recanalization. Note solid fecal scybala within the air shadow of the rectum.

Learn to Study the Plain Film Systematically

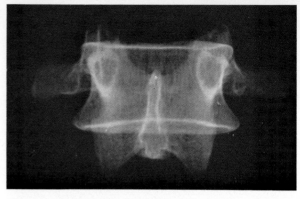

Figure 11-27. Radiograph of a single disarticulated vertebra.

The plain film of the abdomen is important because it is so simple to obtain, involves no danger or discomfort for the patient, and can be immensely informative without complex procedures. So much can be learned, in fact, from plain films of the abdomen in so many different conditions that every physician should be familiar enough with them to study intelligently those on his own patients and recognize some of the common aberrations.

There are many subtleties in the interpretation of abdominal plain films, to be sure, and it is easy to feel, when you first begin to look at them, that you are missing important and obvious changes.

At your stage of learning an orderly manner of approaching the analysis of an abdominal plain film can be strongly recommended. I would suggest that you make a practice of *looking first at the bones* on a plain film of the abdomen (vertebral column, lower ribs, pelvis), excluding from your mind's eye all other structures. (If you do not look at the bones first, you will almost certainly forget them later.)

Then examine carefully *the soft tissues* of a series of smaller areas to include the left upper quadrant, right upper quadrant, both flanks, midabdomen, and pelvis, in that order. In each soft-tissue zone you will be *checking border indicators, organ masses, and fat lines, looking for calcification and for any shift in position or change in shape of the structures you see and identify*.

Then check out the gastrointestinal (GI) tract, accounting for all parts of it in order, whether distended with gas or containing only a small amount, and recognizing some parts of the colon by their content of solid or semisolid feces.

Finally, decide whether there are any gray soft-tissue shadows or radiolucencies not yet accounted for in your survey, and if there are, try to tally them with the patient's history and physical examination.

152

Begin with the spine . . .

The shadows of the *lumbar vertebrae* may appear very confusing when you first look at them, but they will be easy to comprehend and remember once you have analyzed them part for part. To begin with, the box-like body of a vertebra, extending anteriorly, would have a very simple roentgen structure if it could be seen by itself and not superimposed on the complex posterior articulating processes. Because it is literally a flat cylindrical box of dense cortical bone filled with spongy bone, you would expect it to radiograph with a shell of tangentially seen—and therefore denser—bone outlining it, and an interior of many superimposed slender white trabeculae with dark marrow spaces between.

Add to this box outline, now in the PA projection, the two pedicles, cylinders of cortical bone extending straight backward on either side of the spinal canal. Because they too are filled with spongy bone, they will radiograph as cylinders seen end-on and, as you can predict, will appear on the film as two white circles. Now as you look at the vertebrae on any plain film of the abdomen, you can account for the two "eyes" which you see superimposed on the upper part of each vertebral body.

The centrally located white teardrop is the cortical bone investing the spinous process, also filled with spongy bone. The pairs of superior and inferior articulating processes are also to be seen as wings of bone extending upward and downward from each vertebral body to create a butterfly-like shadow behind the vertebral body. Finally, the transverse processes extend out to each side, varying slightly in shape from level to level.

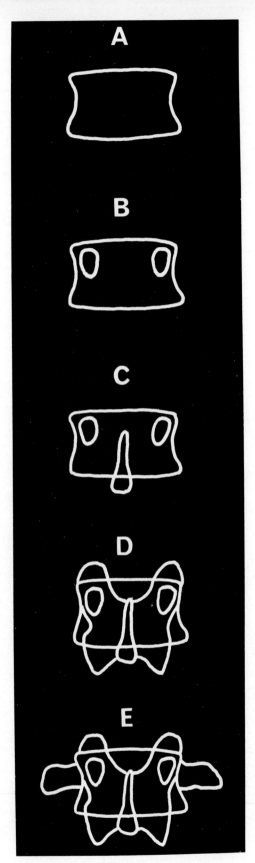

Figure 11-28

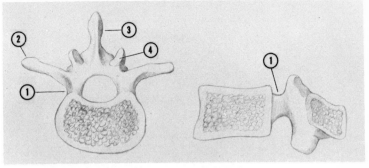

Figure 11-29. Vertebra seen from above and from the side. (1) pedicle, (2) transverse process, (3) spinous process, (4) superior articulating process.

If you always think first of the outline of the vertebral body as you look at the spine on an abdominal film, and then add the posterior structures one by one, you will not be confused by the jumble of overlapping bony parts. A pathologic process which destroys any part of these bony structures will cause the disappearance of a shadow you are now expecting to see and can usually trace because of its symmetry with the same structure on the other side, or above or below at a different level. Thus, if an aneurysm erodes the left lateral surface of the first and second lumbar vertebrae where the aorta lies closely against them, you will see that the cortex on one side is missing, interrupting the smooth squared outline of the body. In the lateral projection some part of the anterior surface of the body will also be missing, the intervertebral discs being better preserved than the bone because they resist pressure erosion better.

By the same token, when an expanding intraspinal tumor destroys the medial bony wall of the pedicles, the radiologist observes that the medial sides of one or more pairs of eyes are flattened and farther apart than those above and below them in the AP view.

The bilateral symmetry of the posterior structures superimposed upon the vertebral body will be useful to you in another way, because it tells you that the ray was passing sagittally through the patient. Routinely, plain films of the abdomen are made AP with the patient supine, but some barium studies and all gallbladder studies are made PA with the patient prone. (Why?) Many types of special procedures are performed in conventional degrees of obliquity, and you will find that the appearance of the vertebrae indicates the direction of the ray.

153

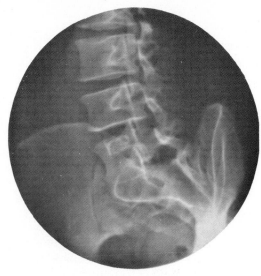

Figure 11-30. Oblique view of the lumbar vertebrae.

Thus if you see the boxy bodies of the vertebrae cleanly separated from their posterior structures, you will know that you are looking at a *lateral* film; but if the bodies and posterior structures are precisely superimposed and bilaterally symmetrical, you are looking at a film made with a *sagittal* ray. *Obliques* will show you the vertebrae about as you see them in Figure 11-30, and note that now you can see through the obliquely directed posterior articulations. All this will have prepared you for the partial obliquity you will often be seeing with scoliosis of the spine, no matter how carefully the technician has tried to position the patient prone or supine.

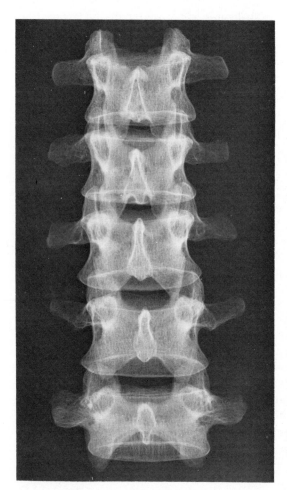
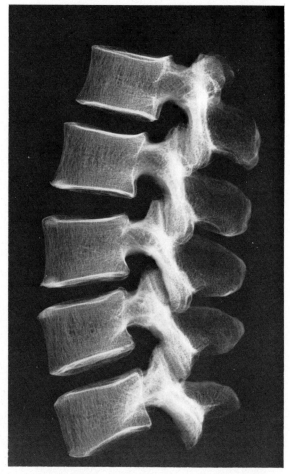

Figure 11-31. AP and lateral views of a disarticulated specimen of lumbar vertebrae. Identify the various parts without turning back.

154

Nearly all the abdominal films you see will have been made with the Bucky diaphragm, and you will observe that you can see the ribs below the diaphragm much better than you do in chest films. The last two ribs arise from their vertebral articulations, extend laterally without being joined to the costal cartilages, and often are not identical.

Calcifications in the costal cartilages (which normally are radiolucent and invisible) may offer some confusion when they are seen superimposed on intra-abdominal calcifications within the gallbladder, kidney, or adrenal gland. Rib calcifications can usually be distinguished by tracing the expected course of the rib anteriorly. Lateral films and body-section studies will afford help when there is reasonable doubt as to the location of such upper abdominal calcifications.

. . . and the pelvis and upper femora . . .

The bones of the *pelvis* differ in the shape of their shadows when the ray passes through PA and AP, as you can anticipate if you think of the structure of the flared and tilted wings of the ilium. These are "flattened out against the film," appearing round and wide on a supine plain film but narrow and more vertical on barium enema films made with the patient prone. This is because the ray which passes through the patient PA is much more nearly tangential to the surface of the iliac wings, so that they are more approximately filmed on edge.

The ray is usually centered on the umbilicus in making a plain film of the abdomen, so that roughly half the air-in-gut shadows will be below this point. You will therefore expect to see (superimposed on the bones of the pelvis and sacrum) the air in the cecum, sigmoid, and rectum, as well as in the small-bowel loops when they do contain air. A loop of air-containing bowel overlying the iliac wing on a supine plain film is often very difficult to differentiate from a round area of bone destruction, and the procedure is to look over several films of the

area: small-bowel air changes in shape and location from film to film, but an area of bone destruction will remain in exactly the same relation to the margins of the bone in which it is present (Figure 11-32).

Note that you see through the cartilaginous part of the anterior portion of the sacroiliac joint and through the symphysis pubis. Identify the spines and tuberosities of the ischia, and note that the hip joint is "seen" because it is bounded on both sides by the cortical bone of acetabulum and femoral head, seen in tangent. Later, when you have read the section on bone, you will look at the bones on a plain film of the abdomen with a more precise eye for abnormalities, but for now leave them and go on to a study of the series of soft-tissue zones.

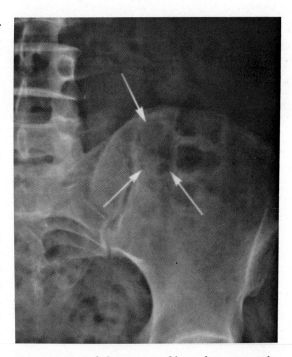

Figure 11-32. Radiolucent area of bone destruction indicated by arrows did not change in relation to the margin of the sacroiliac joint from film to film. The darker air shadows lateral to it did.

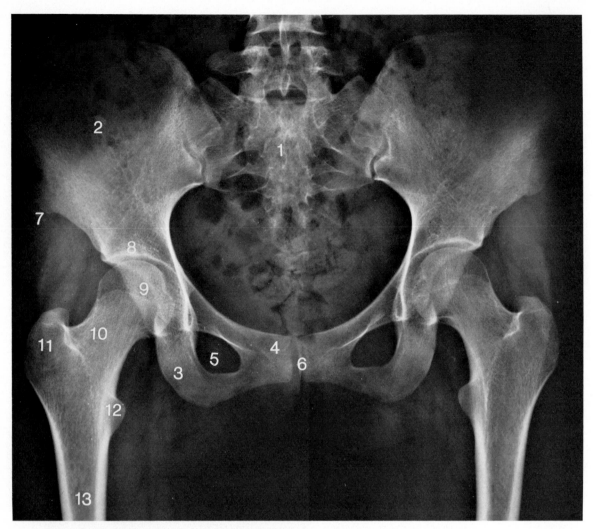

Figure 11-33. Anteroposterior radiograph of the pelvis and upper femora.

(1) Sacrum
(2) Ilium
(3) Ischium
(4) Pubis
(5) Obturator foramen
(6) Symphysis pubis
(7) Anterior superior iliac spine
(8) Acetabulum
(9) Femoral head
(10) Femoral neck
(11) Greater trochanter
(12) Lesser trochanter
(13) Femoral shaft

Abnormality in size or shape of an organ is frequently appreciable from the plain film alone, but there are some differences in the degree of accuracy with which size may be judged by x-ray. The shadow of the *liver* is very misleading as an index to its size, for example, and it must be grossly enlarged before one can assume hepatomegaly from the plain film. Partly because of its shape and partly because of variation in the tilted position of the liver within the abdomen, pronouncements with regard to liver enlargement based on the plain film are risky. You will find that as an assay of the liver size, old-fashioned palpation is a more reliable method.

The liver, so much larger than the spleen, normally tends to depress the organs in this quadrant. Its margin may be seen either as the inferior limit of a gray mass or as a boundary outlined by air in the transverse colon and hepatic flexure. The hepatic flexure is usually lower than the splenic flexure, but may occasionally overlap a part of the liver shadow. Radioisotope scanning techniques are becoming increasingly practicable for routine use in studying the liver, and metastatic lesions may be localized readily within the liver parenchyma. No secretory roentgenographic opacification technique is available at present.

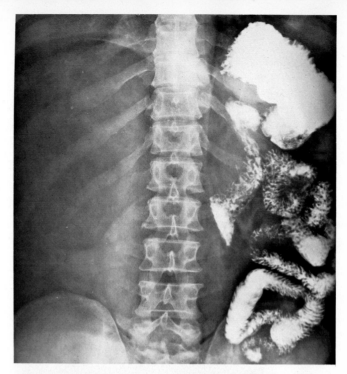

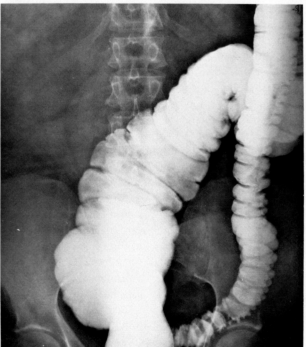

Figures 11-34 and 11-35. Upper GI series and barium enema showing marked displacement of these normal structures by an enormous liposarcoma on the right side.

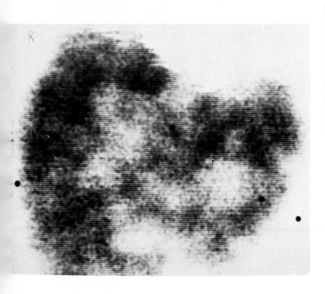

Figure 11-36 (left). Liver isotope scan shows many areas of no uptake in the liver, metastases from carcinoma of the colon.

The *spleen*, on the contrary, may cast a shadow on the plain film which is unquestionably increased in size, although it has not been felt on bimanual examination. In such cases the roentgen method is often vindicated at surgery or postmortem when the spleen is shown to be, in fact, enlarged. You should learn to place a good deal of reliance on a roentgen impression of splenomegaly. A very large spleen is not difficult to recognize and may reach well below the iliac crest and across the midline.

Radioisotope techniques and angiograms carried out by injecting directly into the splenic artery (via a femoral catheter guided fluoroscopically up the aorta and into the celiac artery) readily render the spleen visible—a subcapsular hematoma of the spleen after trauma, for example, being evidenced by a wedge of nonperfused spleen mass, as you would expect.

The *splenic flexure* is quite variable in position. It may be indented by the tip of the spleen, overlap it partly, or extend over it as high as the diaphragm. It should not be hard for you to identify in such cases, since it will have the characteristic smooth haustral indentations of colon as opposed to the crinkled margin of the stomach shadow.

The *stomach* itself is almost never difficult to identify. In the supine film, the air in the stomach will rise into the more anteriorly placed antrum, outlining the heavy rugal folds of gastric mucosa. In the prone position, whatever air is present will rise into the posteriorly placed fundus, so that on a prone plain film made with a sagittal ray the air bubble of the stomach appears as a round dark shadow with a wrinkled margin nearer the diaphragm. These differences, in fact, will also help you to decide whether a film has been made supine or prone. The same principles apply to barium studies of the stomach, as you will see later.

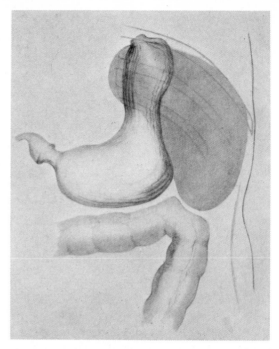

Figure 11-37. The normal stomach indented by an enlarged spleen which depresses the splenic flexure. Shown as it would look if you could see all three structures.

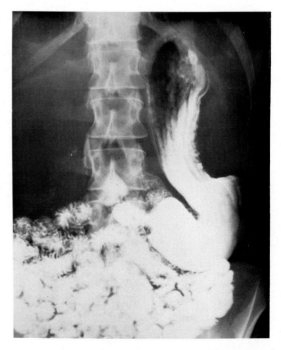

Figure 11-38. The normal stomach filled with barium and indented by an enlarged spleen.

158

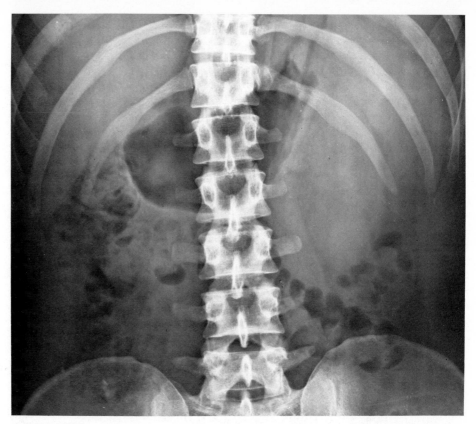

Figure 11-39. Ruptured spleen, thickened through its base, displacing the normal stomach to the right and extending down into the left flank. Note coarse edematous rugal folds of the stomach, which probably shared in the trauma. Was this film made supine or prone?

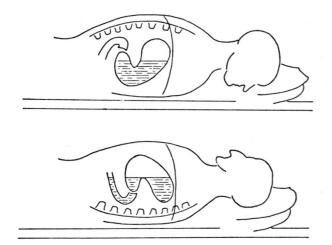

Figure 11-40. Explanation for difference in the stomach air bubble on plain films made with the patient prone (above) and supine (below).

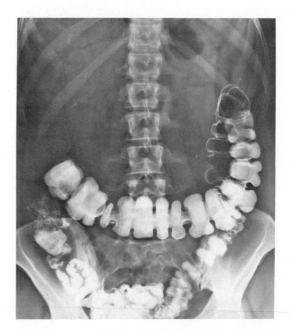

Figure 11-41. Identify splenic and hepatic flexures and tip of liver (not felt on physical examination). Judging from the stomach bubble, was this film made prone or supine?

159

The shadow of the *gallbladder* may occasionally be seen on the plain film as a rounded shadow superimposed over the liver margin and right kidney. It has for many years been successfully rendered visible by administering (by mouth or by vein) radiopaque compounds which are excreted by the liver. These materials do not concentrate sufficiently within the liver cells to visualize them, but the normal gallbladder, by extracting water and concentrating the bile, concentrates the excreted opaque substance so that visualization is possible. This is called *cholecystography*.

Only about 15 percent of gallstones opacify. *The rest are invisible on plain films,* an important fact for you to remember, since we are all brainwashed by the large number of calcified, ring-like, faceted, or laminated gallstones we have been shown. It takes an unusual degree of strength of mind, evidently, for teachers to show students the *common* appearance of something when that appearance is—nothing!

During cholecystography, however, in gallbladders which are still capable of concentrating the opaque substance excreted by the liver, such common radiolucent stones will appear as "filling defects," radiolucent relative to the opacified bile. Unfortunately, poor concentration in chronic cholecystitis has in the past rendered the visualization of such stones difficult or impossible.

More recently the investigation of the gallbladder and biliary tree by ultrasonography and CT has become so successful that cholecystography is being used much less, although in many cases it remains a valuable technique. Sonography of the gallbladder and biliary tree is discussed in Chapters 14 and 15.

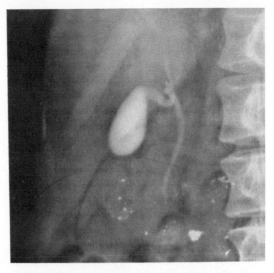

Figure 11-42. The normal gallbladder filled with physiologically concentrated opaque material (cholecystogram). A fatty meal has just been given, and the gallbladder is contracting so that the cystic duct, common bile duct, and, by reflux, a part of the hepatic duct are outlined with contrast material. Scattered flecks of dense white are leftover orally administered opaque material in the gut.

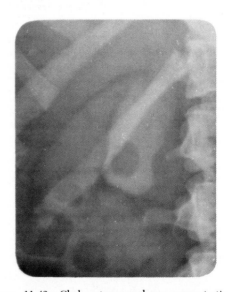

Figure 11-43. Cholecystogram shows concentration of opaque material and an entirely radiolucent stone composed of materials which rendered it invisible on the plain film.

160

Further posteriorly on either side of the spine are situated the *kidneys,* the left a little higher than the right in most patients, the upper poles of both tilted toward the midline and against the psoas muscles. You should trace their outlines as completely as possible. You will have some difficulty outlining the kidneys on a good many plain films because they are nearly always partly obscured by varying amounts of gas in the gut. Make a practice of searching the area for the kidney outline or *any part of it* from which you may be able to resolve the whole shadow. Sometimes you can see the upper and lower poles on one film and the lateral surface on another. If you see no kidney shadow at all on a film of good quality, without too much overlying gas, it may mean that the kidney is very small, has little or no perirenal fat, or that the kidney is ptosed or located ectopically in the pelvis or on the opposite side.

The kidneys, close to the film in the supine patient and outlined by fat, are much better described by the plain-film evidence than they can ever be on physical examination, and you will discover that a difference in size of the two kidneys, for example, or a bulge in the kidney outline is repeatedly brought to your attention first by the radiologist. A difference in length may have significance as an indication of disparity in function. Normally the kidney length should be 3.7 times the height of L2. A parenchymal renal cyst or tumor will enlarge the kidney by ballooning out the pole in which it is present, pushing the perirenal fat before it, so that the change in the dark fat border is perfectly definite from your scrutiny of the plain film.

Ptosis is common and easily recognized when you find the kidney farther down the psoas shadow than normal. Any rotation of the kidney about its long axis will alter the shadow it casts, and this will be apparent to you in the first instance you see of horseshoe, or fused, kidneys. In that anomaly the lower poles of the two kidneys are fused across the midline, and rotation must result from the forward tilting of the lower poles. The kidney shadows will be seen to incline forward at their inferior extremities on lat-

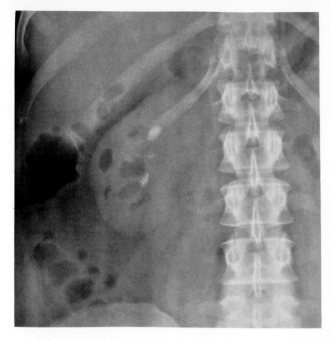

Figure 11-44. The right kidney unusually well seen and apparently containing several stones. Could these possibly be in the gallbladder?

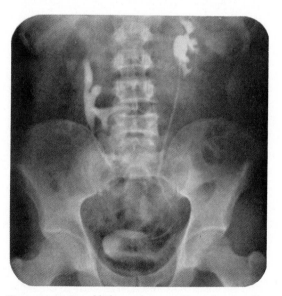

Figure 11-45. Fused kidneys. Suspected from the plain film and confirmed by urography.

eral films, and no well-defined lower poles will be visible. A soft-tissue mass may sometimes be seen across the midline, and the distortion of the draining structures which becomes inevitable produces varying degrees of obstruction.

161

The presence of polycystic kidneys may also be suspected from the plain film because of the large size of the kidney shadows. Their presence is confirmed by pyelograms, which show a characteristic distortion of the calyces, stretched around the many retention cysts. They also have a distinctive appearance at sonography and by CT.

The kidneys are studied specifically by the use of renally excreted radiopaque chemicals (the intravenous urogram), or by injecting similar contrast substances through catheters placed in the ureters during cystoscopy (the retrograde pyelogram). Radiographic study of the kidneys has been revolutionized by sonography, computerized tomography, and other special techniques which are to be discussed in more detail in Chapters 14 and 15. Your concern here is with learning to interpret changes in size, shape, and position of organs you can identify on the plain film. The bilateral enlarged kidney masses in polycystic disease, or the shadow of one mass lying across the midabdomen in horseshoe kidney, exemplify such changes.

The *pancreas*, its head encircled by the loop of the duodenum, lies below and behind the antrum and body of the stomach and against the bodies of the upper lumbar vertebrae as they project forward into the abdomen. The pancreas is invisible on the plain film unless it contains calcifications and stones scattered through it which outline and mark its position. It may be indirectly bounded by organs which normally lie close to it, and a large mass in the head of the pancreas, for example, may expand the duodenal loop and displace the antrum of the stomach forward. As yet no radiographic means of studying the pancreas *functionally* has been developed, the problem being to discover a safely administered radiopaque chemical which is selectively secreted with the pancreatic juices. The pancreas may be "imaged" with isotope scanning techniques, sonography, and CT.

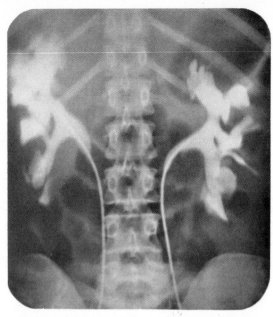

Figure 11-46. Polycystic kidneys, demonstrated by retrograde pyelography, measure 55 millimeters in length on this print compared with 11 millimeters for the height of L2. Normal kidney lenght: 3.7 × height of L2.

Your special survey of the upper *midabdomen*, then, includes some structures which you have "looked for" already, since only an arbitrary division can separate those structures which lie in the upper right and left quadrants from those which, like the pancreas, lie partly also in the midabdomen. Think of the midabdominal structures three-dimensionally, beginning with those most anteriorly placed. The body of the stomach, with its J-shaped streak of air in the supine patient, lies anteriorly against the abdominal wall and just above the curve of the air-containing *transverse colon*. The antrum and duodenal bulb (or cap) turn and point posteriorly so that they are best seen in the lateral view. The bulb and descending limb of the *duodenal loop*, which is partly retroperitoneal, turn downward, passing around the head of the pancreas, to the left and upward again toward the ligament of Treitz to join the jejunum. The duodenum is generally fluid filled and invisibly merged on the plain film with the shadows of other solid or fluid-containing structures near it, although you will see the duodenal loop regularly on barium studies and from it construe the position of the always invisible pancreas. (Chapter 13 covers barium studies.)

162

. . . and finally examine the flanks and lower abdomen.

Examine the *flanks* next, on both sides of the abdomen. The flank stripes may be obscured by the intense black of this area which is often "burned out" at exposures calculated to penetrate the bones of the pelvis and spine. Flank stripes may often be seen well in spite of this by placing the film against a bright light, kept handy by radiologists for the illumination of dark areas on films. The flank stripes will usually be symmetrical bilaterally in thin patients who have been positioned carefully. The dark haustrated colon should be seen lying close against the flank stripe. Free peritoneal fluid will make the flank bulge out and will separate the colon appreciably from the flank stripe. In the presence of inflammation nearby, the flank stripe on that side will be seen to be smudged.

Study the *lower midabdomen* next; follow the known course of the ureters along the psoas shadows down to the bladder, looking for any shadow which could represent a calculus. The ureters are invisible on the plain films, but their shadows outlined with contrast material on pyelograms will help you to learn the variations in their position. Many plain films show small, round, calcium-dense shadows just inside the brim of the bony pelvis. These are calcified thrombi in the pelvic veins, or phleboliths, and generally lie closer to the margin of the bowl of the pelvis than any part of the ureter. Their position, then, will help you to distinguish them from calculi, and you will also be helped by the fact that calculi may be any shape at all and often have jagged points in their shadow profiles, whereas phleboliths are invariably smooth and round and sometimes show a central radiolucency, like a bead ready for stringing (Figure 11-26).

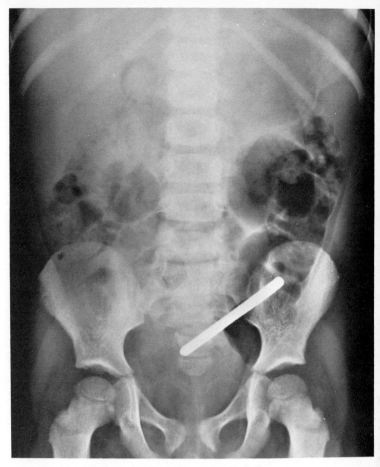

Figure 11-47. Plain film of a child admitted with fever, constipation, periumbilical pain, and an elevated white count. The clinical working diagnosis was appendicitis. At surgery the appendix was found to be retrocecal and perforated. There was inflammation and edema of the tissues of the right gutter and right flank. Note well-seen left and absent right flank stripe. (The broken-off rectal thermometer was recovered and the child made a stormy recovery.)

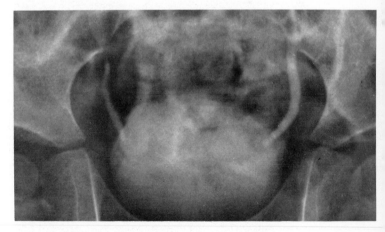

Figure 11-48. Contrast material filling the urinary bladder will help you to recognize the shadow cast by urine-filled bladder on plain films. Note the normal location of the ureters as they enter the bladder.

163

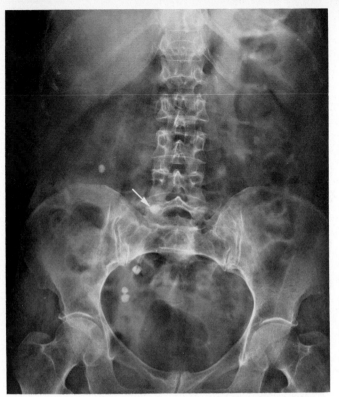

Figure 11-49. Plain film shows several calculi in the lower ureter (arrow to the highest one) and a calcified mesenteric node farther lateral. All stones were passed within ten days, the patient being kept on copious fluid intake. Note air-filled rectum.

The lower midabdomen is a common location for calcified mesenteric nodes, and they will not usually be mistaken for ureteral stones because they tend to look like clusters of small concretions and are somewhat denser than most stones. They vary widely in position from film to film as a rule, because of the mobility of the small-bowel mesentery. They often overlap the bony structures of the vertebral column and sacrum.

The many loops of small bowel are contained for the most part in the lower midabdomen and pelvis. In the normal ambulatory adult, as we have said, they contain fluid and little or no air; but as you will be seeing plain films mostly on patients sick enough to be hospitalized, you will become accustomed to seeing some air-outlined loops of small bowel overlying the lower lumbar vertebrae and pelvis.

The soft tissues within the bowl of the pelvis, finally, include the urinary bladder and lower ureters, the sigmoid and rectum, the uterus and adnexa in the female, and the prostate and seminal vesicles in the male. The bladder, when it contains a moderate amount of urine, is commonly visible on the plain film as a somewhat flattened oval shadow within the pelvis. When it is greatly distended, it may rise up to the umbilicus as a uniformly gray, rounded shadow, not infrequently mistaken for a pathologic mass. The rectum will generally be visible superimposed on the shadow of the bladder and outlined with contained air or feces. The uterus, adnexa, seminal vesicles, and prostate are not visible except by special procedures of various sorts. All may be visualized and studied with injected opaque material, however. Today sonography and CT are widely used to study pelvic masses, as we shall see in Chapter 14.

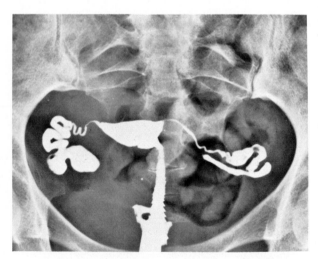

Figure 11-50. A uterosalpingogram. The uterus and fallopian tubes have been filled with a contrast substance as a part of a sterility study. Normally there would be a spill of opaque material from fallopian tubes into the peritoneal cavity, but none is seen here. Conclusion: outer ends of tubes closed.

Unknowns

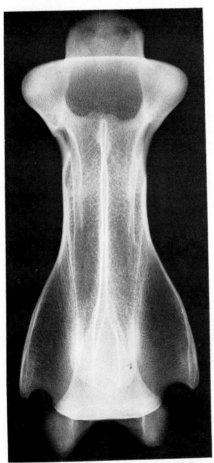

Figure 11-51 (*Unknown 11-1*). Identify. The object radiographed was 9 inches long.

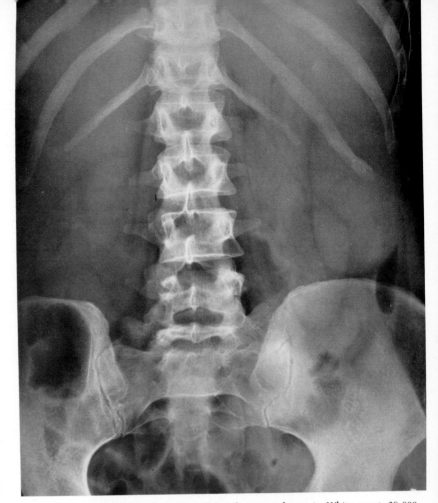

Figure 11-52 (*Unknown 11-2*). Analyze film and propose diagnosis. White count: 28,000.

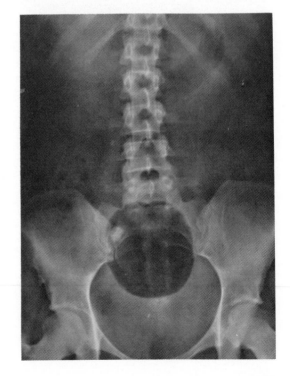

Figure 11-53 (*Unknown 11-3*). Figure out what the radiolucent round mass over the sacrum might be. Patient had a grapefruit-sized pelvic mass on physical exam.

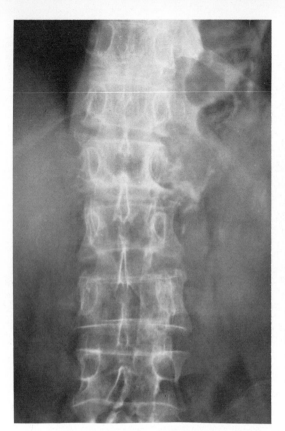
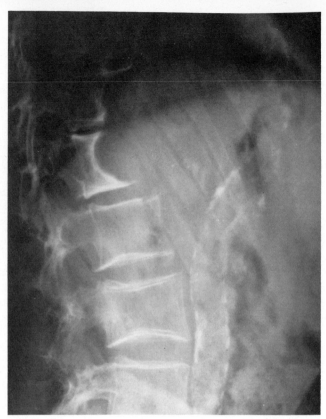

Figure 11-54 (*Unknown 11-4*). Analyze the vertebral shadows, determine any abnormalities, and suggest a diagnosis from the films.

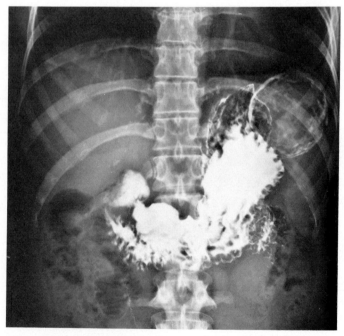

Figure 11-55 (*Unknown 11-5*). You should be able to make a diagnosis from this film.

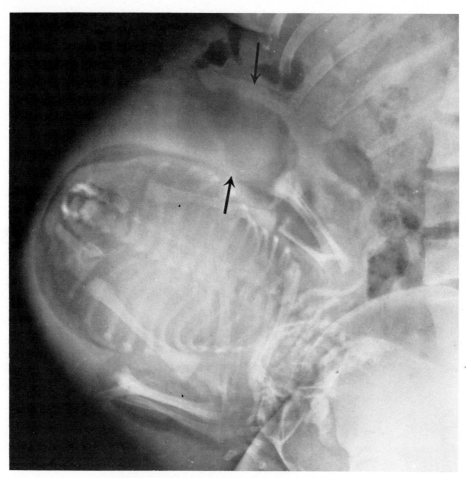

Figure 11-56 (*Unknown 11-6*). This lateral view of the abdomen of a pregnant woman near term shows displacement of air in gut upward and backward by the uterine mass so that the wall of the uterus is bounded by air bubbles scattered at intervals along its surface. What parts of the fetus can you envision better because they are outlined by dark subcutaneous fat? What is the crescentic shadow between the two arrows overlain by a maternal gas shadow?

The Abdominal Plain Film II: Distended Stomach, Large and Small Bowel; Free Fluid and Free Air

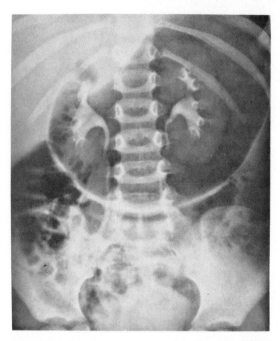

Figure 12-1. Intravenous urogram is seen through air-filled stomach.

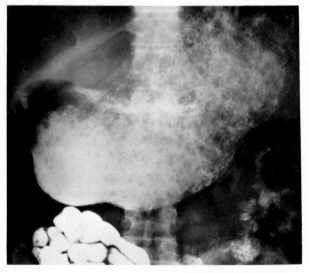

Figure 12-2. The stomach distended with food and barium mixture in a patient with chronic obstruction, the result of scarring after many years of recurrences of his duodenal ulcer. Film was made four hours after administration of the contrast material. Note that there *is* barium in the small bowel, so that some is leaving the stomach intermittently.

The Distended Stomach

To resume your analysis of the plain film, after you have studied the bones and the soft-tissue zones and profiles and decided whether there seems to be evidence for organ enlargement or displacement, you should *look at the whole film at once, directing your entire attention to the gas distribution and content.* Normally the air in the stomach will range from the small, round, wrinkled fundal bubble seen on the prone film to a few oblique streaks of antral air which you will see in supine plain films. Actual visualization of the entire organ filled with swallowed air is not the rule. In Figure 12-1 you see the stomach of a child so outlined, but it was filled intentionally via a nasogastric tube during pyelography in order to displace the confusing gut shadows downward and visualize the kidneys through the stomach bubble.

In pyloric obstruction the stomach may be grossly dilated, of course, and often contains a large amount of food and retained secretions. On the plain films such a stomach will appear as an ill-defined density extending across the upper abdomen, and when the radiologist tries to study it at fluoroscopy, swallowed barium appears to sink into a bog. Attempted examination of such a stomach is futile until the stomach has been emptied. The stomach is also seen distended with air in paralytic ileus and in diabetic coma.

The Distended Colon

As I have said, plain films of hospitalized patients often show a certain amount of air in the small bowel, particularly the ileum, even though there is no clinical evidence to suggest the presence of either ileus or obstruction. You will find that the amount of air in the intestine is increased in plain films made after any kind of painful instrumentation, particularly retrograde catheterization of the ureters. This is unfortunate, since such air usually overlies the kidneys, and the intersecting lines produced by the folded walls of air-filled bowel confuse the details of the shadows of the kidney and its draining structures.

Truly distended loops of small bowel will approach and even exceed the caliber of the normal colon. When they are filled with air, their distinctive mucosal markings will usually identify them; but when they are filled with fluid, they will cast vague, sausage-shaped gray shadows across the midabdomen, often superimposed in the supine film by a bubble of air.

The colon, particularly its distal half, usually contains some air. You may see air outlining solid fecal material within the lumen of the rectum. The cecum and ascending colon more often contain semisolid feces and will be outlined by the characteristic speckled shadow already discussed. Both will show the indented haustrations which generally make identification of the colon easy.

With moderate obstructive distension of the colon, the haustra become shallower but are still visible as serosal indentations, and *more of the colon than is usual will be seen continuously outlined with air.* Thus, when a tumor obstructs at the level of the sigmoid, air may be seen outlining and distending all the colon proximal to that point. With a tumor obstructing at the mid-transverse colon, the proximal half of the transverse colon, hepatic flexure, ascending colon, and cecum will be distended with air. The cecum may eventually balloon to enormous proportions in obstruction of the distal colon, erasing all haustral indentations and appearing as a huge air-filled structure occupying the right side of the abdomen. A neglected patient who

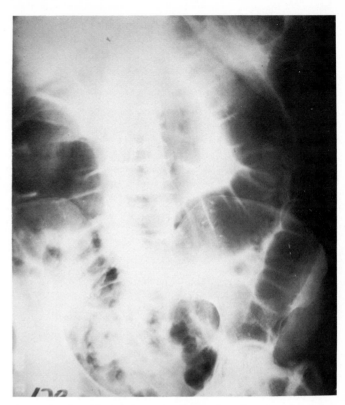

Figure 12-3. Large-bowel obstruction above a sigmoid carcinoma (competent ileocecal valve).

comes into hospital after days of large-bowel obstruction may have ruptured his cecum, in fact, and free air may be detectable in the peritoneal space.

An important point in the diagnosis of all types of mechanical obstruction is that *the compensatory increase in peristalsis which develops is carried beyond the point of obstruction and results in the clearing of air from bowel distal to that point* (that is, from that portion of the gut which can be cleared). Thus, in the obstruction mentioned above at mid transverse colon, you would expect eventually to find the remainder of the transverse colon, the descending colon, and the sigmoid, completely empty and therefore invisible. In this way it is not impossible to make a strong presumptive diagnosis of large-bowel obstruction from a single plain film, with the next step a barium enema and demonstration of the lesion from its distal side.

169

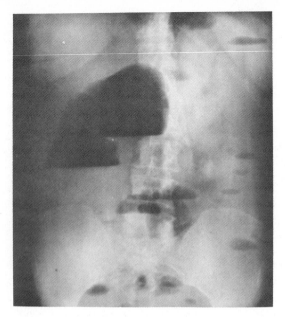

Figure 12-4. Erect film on patient with large-bowel obstruction.

In large-bowel obstruction if the obstruction is *low* in the colon—say, in the sigmoid as in Figure 12-3—only the most distal segment (rectum and distal sigmoid) will be emptied by the increased peristalsis. If the obstruction is *higher* —say, at the splenic flexure as it was in the patient in Figure 12-4—then descending colon, sigmoid, and rectum will be empty and the colon proximal to the obstruction will be seen distended with air. In Figure 12-4 (an erect film) you see the transverse colon and hepatic flexure much distended. The enormously dilated cecum is not seen, since it is filled with fluid, but you can estimate its degree of distension from the length of the air/fluid level crossing the ascending colon.

In low large-bowel obstruction air gradually fills most of the colon and, if the patient is lucky, his ileocecal valve will become incompetent allowing him to decompress his colon backward into his own small bowel. If he is not so fortunate, his valve remains competent and the cecum is likely to become so distended that it may perforate.

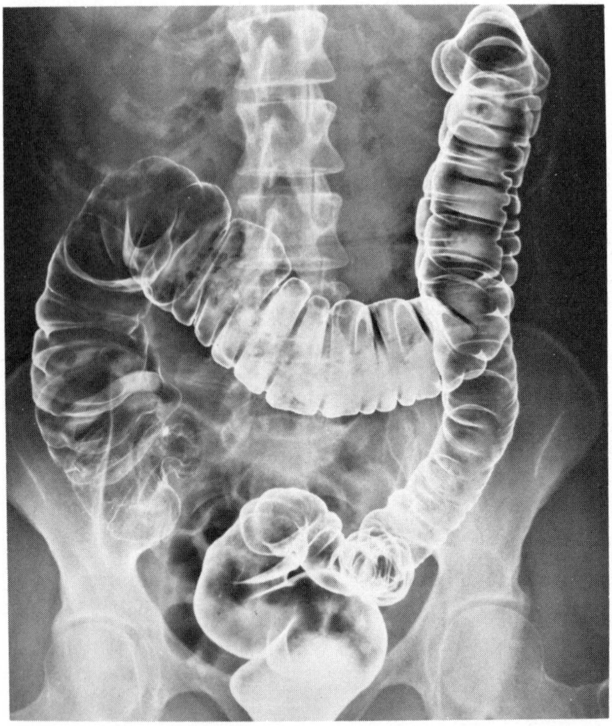

The Distended Small Bowel

Now look at the two films to your right. Figure 12-6 shows you the caliber of the small bowel filled with barium in a normal person and can be compared with Figure 12-7 in which obstructed and distended small bowel is seen visualized with barium and air. The arrow indicates the point of obstruction beyond which no barium passed. This is not a standard procedure; you will *not* be seeing obstructed small bowel outlined with barium, since the addition of insoluble opaque substance to the already retained secretions *above* the obstruction adds to the difficulty of decompression and surgical management. The study of an obstructing colonic lesion by barium enema from its *distal* side is an entirely different matter, since the barium is readily evacuated.

Figure 12-5. Normal colon outlined by a coating of barium on its inner surface and then inflated with air. Use it as a norm in visualizing the accompanying illustrations.

Nevertheless, the film printed here shows you the caliber of moderately distended loops of jejunum with their characteristic cross striations representing the valvulae conniventes. You will say that they resemble haustra, and they do, superficially at least. They differ in their periodicity, however, being more numerous than haustra and more narrowly spaced even when the small bowel is distended. They also cross the gut from one side to the other, as opposed to the haustra, which indent but do not cross the colon and are often not precisely opposite the indentation on the other side. In addition, you will be helped in differentiating between obstructed small bowel and large bowel when you observe that small-bowel loops tend to line up in rows, three and four parallel loops of bowel appearing close beside each other. The colon, when it distends, almost never gives this "arranged" appearance.

In mechanical small-bowel obstruction precisely the same principle applies which was described for the large bowel: clearing of gut beyond the point of obstruction so that it is empty of gas, collapsed, and invisible. If you make a practice of looking for the colon as soon as you recognize distended small bowel, one of these days you will find yourself looking at an unknown plain film on which you can find no haustrated air shadows and you will realize that you *must* be looking at the roentgen findings in mechanical small-bowel obstruction, the entire colon having been swept clear of gas.

In paralytic ileus, on the other hand, both large and small bowel will be seen distended with air, since peristalsis is generally decreased. This is a far less distinctive roentgen picture than that for mechanical obstruction, and you will find that many plain films with quite obviously distended large or small bowel do not fall neatly into one category or the other. This makes for difficulties, indecision, and a sense of confusion in trying to interpret plain films in patients with abdominal symptoms. However, once you have learned to recognize the picture of mechanical obstruction when it is clear, you will feel somewhat more comfortable about studying the equivocal findings so often seen in plain films.

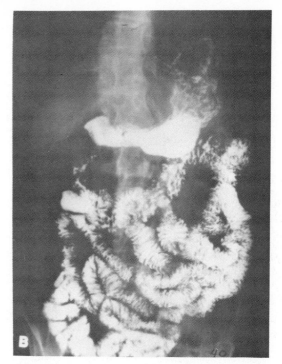

Figure 12-6. Normal small bowel. Barium given by mouth.

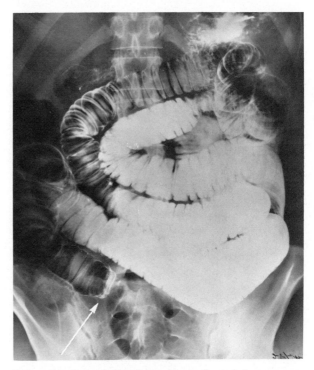

Figure 12-7. Distended small bowel in mechanical obstruction. Note increase in caliber and distinctive markings. It is ill-advised and perhaps dangerous to give barium by mouth to any patient with symptoms suggesting bowel obstruction although, with a tube in place in the small bowel, contrast material may be withdrawn. Feces becomes inspissated only in the colon.

171

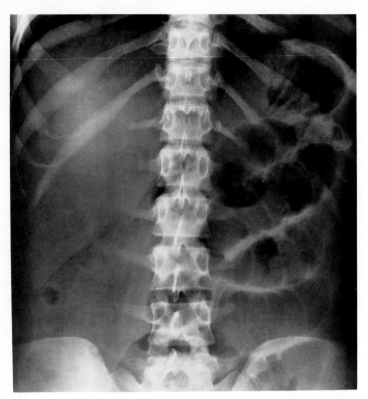

Figure 12-8. Small-bowel obstruction.

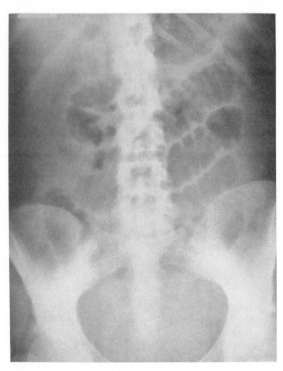

Figure 12-9

Time is the important factor so many of us forget to consider in looking at a single film. It is all too easy, when one is worried about a patient and in quest of diagnostic help, to forget that a single examination is a point on a curve and nothing more, that it represents the state of affairs at only one moment in the course of a patient's illness. *How long* has the obstruction in midtransverse colon been present? Has it been a complete obstruction *long enough* to allow the bowel beyond that point to become cleared of air? If not, then the presence of air in both large and small bowel cannot be distinguished roentgenologically from paralytic ileus, which it will closely resemble. By the same token, an *intermittent obstruction* may allow gas to pass into the distal bowel from time to time. Serial films in patients with abdominal problems are often very informative, indicating the developing change more clearly than any other investigative procedure.

In Figure 12-8 the air-filled stomach is identifiable and several loops of distended small bowel are lined up on the left side of the abdomen, but no air is seen in the colon. This patient had mechanical small-bowel obstruction from an adhesive band in the right lower quadrant, the result of earlier surgery (appendectomy). The other common cause of small-bowel obstruction is hernia (inguinal or femoral) when a knuckle of small bowel is irreducibly caught and compressed.

The patient in Figure 12-9 also has distended loops of small bowel lined up in the central abdomen in a characteristic fashion (which you would expect anyway, since small bowel is anchored to a ruffled central mesentery whereas ascending and descending colon are tethered in the lateral gutters by their mesocolons). Note that there is complete clearing of the colon: QED this *must* be mechanical small-bowel obstruction. In this patient it was caused by stenosing terminal ileitis; the blankness of the pelvis is due to the fact that it is full of fluid-filled obstructed ileal loops and collapsed rectum and sigmoid.

172

Too Much Air in the Intestine: two categories of plain-film findings to help you

I. *Too much air in either colon or small bowel, but none in the other part*

—is either:
A. Small-bowel obstruction old enough to have allowed the colon to clear, or
B. Large-bowel obstruction with a competent (tight) ileocecal valve.

II. *Too much air in both parts of the bowel*

—is one of the following:
A. Paralytic ileus
B. Large-bowel obstruction with an incompetent ileocecal valve, allowing the patient to decompress his distended colon backward into his small bowel
C. Small-bowel obstruction which is—
   (1) Early (colon has not had time to clear), or
   (2) Intermittent (knuckle of small bowel caught in hernia or behind adhesion from time to time).

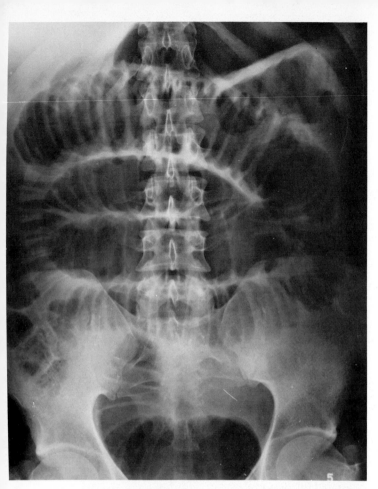

Large or Small bowel?

*Analyze the figures to the left before
you read the legend.*

Figure 12-10 (left above) shows many parallel loops of
widely distended jejunum stretched across the abdomen, air
in the stomach and cecum, but none in the rest of the colon.
Mechanical small intestinal obstruction. Figure 12-11 shows
an immense loop of widely distended and still visibly haustrated large bowel, and no air in the rectum. This proved at
surgery to be a volvulus of the sigmoid colon, twisted several times and gangrenous. Figure 12-12 shows operative
delivery of the volvulus. Arrow indicates the twisted area,
the lower part of which can often be shown on the barium
enema as a twisted spiral of opaque streaks beyond which no
barium will flow.

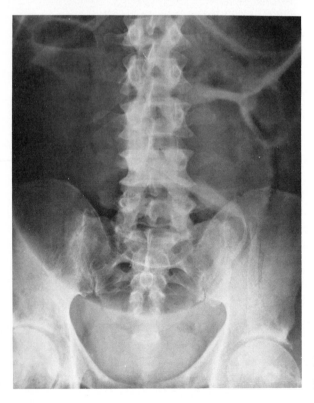

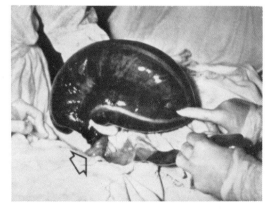

Figure 12-11 (left)

Figure 12-12 (above)

174

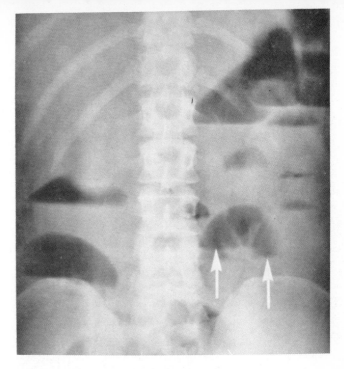

Figure 12-13. Standing film of a patient with low small-bowel obstruction. Arrows indicate a hairpin loop.

When a patient is admitted with abdominal pain and his initial plain film shows both large and small bowel to be distended, the findings are equivocal, as we have said, in that they may represent either paralytic ileus or an early or intermittent obstruction, for example. The activity of the bowel sounds, repeatedly observed over a period of time, may or may not clarify the issue. Serial films may show changes in the roentgen findings which provide helpful clues. If the patient is well enough to stand, the erect film is sometimes informative. One must always bear in mind that a patient with small-bowel obstruction and a cleared colon at home the day before yesterday may have developed peritonitis and secondary ileus by the time he is admitted to the hospital. The plain film, like any other roentgen study, can only be interpreted intelligently in the light of a good clinical history.

Although its value has been overrated, the standing film may provide some additional clues. The small intestine always contains fluid, and when obstructed or paralyzed it accumulates additional fluid and air. On the erect plain film, the air-fluid interfaces inside distended loops of gut will appear as fluid levels, varying in length according to their size and the relative quantities of air and fluid within them. Loops entirely filled with fluid will cast ill-defined gray shadows in both the supine and erect positions. Loops with little fluid and a great deal of air will appear like those in Figure 12-10. Loops three-quarters full of fluid and containing a relatively small amount of air may be very deceptive, since in the erect film they will show short fluid levels and in the supine plain film rather unimpressive bubbles of air superimposed on the indefinite gray of the fluid. You can appreciate the fact that such a patient may not have so startling an initial plain film, and yet be sicker and in a more advanced stage of obstruction than the patient in Figure 12-10. You cannot depend entirely upon the size and appearance of the air-distended gut as an index to the degree of obstruction or to its duration. Moreover, the possibility of the additional presence of free peritoneal air or fluid should always be entertained in these patients.

One helpful detail about the comparison of standing and supine plain films on the same patient is that to some extent the tone of the bowel and its peristaltic activity are evident from the plain films. In the patient with paralytic ileus and decreased peristalsis, the loops in either film will *tend* to appear flaccid and of wide caliber with long fluid levels in the erect film. The patient with mechanical obstruction and increased bowel sounds, on the other hand, *tends* to show occasional "hairpin" loops in the erect film. These are so called because ascending and descending limbs are seen filled with air, having short fluid levels on either side but at different levels, indicating rushes of peristalsis which have dumped fluid from one side of the hairpin into the other (Figure 12-13).

This finding is meaningful only when distinct on the plain film of a patient with clinical signs of markedly increased peristaltic activity who has supine plain films which indicate obstruction. *Its absence means nothing and does not in any way contradict the findings of obstruction suggested by the supine film, since hairpin loops are well known to be inconstantly present in obstructed patients.* Taken together with the bowel sounds heard clinically, such observations may be useful: for example, the development of a suddenly silent abdomen after the roentgen observation of hairpin loops in the standing film might presage bowel perforation and the beginning of peritonitis.

175

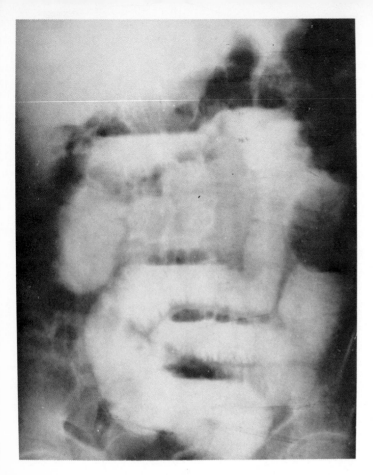

Figure 12-14. Standing film of a patient with low ileal obstruction whose distended small bowel is visualized because she has been given a water-soluble contrast substance. Note the small air bubbles in relation to the large amount of fluid in the loops.

Free Peritoneal Fluid

The overall grayness of standing films results partly from the difficulty of obtaining penetration with the usual exposures, since the abdomen is pendulous and much thicker erect than it is supine. The gray density of such films is also partly due to the presence of retained fluid within the obstructed loops. You will have noted that in erect films the outlines of kidneys and psoas muscles usually disappear. The same grayness and the same absence of outlines would be seen in a supine plain film on a patient with free peritoneal fluid.

After making any decisions you can with regard to the amount of air-in-gut and its distribution, direct your attention to the *general density* of the plain film. To state the oversimplified extremes first, as usual: large amounts of free *air* in the peritoneal space will increase the radiolucency of the abdomen, just as you would expect, and the film will look darker. Large amounts of free *fluid* will add to the radiodensity of the abdomen and the film will appear lighter gray than usual. These statements are true for the conven-

tional exposure techniques used for radiography of the abdomen. Obviously, a film which has been exposed with a relatively more penetrating x-ray beam will have a more uniformly gray appearance, since every structure interposed will have been penetrated effectively. The blackness of any radiograph, however, is a function of total exposure in milliampere-seconds, plus secondary radiation, as well as of the penetration of the beam (kilovoltage). If the intestinal loops are filled with fluid, the effect is that of adding more thickness to the patient, and for the same exposure factors, such a film will be gray and indistinct. This tends to obscure other structures such as the bones. Look at *them*, then, and decide whether they are as well and as clearly shown in their detail as usual; look at the peripheral soft tissues, deciding whether they are overexposed (too black). If these areas are not unusual, then an overall grayness is meaningful and suggests abdominal fluid.

When there is a small amount of fluid free in the peritoneal space, it will gravitate to the most dependent part of the abdominal cavity, which, in the supine patient, is the bowl of the pelvis, as you see in the diagram in Figure 12-15. Such relatively *small amounts of free fluid* probably go unobserved often, because we are more or less accustomed to seeing the pelvis filled with the density of a distended bladder or fluid-containing loops of bowel.

Larger quantities of peritoneal fluid will spill over into the abdominal cavity, flowing up the flanks on either side of the high midline ridge of the spine. Fluid collected in the flank displaces the colon medially away from the flank stripe, and with even greater accumulations, air-filled loops of bowel float up under the arched anterior abdominal wall. They are seen on the supine plain film as a cluster of radiolucent shadows in the central abdomen surrounded by the uniform gray of the peritoneal fluid (Figure 12-19 on the next page).

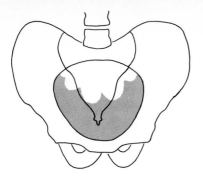

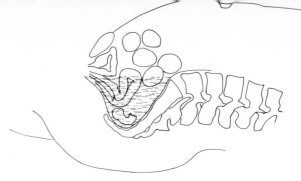

Figure 12-15 (above). Half-moon of gray in the pelvis may mean free fluid (in a patient you *know* had just been catherized). Scalloped undermargin due to loops of ileum dipping into fluid.

Figure 12-16 (above). Lateral diagram of a supine patient with free peritoneal fluid accumulating in the most dependent part of the abdominal cavity, the pelvic bowl.

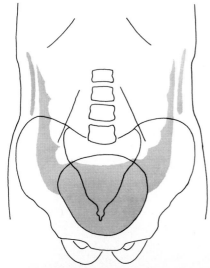

Figure 12-17 (left). Increasing amounts of fluid flow into the flanks and could be shown to shift freely with change in position of the patient.

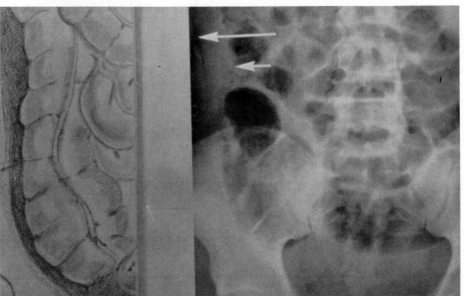

Figure 12-18. Liver rupture with blood in the flank following an automobile accident. Note that the colon is displaced medially away from the flank stripe by the distance between the points of the arrows. Surgery disclosed a tear in the dome of the liver and free blood throughout the abdomen.

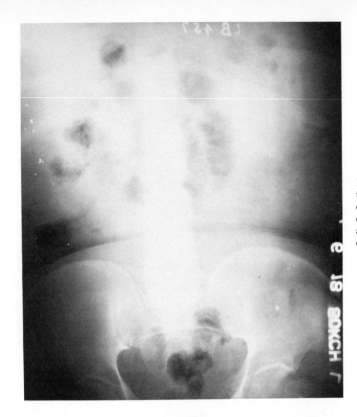

Figure 12-19 (left). Cirrhotic patient with ascites. This patient has the classic roentgen findings of *ascites* with a general grayness and loss of landmarks due to the addition of the density of free peritoneal fluid concentrated in the pelvis and flanks. Now study Figure 12-20 before you read the legend. Is this ascites?

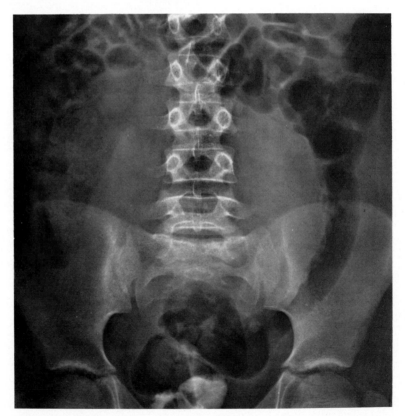

Figure 12-20. No, this could not be ascites. The colon is displaced out of the midabdomen, curving around a central fluid-density mass which is too round and too high to be a distended bladder, did not disappear on catheterization, and proved at surgery to be an ovarian cyst.

178

Free Peritoneal Air

Free peritoneal air, on the other hand, fills the highest part of the abdominal cavity (which in the supine position is the anterior part), and massive amounts of peritoneal air strikingly outline the organ masses of liver and spleen including their lateral and superior (diaphragmatic) surfaces. A large amount of free peritoneal air forms a quite distinctive, radiolucent, pear-shaped shadow of the whole abdominal cavity which is hard to forget once you have seen it. Small amounts of free air may be quite as important to detect as larger amounts, since they are seen most frequently with perforation of a hollow viscus.

A patient well enough to stand will show crescents of radiolucent air interposed between his diaphragm and liver and spleen, and such a finding is occasionally first detected on an admission chest film.

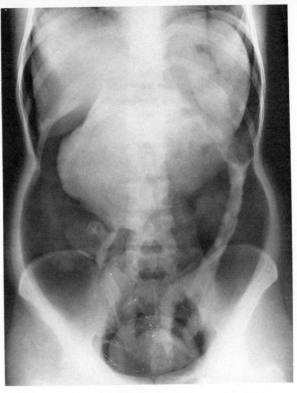

Figure 12-21. Large amount of free peritoneal air fills out the flanks and pelvis, casting a peculiar and distinctive pear-shaped shadow (pear inverted, of course!).

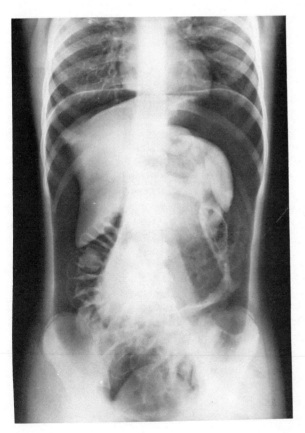

Figure 12-22. Free peritoneal air. Note that you see both sides of the wall of the ascending colon. Why?

179

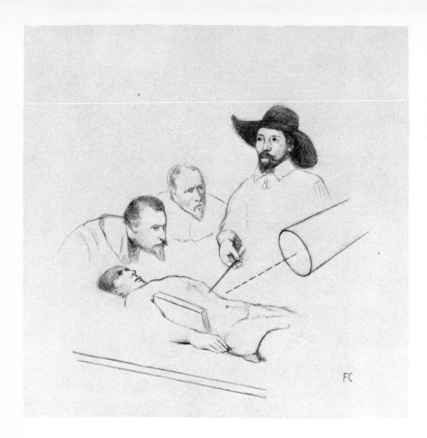

Figure 12-23. Lateral abdominal radiography with the patient supine. Question: Has the patient free peritoneal air? Dr. Tulp indicates the direction of the beam to two eager residents.

FC

The patient with a perforated viscus is often too ill to stand, and in any event ought not to be disturbed any more than is absolutely vital to a diagnosis. For this reason the search for free air is much more often carried out by decubitus and horizontal beam radiography. The horizontal beam method is demonstrated in Figure 12-23, in which the patient lies supine and is radiographed from side to side, a cassette being placed vertically against his flank. In this way air free against the underside of the abdominal wall will be appreciable, even in small amounts. A useful variation on this technique places the patient on his left side in his bed or on the examining table, and he is radiographed anteroposteriorly with a horizontal beam. Free air will rise over the lateral surface of the liver. This is called a *lateral decubitus film* (Figure 12-26).

You have seen the gut because of air contained within it, in other words because its *inner* surface is rendered visible. With free air in the peritoneal space, *both the inside and the outside of the gut wall may be seen.* This is easy to imagine with a large amount of free air into which protrude loops of air-filled bowel (Figure 12-24). *Both* sides of the wall of a loop of gut may also be seen on a regular supine plain film of the same

patient, made, let us say, before there was any suspicion of a perforated viscus (Figure 12-25). This phenomenon is not seen on a normal film.

Finally, you will occasionally see both free fluid and free air in abundant quantities in the abdomen, and their roentgen appearance differs only slightly from what has been described for each. In the supine plain film, the air floats on top of the fluid anteriorly under the abdominal wall and is seen on the film as a large, well-defined bubble (Figure 12-27). In the erect film, the fluid-air interface will be seen as a long, startling fluid level, obviously not within any part of the bowel. The terms "contained" and "uncontained" air-fluid levels are sometimes employed to differentiate the air above fluid levels which are limited by gut wall (in intestinal obstruction) and those which go straight to the abdominal wall and are not confined in any way. "Uncontained air" may also be used to describe air in abscess cavities or fistulous tracts which does not take the shape of any hollow viscus.

180

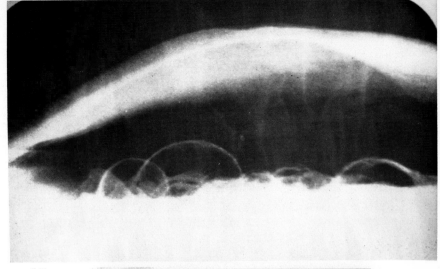

Figure 12-24. Lateral radiograph of the abdomen made with the patient supine. Abundant quantities of free air collected under the abdominal wall outline the serosal side of the loops of bowel.

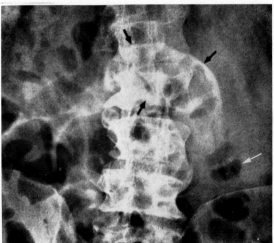

Figure 12-25 (right). Supine plain film on a patient who had free peritoneal air. Note that in this view also, both sides of the bowel wall may occasionally be seen. Contrast the loop indicated with black arrows, which is outlined with free air, and others which are not (white arrow).

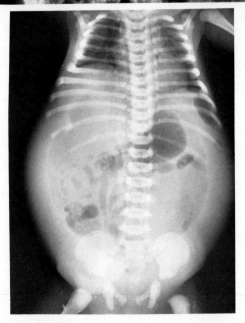

Figure 12-26. Lateral decubitus film in a patient with perforated viscus and a small amount of free air. Patient lying on his left side and filmed sagittally with a horizontal beam.

Figure 12-27. Free peritoneal air and fluid seen on a supine film in an infant with meconium obstruction and perforation of the small bowel.

181

CHAPTER 13 Contrast Study of the Gastrointestinal Tract

Diagnostic radiology is entirely based on contrasting the density of adjoining structures. Up to now you have been thinking mostly in terms of naturally occurring density contrasts, and wherever they can be relied upon to produce the desired information they are preferable to any artificial contrast study. In fact, in the heady and exciting development of modern intracavitary contrast work, the great value of naturally occurring contrast substances like fat and air tends to be overlooked. As dedicated workers in the field of pediatric roentgenology have pointed out, very nearly the same information about, for example, the gastrointestinal tract of an infant is available from deductive reasoning about *air* shadows as from barium shadows, and the chances of causing inhalation of vomitus are minimized.

Soon after the discovery of the roentgen ray the idea of augmenting natural contrast occurred to physicians working in different parts of the world. The ramifications of the many methods of study which were begun even before the turn of the century are still unfolding before us, and the possibilities of new contrast studies seem limitless. The training of a radiologist in these many methods of investigation is lengthy and complex; yet it should always be his concern to examine the patient by the least harmful means available which will produce the information needed. The experienced physician-radiologist knows that complex methods of investigation requiring highly specialized machinery and trained personnel are not *invariably* those best suited to the individual problem, nor will they *invariably* produce more information. While such reservations must influence the choice of the type of examination

planned, one can never lose sight of the fact that a particularly suitable investigative method may be undertaken *in spite of some potential secondary side effect*, as a deliberate risk, in order to make a diagnosis and ultimately secure appropriate treatment for the patient.

Some contrast studies are virtually harmless; others have well-recognized contraindications. Air itself, artificially introduced as in the visualization of the ventricles and outer surface of the brain, is not without discomfort and some hazard to the patient. So many studies incur little risk and minimal discomfort and have become so routinely a part of the diagnostic plan, however, that perhaps too few physicians could list half a dozen conditions in which a gastrointestinal series, for example, should *not* be carried out, or in which it would be better to postpone the procedure. Barium sulfate in water suspension is itself inert, and none of it is absorbed during its passage through the gastrointestinal tract, but almost any such study involves the taking of numerous films and perhaps repeated fluoroscopic inspections over a period of several hours. The process is fatiguing for the patient, particularly the acutely ill patient. The anxiety of the patient is always an important part of the hazard of the procedure. Such anxiety is allayed to an appreciable extent by intelligent preparation: a referring physician, if he will take the time, can always explain a little about the procedure in advance. The patient suspected of having a recent coronary occlusion should *not* be sent to the radiology department prematurely for an extended and fatiguing procedure, and the patient with symptoms suggesting any kind of large-bowel obstruction should not be given barium by mouth, as it becomes dehy-

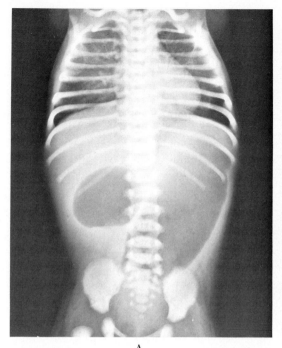 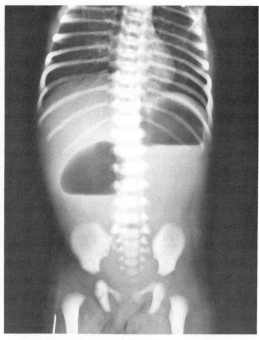

A   B

Figure 13-1. The "double-bubble" phenomenon in duodenal atresia. In this 4-day-old girl with persistent vomiting since birth, the naturally occurring substance, air, provides all the necessary information. There is no need to add barium or other opaque substance. The air shadows alone provide evidence that nothing has passed beyond the duodenum, the remainder of the abdomen showing a blank, uniform gray shadow. The obstruction is not at the pylorus because there are two distinct bubbles of air-distended gut and, in the erect film, two distinct fluid levels. The obstruction must therefore be in the duodenal loop; surgical correction is mandatory. The addition of barium or other opaque substances is pointless, will not alter the indicated treatment, and might be vomited during anesthesia. (A made supine, B erect.)

drated in the colon. The very preparation of the patient for a colon study requires thorough cleansing of the bowel usually by catharsis, and such measures would sometimes be contraindicated clinically in the debilitated or dehydrated patient, or one in severe electrolyte imbalance.

In sum, then, the complex contrast study should not be requisitioned without consideration of the entire clinical problem, nor should it be undertaken when the patient is not in a reasonably safe condition to undergo it. You would do well to observe one example of each of the major investigative procedures for yourself, so that you will understand not only what it will require of your patient in terms of energy and stamina but also the degree to which the patient's cooperation may be required for the success of the procedure. A patient who is paralyzed may not be able to stand for certain parts of a gastrointestinal examination which are usually carried out in that position. A patient who speaks no English will be particularly difficult to examine because he must hold his breath on command during the exposure of films, and if he does not understand and continues to breathe, the films obtained will often be valueless. Obviously, this kind of difficulty may be prevented by your discussing the procedure with the radiologist before it is carried out. The examination of the paralyzed patient may be modified, and a patient with a language problem may be attended in the fluoroscopic room by someone who can translate and reassure. *If intelligent consideration for the patient is the major concern of both radiologist and referring physician, undersirable developments resulting from any sort of procedure will be kept to a minimum.* (Needless to say, this applies no more to radiology than to any other branch of medicine.)

Principles of Barium Work

Having warned you that clinical judgment must be applied to the selection of contrast procedures, let me give you a somewhat fuller appreciation of what such procedures have to offer as diagnostic tools. Early investigators used a rubber-coated metal wire passed into the stomach with a view to "outlining the curvatures." From such a crude beginning the polished refinements of modern gastrointestinal studies now constitute a whole branch of radiology. They involve the interpretation of shadows not only of whole casts of hollow structures but also of the far more complex shadows of thin films of opaque substance caught against the mucosal irregularities of the inner surface of the gut. Such *mucosal relief studies*, as they are often called, are carried out with minimal amounts of opaque material, manipulated and spread over the surface of the clean mucosa during fluoroscopic study, *spot films* being obtained at frequent intervals by mechanically substituting a small cassette for the fluoroscopic screen. The technical expertise required by the procedure and the judgment and experience needed for interpreting correctly the observed shadows constitute one of the most sophisticated accomplishments of the radiologist.

Nevertheless the conclusions he draws are basically no less logical than everything else you have been learning to appreciate about the field, and in order to comprehend the reliability of the evidence offered by roentgen data obtained from barium studies, you should understand some of the fundamental implications of the various kinds of roentgen observations based on such procedures. To that end, examine the hypothetical drawings in Figure 13-2 and 13-3. The gastrointestinal tract is essentially a tube, and the roentgen principles for examining it vary only in degree, even in the stomach, cecum, and rectum, where its tubular structure has been modified by nature. The simple tube in *A*, filled with an opaque substance and radiographed, would produce a shadow like the one you see in *a*, smooth-bordered and uniformly dense. A polyp protruding into its lumen upon a stalk like that in *B* would produce a barium cast-shadow like the one in *b*. A solid tumor growing in its wall like that in *C*, and protruding into the

lumen as a sessile growth, would produce a shadow like *c*.

Both of these alterations in the original normal tubular shadow are what are referred to as *filling defects*, or, as they were called earlier, subtraction shadows. This last term for filling defect has been virtually abandoned in radiologic parlance, yet it is an excellent term that describes succinctly the change in the shadow. A part of the expected luminal shadow has been subtracted, because barium has been displaced by radiolucent soft tissue.

The growth you see in *D* has entirely encircled the tubular structure being examined, so that a constriction of the lumen is produced. This is often called a *napkin-ring defect*, but times change and the napkin ring has vanished from the dining table, so that possibly we ought to equate this type of filling defect with some more familiar object like a doughnut. If you prefer, the term *annular lesion* is commonly employed and less gastronomic. In any event, whenever you see a barium shadow like that in *d*, you ought to *reconstruct mentally the rigid annular lesion which has produced it, supplying tumor or other soft tissue wherever the barium has been displaced.* The abrupt and often angular change in the shadow where normal luminal wall meets the margin of a tumor is frequently and aptly referred to as a *shelf*, and its consistent appearance on film after film in the same location is to be interpreted as reliable evidence of rigidity of some sort in the otherwise distensible wall of the gut. (*Aa*, *Cc*, and *Dd* in Figure 13-4 represent the shadows which would be cast if the related segments of gut were *distended* as opposed to being gently filled. Note that the rigid areas remain rigid.)

Figures 13-2 (top), 13-3 (middle), and 13-4 (bottom) (opposite page). Hypothetical examples of gastrointestinal pathology and the changes in the barium cast-shadow produced in each (see text).

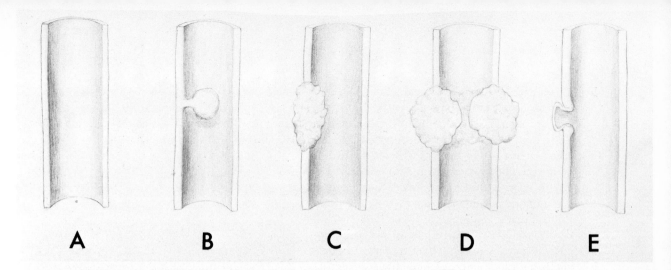

A   B   C   D   E

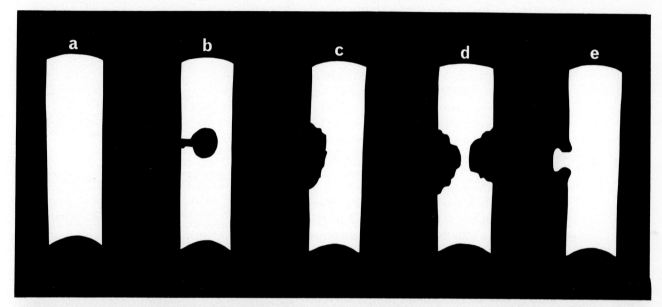

a   b   c   d   e

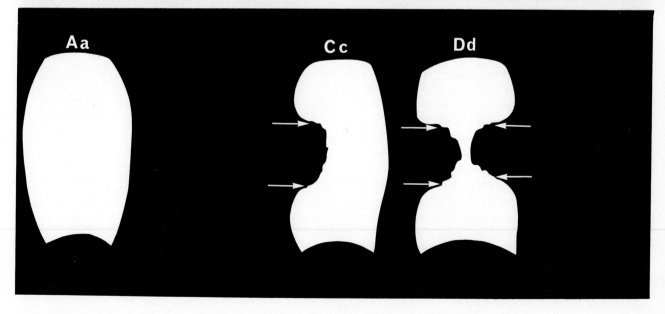

Aa   Cc   Dd

You will find that a filling defect and its shelf-like margin are often so precisely the same from film to film in a series made during the barium study that they may be superimposed on each other over a bright light. Try it. If on two or more such films you can bring into perfect register the margin of a filling defect suspected of representing a malignant tumor, then the probabilities that it *is* a tumor are greatly enhanced. If, of course, two such films do *not* superimpose, it may mean either that the area in question is not rigid, and therefore changes slightly, or that the two films were made in different projections.

In *Aa*, *Cc*, and *Dd* the barium casts of our stylized tubular structures are represented as having been distended with fluid. The normal (and therefore normally elastic) tube in *Aa* has distended evenly according to the evenly distributed fluid pressures within it. The sessile lesion in one wall in *Cc* is rigid, although the wall above and below it can and does distend. Its barium-outlined profile between the two arrows would be superimposable, bump for bump.

The annular lesion in *Dd* is also rigid and superimposable, although the lumen on both sides of it balloons out with the increase in fluid pressure. Moreover, no change in this demonstrably rigid area would occur in the course of the entire study.

If up to now barium studies have tended to confuse you, if you have wondered how any firm conclusions can ever be derived from them at all, this is the time to tell you that the sobriety and assurance of his interpretations are possible to the radiologist largely because he has been able to demonstrate a finding *repeatedly*. No finding present on a single film only is worth very much, and the resident in training in radiology soon finds that positive diagnostic observations made from barium studies must be consistently demonstrable if they are to be believed. So variable and shifting are the shadows presented by opaque substances within the gastrointestinal tract that it is right that only those *consistently present* should be taken seriously. This is no less true for other spheres of roentgen investigation, to be sure, nor for that matter for other branches of medicine. Any

single positive test, always negative thereafter, is unlikely to weigh much in the balance of evidence, and the principle is no different for more complex investigative procedures.

A

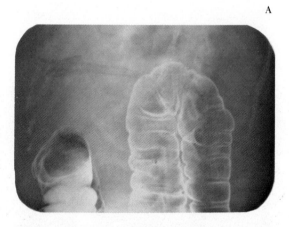

B

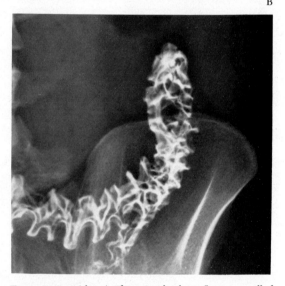

Figure 13-5. A (above): The normal splenic flexure unrolled by turning the patient so that there is no overlap. Colon has been filled with barium, evacuated, and inflated with air. B (below): The normal mucosal relief pattern of the splenic flexure after evacuation of barium. The collapsed colon shows a wrinkled mucosal lining, and the haustra are closer together.

Constriction: Constant
and Inconstant

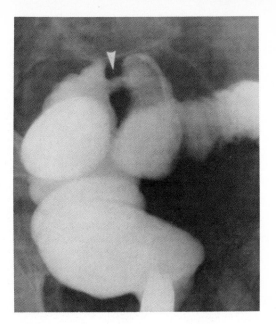

Inconstant

Figure 13-6. A convincing annular constriction near the rectosigmoid junction could not be redemonstrated either fluoroscopically or on films. This is a notorious area for overlap, however, and the patient came to surgery. No lesion was found.

Constant

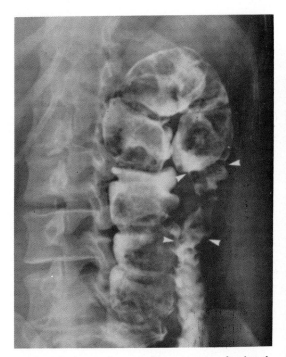

Figure 13-7. An annular area of narrowing just distal to the splenic flexure was constant on all films obtained during a barium enema. Note evidence of low-grade obstruction in the relative dilatation of the transverse colon and splenic flexure, which contain fecal boluses and barium. The descending colon below the lesion shows the pattern expected from collapse of empty colon. Carcinoma was found at surgery.

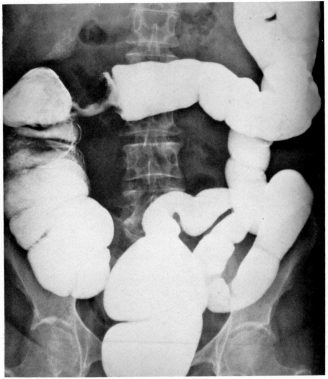

Figure 13-8. Constant annular lesion near the hepatic flexure proved to be carcinoma as expected.

187

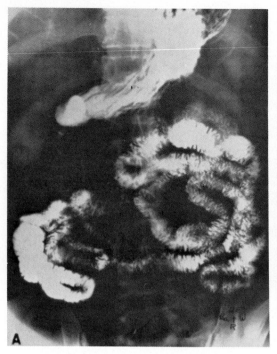

A

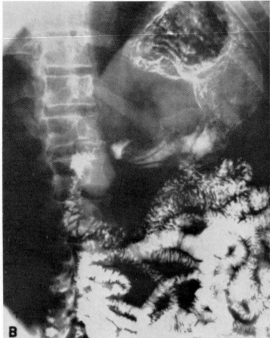

B

The variation of barium shadows within the gastrointestinal tract is well illustrated by the films made during the *upper GI series* which you see in Figure 13-9. A, made prone half an hour after 10 ounces of barium suspension had been swallowed, shows the stomach nearly empty and the jejunum and upper ileum filled. B, made 15 minutes later in an oblique position, shows most of the small bowel, and C, made an hour after the administration of barium, shows the right colon filling. Note the haustrated faint shadows beneath the shadow of the gallbladder: these are colon in which barium is mixed with fecal material. Cholecystography had been done that morning and the patient kept fasting. There is a single round filling defect within the gallbladder shadow representing the displacement of opaque material by a solitary calculus of lesser density.

You may be inclined to reject the possibility of demonstrating any structure consistently in so changeable a barium pattern, but look carefully at Figure 13-10 (*Unknown 13-1*), four spot films of the stomach and duodenum of a patient who had guaiac-positive stools. She had no hemorrhoids, negative findings on sigmoidoscopic and barium enema study, was not anemic, and enjoyed excellent health.

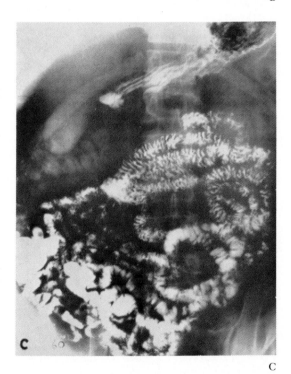

C

Figure 13-9. Normal upper gastrointestinal series, large films only. Smaller films made in several conventional projections of the stomach and duodenal bulb, and spot films made during fluoroscopy, would complete the series (see text).

188

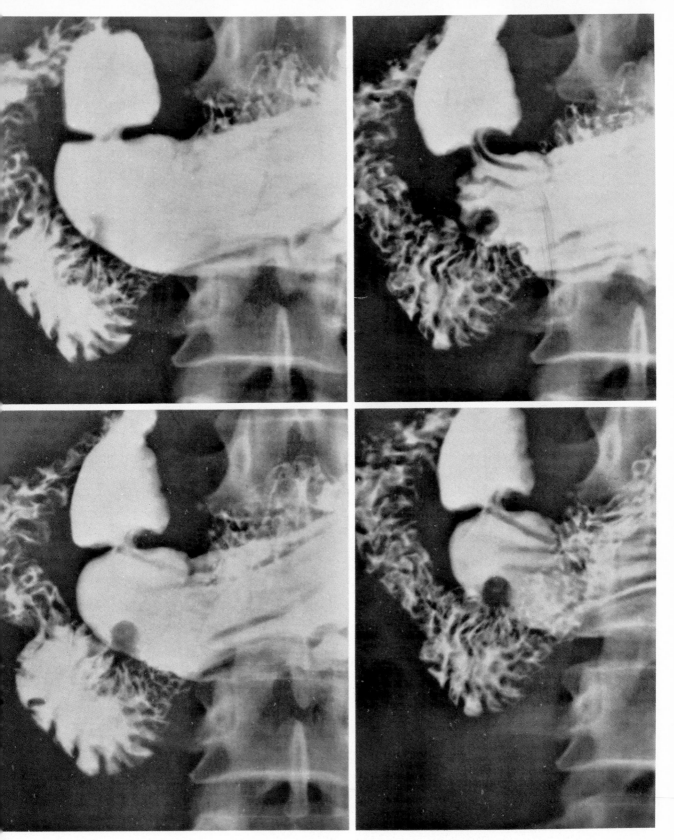

Figure 13-10 (*Unknown 13-1*). Can you spot the consistently present filling defect?

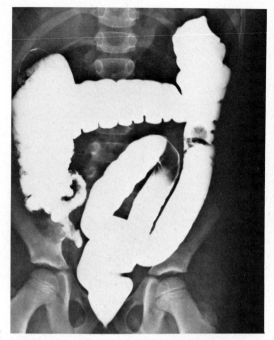

A

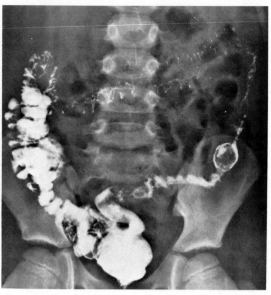

B

Figure 13-11. Polyp in the descending colon in a boy with bloody stools and crampy left abdominal pain. Note that the polyp is seen demonstrated in three different ways, always in the same location. In A it is seen as a radiolucent filling defect in the opaque barium column. In B, after evacuation, the polyp is seen because it prevents the collapse of the barium-coated walls of the colon, a regular finding in intraluminal soft-tissue masses. In C the polyp, coated with opaque material, is seen outlined by air.

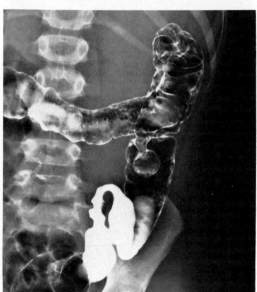

C

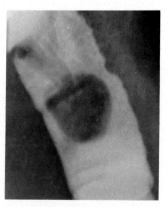

Figure 13-12. Polyps within the colon may be demonstrated as radiolucent filling defects displacing the contrast substance. Note stalk, which is well seen.

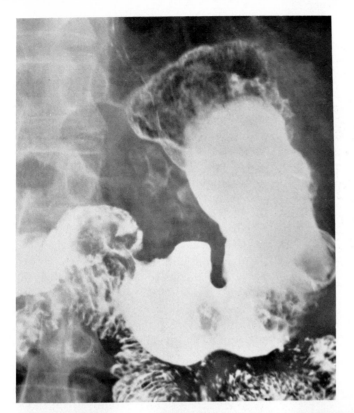

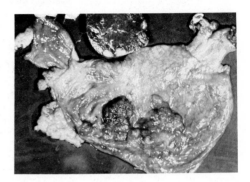

Figure 13-13 (left). Filling defects along the greater curvature in a patient with "pernicious anemia." There is also a defect inside the duodenal bulb. The patient refused surgery and endoscopy. Figure 13-14 (below). The open stomach at postmortem. Polypoid lesions along the greater curvature proved to be adenocarcinoma. There was also a larger carcinomatous polyp prolapsed into the bulb.

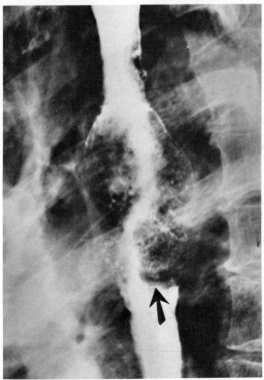

Figure 13-15. Another patient with carcinoma in midesophagus. Note irregular rigid lumen. Arrow indicates shelf of tumor.

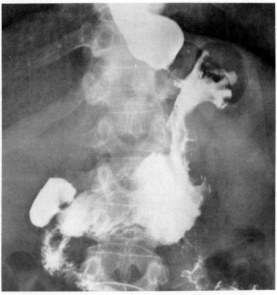

Figure 13-16. Constant rigid filling defect on the upper part of the greater curvature. Note infiltration of cardia. Esophagus does not empty. At postmortem: adenocarcinoma, primary, in the stomach.

191

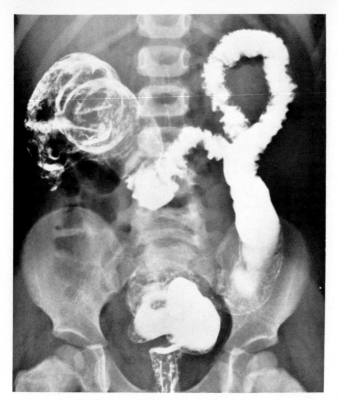

Figure 13-17. Intussusception. Intraluminal mass composed of the patient's own cecum and terminal ileum which have been telescoped inside the lumen of the ascending colon and hepatic flexure, waves of peristalsis forcing it farther along the lumen of the large bowel. Early in the illness, intussusception may often be safely reduced by barium enema without manipulation. In cases of longer duration or in patients with peritoneal signs suggesting a compromised vascular supply, surgery is the treatment of choice.

Intraluminal masses, which you see illustrated on these pages, may take many forms. Polyps range in size from a millimeter to several centimeters. Polypoid tumors may fill up the lumen of the gut. Barium passing between the tumor and the normally distensible wall of the gut will outline the tumor, showing the normal mucosal markings stretched over the tumor. The barium shadows so formed will reflect the irregularities, if any, of the surface of the tumor as well as those of the muscosa lining the bowel. These can often be seen as a double moulage, the one distinguishable from the other, like those in Figure 13-19.

Intraluminal masses can sometimes be seen to be free floating in the barium, unattached to any wall. Occasionally, matted intraluminal masses are formed of foreign substances like hair or vegetable fibers, becoming too large to be passed and eventually causing symptoms. These are called bezoars (Figure 13-18) and are similar to the hair balls animals vomit. They can usually be differentiated from intraluminal soft-tissue masses because barium mixes itself within the matted bezoar, giving an appearance quite different from tumor coated with barium. Figure 13-20 shows another sort of intraluminal mass. You can see now why it is so vital to have the patient fasting overnight before a gastrointestinal examination with barium: the mucosa must be perfectly clean and the lumen clear of food and feces.

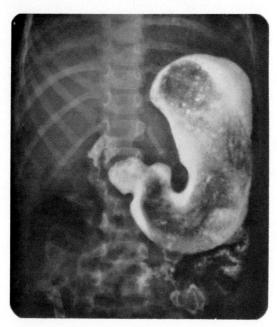

Figure 13-18. Bezoar in the stomach, composed of matted hair, in a little girl known to chew the ends of her pigtails.

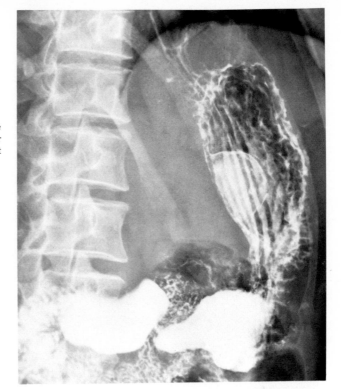

Figure 13-19 (right). Benign tumor projecting into the lumen of the stomach from its sessile base high on the lesser curvature. The normal rugal folds either behind it or in front of it are seen outlined with barium.

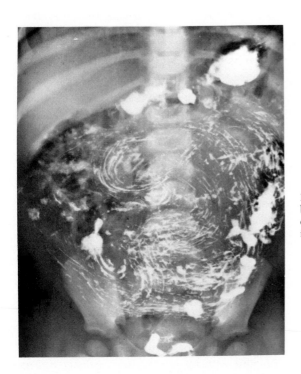

Figure 13-20 (left). Numerous ascarid worms outlined with barium are seen filling the small bowel as intraluminal filling defects. A film made the following day will often show a barium study of the gastrointestinal tract of the worm!

Gastric Ulcer

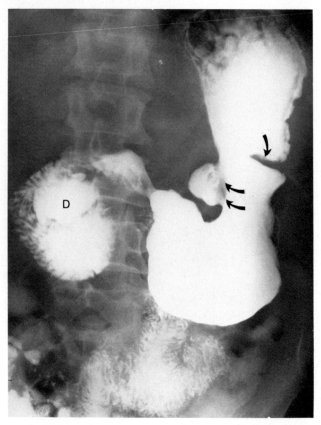

Figure 13-21. Large ulcer crater projecting from the midlesser curvature. Note radiolucent collar of granulation tissue (Hamptons's line, twin arrows) across the base of the ulcer. Upper arrow indicates a partial constriction of the lumen by an area of spasm along the greater curvature in response to the large active ulcer. *D* is a diverticulum arising from the medial wall of the descending limb of the duodenal loop.

The last of the five hypothetical tubular structures in Figure 13-2 shows what might be called an "addition shadow," although that term is not actually used. An ulceration has occurred in the wall of the tube, forming a small additional hollow space into which the opaque substance can flow. The term generally applied to this type of shadow in radiologic parlance is a *niche*, and you will find that term used commonly in reference to the projecting shadow of a barium-filled ulcer crater in the stomach or duodenum. Only when seen in profile, of course, will it be a projection from the normal margin of the gut wall. When a barium-filled ulcer crater is seen en face, it appears as a spot of white more dense than the surrounding shadow because it is frequently encir-

cled by a rolled-up margin of granulation tissue (or tumor, as the case may be). Ulcer craters which are filled with blood clot or food particles at the time of examination with barium will not be visualized at all. As they heal they fill in from the sides, becoming sharp and thorn-shaped in profile and finally disappearing altogether.

Because the tubular gastrointestinal tract is flexible, fills and empties in response to waves of peristalsis, and has opposing walls coated with barium, there are myriads of small angular barium shadows in most of the films you examine. To find among them one which can with confidence be labeled a niche requires that it have certain characteristics. In the first place, a niche is deeper than most of the valleys between the folds of mucosa. Therefore its shadow will be *denser*, because it represents a slightly greater thickness of barium. Because it is an ulcer it will have no mucosal pattern, and because it is generally surrounded by inflammatory reaction it will be less flexible than the rest of the gut wall. The shadow of the niche accordingly will be *constant in shape and size*. It will be *consistently demonstrable* in the same place from film to film, and all these characteristics enable the radiologist to find and identify it in the course of his study.

There are numerous other details which help him in interpreting his findings. For example, when he observes that the nearby mucosal folds in the stomach converge toward a demonstrable ulcer crater, he may report that the ulcer is almost unquestionably benign, because in differentiating the two types of ulcer in the stomach, the *convergence of folds* has proved to be the most reliable indication of benignity. You will hear much about the differentiation of benign and malignant ulcers in the stomach, and you will find that a few craters seem probably benign and turn out to be malignant, while a few benign ulcers of long standing are so embedded in scar tissue, so rigid, and so reluctant to heal on medical management that they are believed to be malignant by the referring physician, radiologist, and surgeon, and only the pathologist with his microscopic evidence can establish the facts.

194

To give you some easily remembered (if somewhat streamlined) statistics on benign and malignant gastric ulcers and their diagnosis by x-ray, you should anticipate that in the hands of a well-trained radiologist:

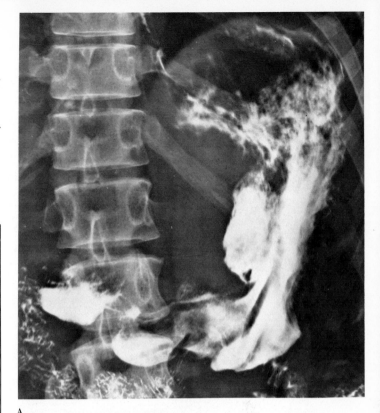

A

Of 100 benign gastric ulcers:
  75 will be clearly benign from the first examination with barium
  25 will be less definite in character and may require one or more additional roentgen examinations before diagnosis is possible
  A few will be impossible to diagnose without endoscopy, biopsy, or surgery.
Of 100 malignant gastric ulcers:
  75 will be clearly malignant and will need biopsy
  25 will require further study, endoscopy, biopsy, or surgery.

Keep in mind that:

(a) Most gastric ulcers are benign (90 percent).

(b) Size and location of an ulcer crater are *not* an index to determining malignancy, no matter what some surgery textbooks still say.

(c) Every "benign" gastric ulcer must be followed by x-ray until it has disappeared because failure to heal may be a sign of *carcinoma in situ.*

(d) There is no need to gastroscope the large number of gastric ulcers which are *convincingly benign by x-ray* (68 percent of all ulcers); only the problematic or clearly malignant ones require endoscopy and biopsy.

In the anxiety produced by today's spiraling hospital costs, many physicians order endoscopy for patients who do not really require that procedure for diagnosis. Most upper GI bleeders stop bleeding spontaneously, but gastroscopy is certainly indicated if they do not.

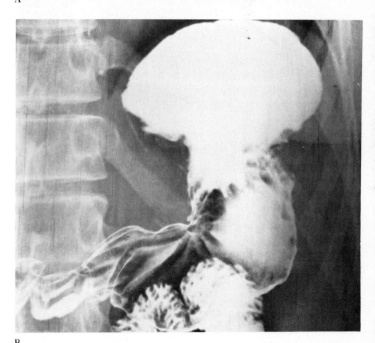

B

Figure 13-22. Natural history of healing in a large benign gastric ulcer, A. In B, six weeks later, the healing thorn-shaped crater might easily be missed. The convergence of folds toward the small remaining crater reinforces its probable benign character, but it must be followed by x-ray until completely healed.

195

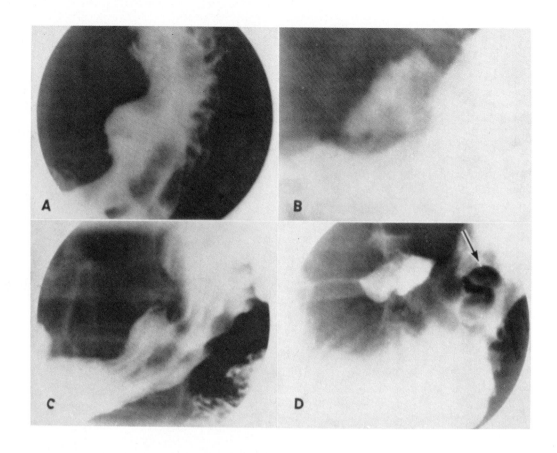

Figure 13-23. Four proved malignant lesser curvature ulcers. A: The ulcer is *within a mass*, and there is marked distortion and infiltration of the surrounding mucosa. A, B, and C would probably be labeled malignant by most radiologists. D is more difficult, but the nodularity of the fold indicated by the arrow is suspicious. No real pronouncements should ever be made from films alone without knowing the dynamic behavior of the stomach at fluoroscopy. These craters would all be confirmed at endoscopy and biopsied.

196

Duodenal Ulcer

What is true about the identification of stomach ulcers is true about duodenal ulcer craters, in that they are consistently demonstrable denser flecks of barium. However, in the duodenum the problem is somewhat different, since instead of a wide sac the structure to be examined is now a narrow tube with a bulb or ampulla at its commencement distal to the pyloric canal. Although the crater itself is demonstrated in much the same way as it is in the stomach, still more important and informative in the long run are the changes due to scar tissue formation in this characteristically recurrent condition.

The most common location by far for the crater is in the center of the posterior wall of the bulb. After several episodes of ulceration and healing, permanent strands of scar tissue develop which constrict the lumen of the duodenal bulb and limit its free distensibility after the fashion of a reefed sail. These limiting bands of scar tissue produce distinctive changes in the shape of the shadow of the barium-filled bulb, so that its cavity seems to be divided into several cavities bulging outward from the central point at which the ulcer crater has been present or may still be seen. This appearance has been called the *clover-leaf deformity* of the duodenal bulb or cap (Figure 13-24).

However, it is only one of the more advanced scarring patterns in long-standing duodenal ulcer disease and is present in by no means all of the advanced cases you will see. Another common pattern of scarring is a gradual development of a stenosed apex of the cap, eventually producing a high degree of obstruction and usually caused by ulcers which are located at the apex of the cap, where it normally narrows to become the descending limb of the duodenum. Still other patterns of scarring are produced by eccentric ulcers which for some reason occur less frequently or heal more readily. In these the bulb is seen to be deformed by a reef of scar tissue on only one side, and the barium-filled bulb will appear quite asymmetrical.

Several chapters could be written on the subject of duodenal ulcer disease, and you will gradually become familiar with the problems of diagnosing this entity radiologically. One very important point to remember is that a duodenal ulcer crater is fairly easy to demonstrate with barium in its early episodes. After scar formation has become fairly well advanced, however, the crater itself becomes more and more difficult to visualize with each successive attack, and at length the radiologist will find it almost impossible to demonstrate in spite of unquestioned reactivation suggested by the patient's symptoms. For this reason, *reexamination with barium is not at all indicated with each new attack* in a patient with a well-established diagnosis of duodenal ulcer crater or typical scarring, (duodenal ulcer disease). Once the diagnosis has been made, the clinician does well to be guided by the patient's symptoms alone. Only with the appearance of a significant change in the patient's long-standing symptoms, or increasing evidence of obstruction, need reexamination be carried out.

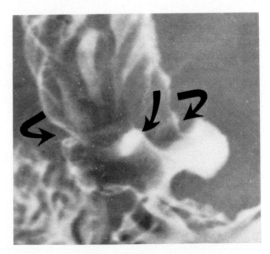

Figure 13-24. Classic location for duodenal ulcer on the posterior wall in midcap. Note indentations on greater and lesser curvature sides of cap (bent arrows), the beginning of scarring that will produce a typical "cloverleaf" deformity as the proximal and distal portions of the cap distend.

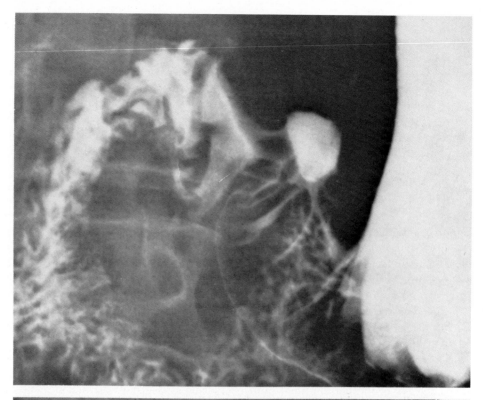

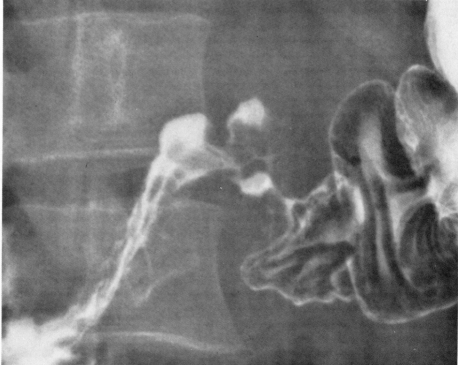

Figure 13-25 (above) and Figure 13-26 (below). Two patients with cloverleaf deformity of the duodenal cap. Because of the advanced scarring it would be impossible to say from these two films whether there was an active crater present. The behavior of the duodenum under the fluoroscope and the appearance of additional spot films might or might not decide the matter.

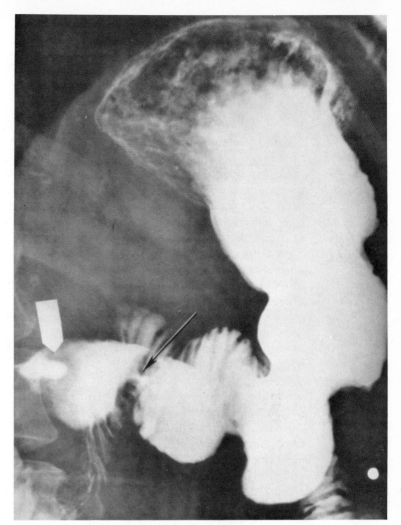

Figure 13-27. Large ulcer crater (white arrow) at the apex of the duodenal bulb. The scarring produced by craters in this location is likely to lead eventually to obstruction. Pylorus is indicated by black arrow.

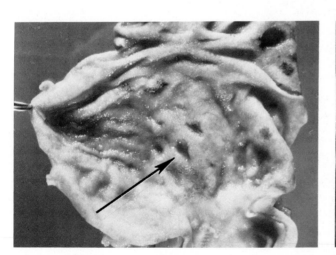 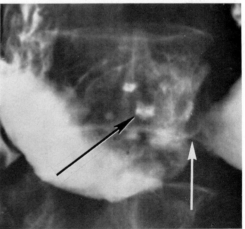

Figure 13-28 (left) and Figure 13-29 (right). Surgical specimen and radiographic spot film of a patient with multiple ulcer craters on the posterior wall of the duodenal bulb. In both the black arrow indicates the largest central crater, around which the others are arranged in a circle. White arrow indicates the pylorus. The duodenal bulb is filling with air, so that barium remaining in the craters on the posterior wall is clearly seen.

199

The GI Series

The student who looks at radiographs of the barium-filled stomach for the first time often has some difficulty identifying the various parts of the stomach, in particular the pylorus, and this difficulty generally stems from the fact that each of the conventional views of the stomach is made in a different projection with the patient differently positioned. The fluoroscopist usually begins with the patient standing, and examines the esophagus and stomach with a small amount of barium to study the mucosal relief pattern. Then he tilts the power-driven fluoroscopy table into the horizontal position, arranges the patient prone and turned slightly up on his right side. The patient drinks more barium and is turned into the supine position. Spot films are made at intervals whenever the radiologist sees anything on the screen he wishes recorded. Next, large films are made by a technician in a series of specified projections. These generally include one made straight prone, one prone but turned slightly to the right (the right anterior oblique), one made in a straight lateral projection with the patient on his right side, and one made supine with the patient rolled to the left slightly so as to fill the antrum of the stomach with air.

Study the following series of normal stomachs in various positions, in many of which the pylorus is identified by a black arrow. Note in each the varying shape of the stomach and of the duodenal bulb, as well as the deep indentations in both curvatures (peristaltic waves which progress when seen at fluoroscopy).

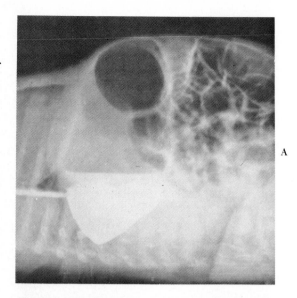

A

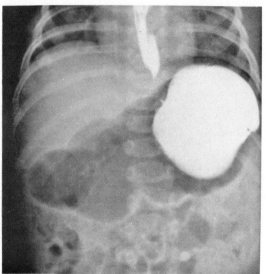

B

Figure 13-30. A baby lying on his back is being fed barium. Note that, just as you saw it in the supine plain films, the antrum of the stomach is filled with air, while the pool of barium collects in the more posteriorly placed fundus of the stomach. It is easy to understand from these films why babies more readily vomit their feedings when left lying on their backs, and why they are burped upright against the mother's shoulder with the undesirable swallowed air in the fundus.

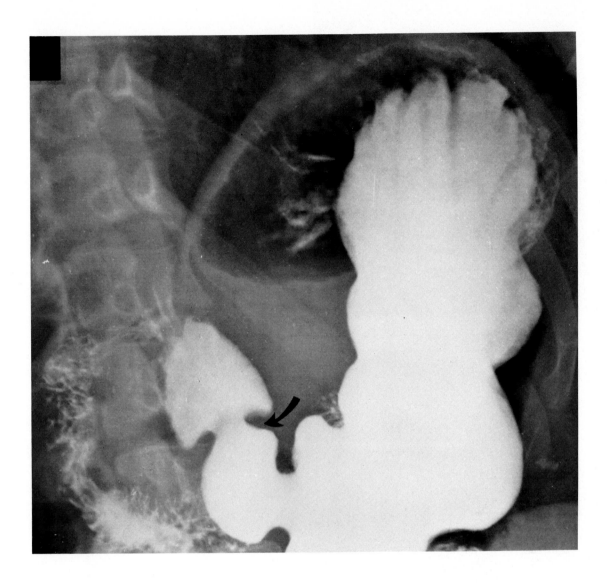

Figure 13-31. Another patient, prone but turned slightly to the right. Pylorus is seen as barium passes through it. The standard right anterior oblique projection "unrolls" the antrum, duodenal bulb, and loop. Note obliquity of the vertebrae as a clue to the position. Although film is made prone, it is always viewed as though the patient were facing you.

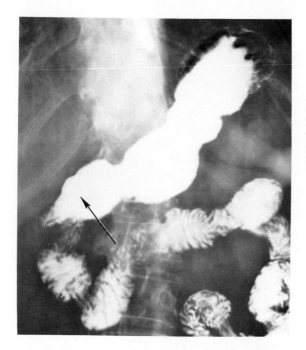

Figure 13-32. Prone film from a gastrointestinal series in an adult. Arrow indicates the position of the pylorus, although you cannot see it because of the overlap from barium in the antrum. Note the well-seen duodenal loop, often partly hidden by the antral barium.

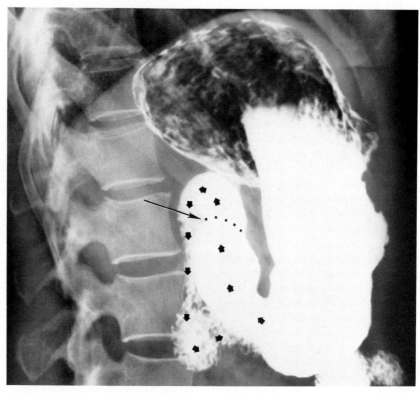

Figure 13-33. Lateral view, the patient now turned straight onto his right side, as you can see from the vertebrae. Arrow indicates position of the pylorus. Base of the cap is indicated by dots. Flow of barium from antrum to duodenal bulb, down the descending limb of the loop, and then forward and to the left is marked with small dark arrows. The descending duodenum in this view usually lies along the anterior borders of the vertebral bodies or overlaps them slightly. Retroperitoneal or pancreatic masses often displace the duodenum forward, a fact best appreciated in this view. Ulcer craters on the *posterior* wall of the stomach are frequently difficult to visualize except in this view.

202

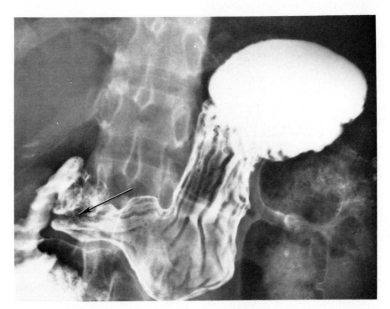

Figure 13-34. This patient has been turned from the right lateral position onto his back and a supine film has been made. Air from the fundus has ballooned out the barium-coated antrum. Pylorus indicated by an arrow. Most of the remaining barium rolls back into the fundus.

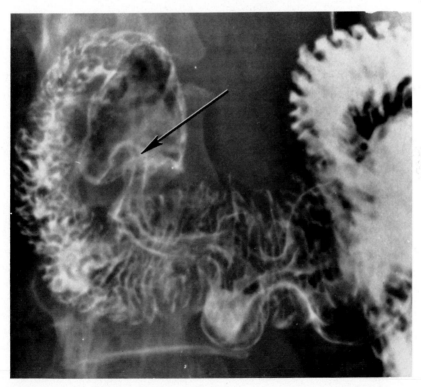

Figure 13-35. Another example of the supine left oblique, a means of studying the stomach antrum and often the duodenal bulb by double contrast, that is, coated with opaque barium and then inflated with air. The antrum is seen here superimposed on the barium-coated mucosa of the duodenal loop. Each can be distinguished by its relief markings. Note deep peristaltic waves in the antrum. Arrow indicates the pylorus.

203

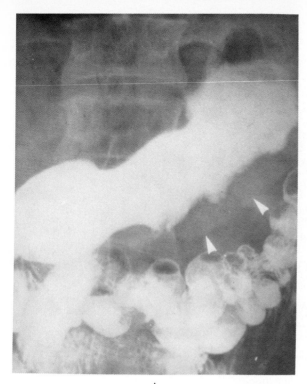

A

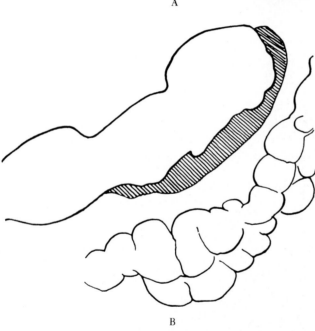

B

Figure 13-36. Radiograph, A, shows stomach wall thickened and rigid due to infiltrating carcinoma. Drawing, B, indicates the way you should try to supply the tumor in imagination when looking at such radiographs. At fluoroscopy no peristaltic waves at all would pass through a rigid segment of this type.

Rigidity of the Wall

In studying the gastrointestinal tract, then, the radiologist looks for a mucosal relief pattern which seems to him to be within normal limits of variation. He searches specifically for crater niches while manipulating the gut through the abdominal wall, his hand protected by a leaded glove. He then fills the succeeding parts of the gut with barium, testing their distensibility and looking for areas of *rigidity*, which may indicate even without any apparent ulceration that the wall is invaded by new growth or scarred by inflammation.

The recognition of an area of rigidity in gut wall is more difficult in many ways than the recognition of a crater, because the wall of the gut varies so much from part to part normally and because early infiltration with sheets of tumor cells does not render the wall entirely rigid but rather limits it elasticity, much in the way a sheet of rubber changes with age. If you can imagine a remarkably distensible organ like the stomach, into the wall of which has been set a piece of rubber which has lost some of its elasticity, you will have a fair idea of the behavior which can be expected from such a segment under the fluoroscope. Barium pushed against it with the gloved hand will fail to produce quite the prompt bulging expected. Barium pushed upward by the examining hand into normal gut shows a marginal pattern of wrinkles or folds as the flexible wall is mechanically displaced; the rigid or infiltrated segment will fold sluggishly and less deeply. Peristalsis too will be altered, and as one watches the normal passage of ring-like constrictions along the organ, one sees that they are resisted by the suspicious segment, which indents less readily with the passage of the wave. This is perfectly logical, since the contraction of sheets of muscle in the wall is limited by the infiltration of tumor cells, by edema, or by postinflammatory changes, as the case may be.

Decisions with regard to the flexibility of the gut wall, then, are based on the manner in which it is seen to distend with barium, to respond to manipulation, and to contract physiologically.

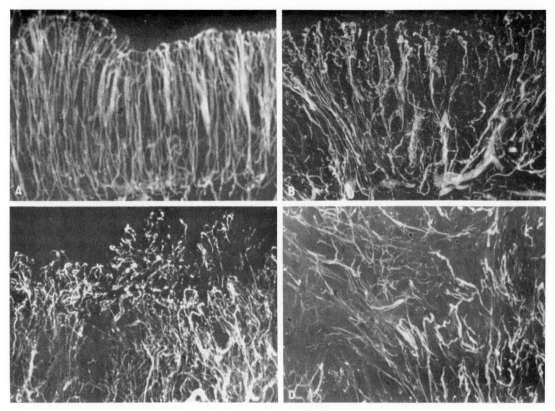

Figure 13-37. (See text.)

Rigidity in the wall of the gut, increasing as invasion by tumor advances, can be even better comprehended by examining the four illustrations above. They are *microangiograms*, in which specimens of gut removed at surgery are injected via their arteries with a radiopaque medium and radiographs made of the frozen sections. Here you see in A the normal pattern of the arterioles in the intestinal mucosa, with their narrow straight vessels, terminal arcades, and branching. The other three cuts show this architecture distorted by the invasion of carcinoma in the wall of the gut.

Inflammation in the bowel may result in ulceration or in total loss of mucosa, as seen in regional enteritis with serial barium studies of the small bowel. After long-standing chronic inflammation, scarring and fibrosis may result in localized constriction and intestinal obstruction or in general loss of elasticity with demonstrable shortening of the involved bowel. This occurs in late ulcerative colitis of the colon as well.

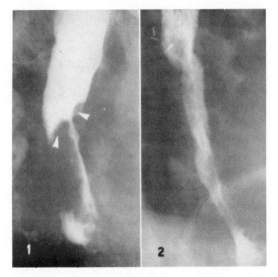

Figure 13-38. Patient with dysphagia. 1: Carcinoma of the esophagus narrowed the lumen to a tunnel a few millimeters wide and 10 centimeters in length, a rigid segment which never changed either at fluoroscopy or on the other films. Arrows indicate shelf. 2: Appearance after radiation therapy.

205

The Barium Enema

The cecum and rectum, like the stomach expanded sections of the gut, are difficult to examine and present special problems for the radiologist. The colon can only be examined properly with a clean mucosa after it has been thoroughly cleansed. This usually requires catharsis, although patients in whom catharsis is contraindicated may be studied after two days on a low-residue diet followed by two days on a liquid diet and cleansing enemas. The cecum should not be considered seen in its entirety until there is retrograde filling of either the appendix or the terminal ileum. This is a vital point in patients with unexplained anemia in whom carcinoma of the cecum must be ruled out.

Carcinoma of the rectum should be diagnosed by the clinician on physical examination. The radiologist knows that because of the great distensibility of the rectal ampulla it is easy for him to miss entirely a sizable carcinoma in this location, obscured by the barium surrounding and concealing it.

During the barium enema patients are examined as the barium is being instilled by gravity into the rectum, sigmoid, descending colon, transverse and ascending colon, and cecum. In the supine position the flexures are studied in various degrees of obliquity. When the colon is filled, a prone film is obtained and the patient is allowed to evacuate the barium, after which a second film is made to show the emptied large bowel and its mucosal relief pattern.

The rectosigmoid colon, because of its great redundancy and overlap in the pelvis, is very difficult to "unroll" and therefore to visualize in every part. A number of ingenious maneuvers have been designed by radiologists to help locate malignant lesions in the sigmoid. Patients have been examined at a sharp incline on a table with the head down, so that the loops of bowel will be pulled up out of the pelvis by their own heavy barium content and the sigmoid will be straightened. Patients are routinely examined in oblique projections and laterally, and many radiologists use a view in which the central ray is directed obliquely caudad in the sagittal plane in a prone patient (see next page spread, Figure 13-42). The patient may also be examined sitting up, the ray directed downward through the back as in Figure 13-40. New projections are constantly being evolved for the better visualization of opaque-filled structures. The cooperation of the patient makes a great deal of difference in the success of these procedures. For this reason, it seems to me that it ought to be a rule of thumb with physicians to explain to the patient briefly beforehand approximately what is going to be done.

The radiologist searching for intraluminal tumor masses in the colon often allows the patient to evacuate most of the barium and then insufflates the colon with air so that a *double contrast* study can be filmed. Or he may elect to use the double contrast method from the start of the examination, instilling a small amount of barium and then air as needed.

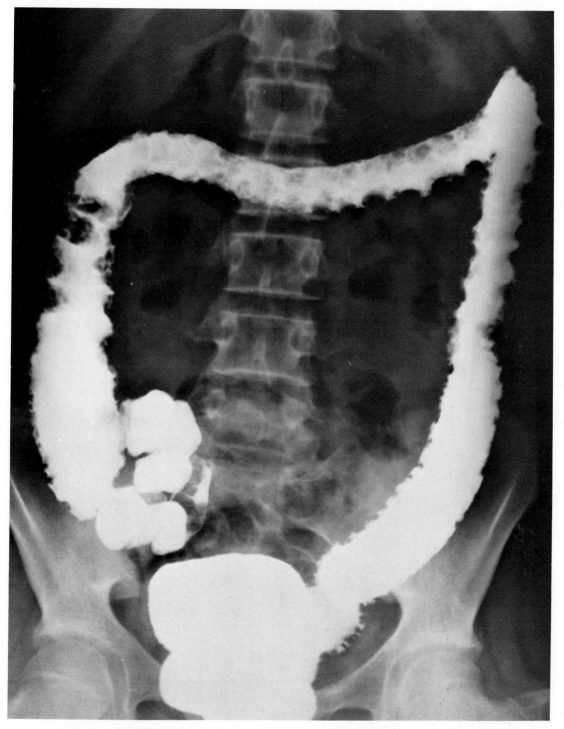

Figure 13-39. Ulcerative colitis in a young boy. Here ulceration is seen throughout the colon from cecum to anus. Scar tissue formation with disappearance of normal haustration and some shortening in length of the colon is evident. Note absence of usual redundancy at flexures and classic collar button ulcers.

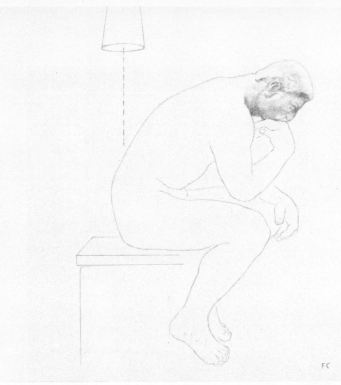

Figure 13-40 (left). A special position in which the patient may be examined in order to unroll the sigmoid colon.

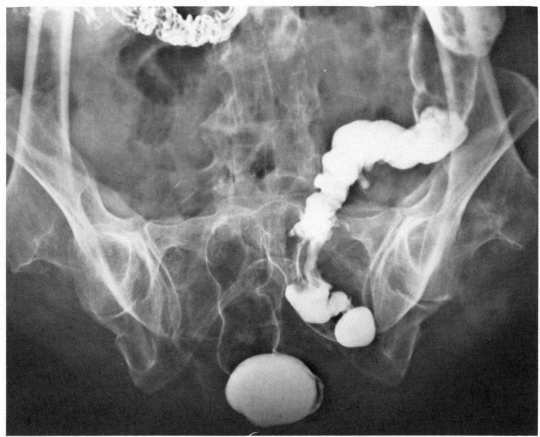

Figure 13-41. Annular lesion at the sigmoid flexure visualized in this fashion. Note bony structures.

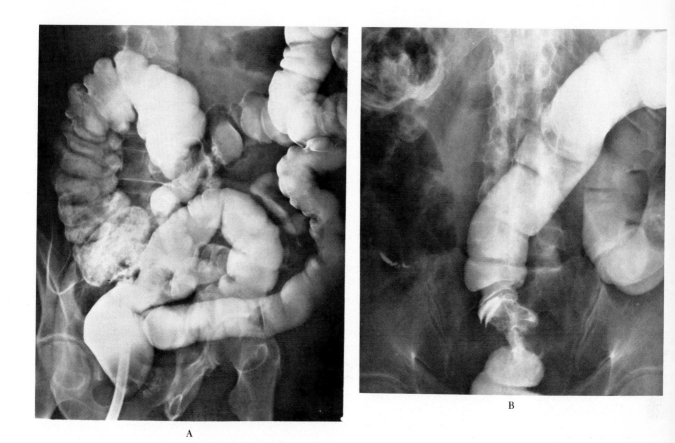

A   B

Figure 13-42. A: Conventional barium enema examination
fails to show the lesion at the rectosigmoid junction, a carcinoma producing annular constriction which is well seen in
the special view, B, made with an oblique sagittal ray.

Radiation Hazard

If you go into orthopedics, internal medicine, or general practice as a speciality, the question is sure to arise whether or not you should own x-ray equipment, and perhaps a fluoroscope. As Dr. George Holmes once said, "The ownership of a fluoroscope does not make one a fluoroscopist!" Even the limited information I have just given you about the ways in which the trained radiologist arrives at decisions, based on films and fluoroscopic study together, may have convinced you that highly specialized training is required for many phases of a radiologist's work. *What you may not have appreciated is the fact that a fluoroscope is a dangerous instrument in the hands of the inexperienced.*

It is true that there is something dazzling and magical about being able to see through human tissues; it is true that patients are impressed with the procedure. But when you also consider that good judgment in the manipulation of living tissues under the fluoroscope (as well as interpretation of the usually vague shadows seen there) is obtainable only after years of training and practice, then it must strike you that this phase of medical diagnosis is best left to the radiologist.

It is a fact that reconditioned, second-hand fluoroscopes of obsolete design have been for years passed on as "bargains" to general practitioners, and that these machines constitute a very real danger to doctors, nurse-technicians, and their patients. This is particularly true in the unfortunate practice of substituting "a quick fluoroscopy of the chest" for a properly obtained chest film. Careful studies have shown that some types of lung pathology which are obvious and well-documented on the chest film are routinely missed at fluoroscopy, even by experts. The first lung cancer you see on a chest film and know to have been overlooked in its earlier stages because of this careless practice will certainly affect you very deeply. Only up-to-date (and many times more expensive) fluoroscopes with modern high-gain image amplification should ever be used in the roentgen diagnosis of disease.

The use of even such modern fluoroscopic machines, however, has certain built-in dangers about which you ought to be informed. Much has been written about the hazards of radiation, and there can be no question that *any* radiation that is unnecessary is ill used. Remember in general (so that you will have things in proportion) *that fluoroscopy exposes the patient and physician to a much greater amount of radiation, per single procedure, than examinations involving simply the making of films.*

The radiologist has been specifically trained to limit fluoroscopic exposure in a variety of ways to the smallest amount of radiation that will provide the required information. Studies have been made comparing measurements of radiation exposure to both patient and physician (1) when an expert trained in the work is operating the fluoroscope, and (2) when a physician unfamiliar with the expected norms and technical maneuvers is fluoroscoping. These studies show that *training cuts exposure to a very small fraction.* Those who train fluoroscopists feel that it takes up to five years to develop proficiency and dependability in the techniques required.

Radiologists in training centers have strict procedural rules, which their residents must learn to observe as they develop diagnostic acumen. For example, they *never* stand in a room in which a film exposure is being made. Nor do they *ever* put an unprotected hand into the x-ray beam. In some training centers they are required to limit and record the total clocked fluoroscopic time for any single procedure like a GI series or a barium enema. This means they must learn to use an interrupted beam for brief intervals, making the necessary fluoroscopic observations efficiently in the shortest possible time. They must also use a well-collimated, narrow beam in order to limit scattered secondary radiation from the patient's body and the equipment. This practice also improves the image clarity.

When today's radiologists observe all the rules carefully, they are themselves in no danger of a decreased life expectancy at all, and

210

they have the satisfaction of knowing that the patient has received minimal exposure. Current statistical studies show that the shortened life span that used to be found among radiologists was related to ignorance of the dangers of radiation and no longer obtains. In an excellent review of the whole problem of the hazards of ionizing radiation in roentgen diagnosis, the Department of Health, Education, and Welfare issued regulations for minimum standards as of August 1, 1974, for all equipment purchased new. These regulations should minimize the danger to both patients and physicians.

The publicity that radiation hazard has received in the lay press in the past two decades (although some of it is quite inaccurate) must be considered a good thing, since it has made both patient and physician aware of the fact that any unnecessary x-ray exposure is to be avoided. However, the valuable, lifesaving information available through roentgen diagnosis must always be balanced against the implicit dangers. Ignorance is deplorable where so much is at stake. The family of a leukemic child, a patient of mine, who rejected palliative therapy "because we have read that those x-rays are dangerous," was pitiably misinformed. Equally misinformed was the house officer in one hospital who asked us whether his wife should have an abortion because she had had a preemployment chest film before she knew she was pregnant. The exposure to the female pelvis from a chest film is so small as to be negligible. On the other hand, if a young woman early in her pregnancy developed cramps and bloody diarrhea, raising the question of ulcerative colitis, one would most certainly delay as long as possible before doing a barium enema, unless the hemorrhage became truly dangerous.

Experts are still trying to determine the safe lifetime exposure. It must include basic cosmic radiation, to which even primitive man was exposed. Such background radiation is impossible to avoid, but certainly one can avoid or reduce the hazard of medical irradiation by limiting the use of all fluoroscopic radiographic procedures to those in which the advantage to the patient outweighs the risk. You should begin by remembering to order abdominal radiographic procedures on women in the childbearing years *only* during the first ten days after the commencement of the last menstrual period, thus limiting the chance of injury to a fetus at its most vulnerable period of growth.

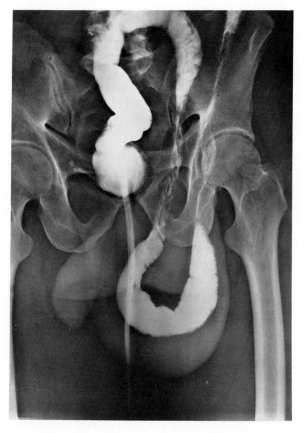

Figure 13-43 (*Unknown 13-2*). Make a diagnosis.

211

14 Newer Imaging Methods: Ultrasonography and Computerized Tomography

Now that you have addressed yourself to the study of the plain film and to the principles of radiographic contrast studies, you have certainly acquired an even more expert stereotactic feeling for considering body structures always in three dimensions. Even if you were blind, had therefore never seen an *apple* or known that such a shape existed, you would be able intellectually to reconstruct its three-dimensional form precisely from assembled slices which you had been able to touch-examine with your fingers.

Modalities of imaging in modern medicine offer you such information about organs and structures inside your patient. Two of these modalities are gaining widespread usefulness so rapidly that you will need to learn to accept the data they provide if you are to function efficiently as a doctor.

Ultrasonography

It is a curious fact that high-energy sound waves beyond the range of the human ear were produced experimentally some 15 years before Roentgen discovered the x-ray. No attempt was made to develop ultrasonography for medical use until after the stimulus of its use during World War II in the underwater detection of submarines. Since the 1950s, however, sonography has earned an important place in medical diagnosis and physicians find they employ it on some of their patients practically every day.

The fact that sound waves are absorbed by many solid substances but transmitted readily by water meant that a beam of sound could be projected through the water toward a submarine and its reflection from the surface of the ship timed so that the presence of the ship, and its distance, were known.

Translated to medical use, this means that a beam of sound waves projected into the body from the surface of the skin will be transmitted forward by *sonolucent* (fluid) substances, a part of the beam being reflected back when it encounters an interface with a substance or structure of different *acoustic character*. The time needed for the signal to return *locates* the depth and describes for us the interface from which it was reflected. The rest of the initial beam continues on into and through the encountered organ or mass, reflecting more and more of the beam from other interfaces at measurable distances, until finally the last of the beam is absorbed.

Whenever the beam encounters a fluid-filled (cystic) structure inside the body, the sound is transmitted with negligible absorption until it reaches the interface of the far wall of the cystic structure from which it is first reflected.

Sound is transmitted well through any fluid, but poorly or not at all through bone, air, and barium. In examining a patient, we exclude the air/skin interface by applying an oil or jelly to the skin of the patient and stroking the sound source, or *transducer*, in contact with and across the surface of the skin along the edge of an imaginary slice of the patient for which one wishes to obtain depth soundings.

The beam of sound is produced in pulses or periodic bursts, very brief in duration, and the same transducer then "listens" for the returning echoes until the next burst of outgoing sound. The transducer listens 99.9 percent of the time and emits sound in the remaining fraction. Thus it is a listening device much more of the time than it is an emitting device.

Returning echoes are converted into electric energy and reproduced on a video monitor, where they appear as dots of varying brightness and remain there until they are "erased." Thus the sonographer "builds up" information in the course of a few seconds of sound emission and reception which gives us a picture on the screen composed of dots of light, the location of which are determined by a special localization system. This therefore appears as a *picture of a slice of the patient.* It is easy to tally such pictures with one's intellectual awareness of cross-sectional anatomy.

Unlike the important tissue injury of ionizing radiation, which has to be taken into consideration in electing to carry out any radiographic study, pulsed diagnostic ultrasound seems to have no injurious effect whatever in the range used for medical technology. This makes ultrasound a particularly valuable tool, especially in imaging pelvic structures in obstetrical and gynecological practice—and it is there that we will illustrate first the practical principles of ultrasonography.

A patient being prepared for pelvic ultrasonography is instructed not to void for sometime beforehand, a full urinary bladder providing a sonolucent mass in the lower abdomen which displaces undesirable air-containing loops of bowel up out of the pelvis, so that a good beam of sound transmitted through the bladder will encounter the pelvic organs behind it.

In Figure 14-1 you are looking at a *transverse* cross section just above the symphysis pubis (bone interferes by absorbing the beam, remember). The beam of sound has entered through the lower abdominal wall (top of the figure). You are looking up at the slice from the patient's feet, a conventional point of view for both sonograms and CT scans in the transaxial plane. The large uniformly black structure is the urine-filled sonolucent bladder. Posterior to it you see an oval mass which is the normal uterus. Note the many dots representing echoes from the muscular wall, and the slit-like uterine cavity with its darker ring of endometrium.

Compare now the information which even a beginner can derive from Figure 14-2. This is another exactly similar cross-sectional slice. You can identify the urine-distended bladder, the uterus, and on either side the adnexa, suspended in the broad ligament. Behind the uterus is a sonolucent black area similar to the

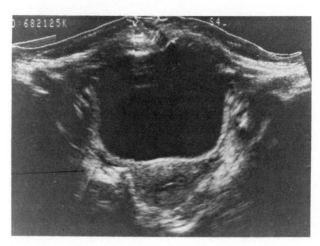

Figure 14-1. Normal transverse sonogram, female pelvis.

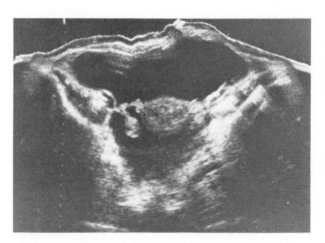

Figure 14-2. Transverse sonogram, female patient with ascites.

bladder, which is a collection of (ascitic) fluid in the cul de sac. The patient is, of course, lying supine on the examining table so that the bowl of the pelvis is the most dependent part of the abdomen.

213

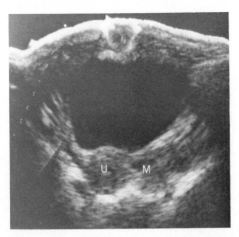

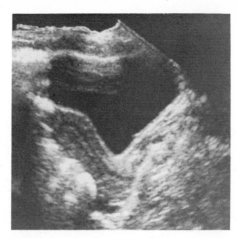

Figure 14-3. Transverse pelvic sonogram on female patient with abdominal pain and vaginal bleeding. (See text.)

Figure 14-4. Normal longitudinal midline pelvic sonogram on female patient.

Now look at Figure 14-3, also a sonogram made in the transverse direction. Remembering that, since you are looking from the patient's feet, her left is on your right, you will be able to make out a round mass (*M*) on the left side of the pelvis adjoining the uterus (*U*). The uterus with its central cavity is easy to identify. Note that there is nothing like the "mass" on the right side of the patient's pelvis. This patient was pregnant and began to bleed suddenly after experiencing some lower abdominal pain. The mass you see here turned out to be an ectopic pregnancy in the left Fallopian tube requiring emergency surgery.

Note that plenty of echoes are being reflected from the mass, telling you that it is not cystic like the bladder at all. Ectopic pregnancy usually produces *complex masses*, that is, partly cystic and partly solid. Any such pelvic mass imaged sonographically is assumed to be an ectopic pregnancy in a pregnant patient who is bleeding and who does not have an intrauterine gestational sac visualized.

As early as five weeks past the start of the last menstrual period a highly echogenic area may be seen inside the uterus, and by seven weeks the gestational sac is clearly visualized. At about eleven weeks the fetal head can be seen (easy to measure from the widest biparietal diameter), and with certain other sonographic findings gestational age can be determined. Fetal death may be suggested by failure of these dimensions to increase normally on serial sonograms. By nine weeks the placenta can be seen lining a part of the uterine cavity, and a low placenta would be easy to diagnose in a patient in the third trimester with bleeding.

A pregnant patient who is "large for her dates" should be examined by ultrasound. It may become apparent that the expected date of confinement is miscalculated. Polyhydramnios is, as you could anticipate, easy to detect, the fetus floating in a too-abundant pool of sonolucent fluid. Ovarian tumors or cysts, multiparity, myoma, or hydatidiform mole all have clear-cut sonographic appearances.

Pelvic sonography is usually carried out in two planes at right angles, the *transverse* one you have been looking at and a *longitudinal* one in the sagittal plane. In Figure 14-4 you are looking at a normal longitudinal midline sonogram, the beam entering at the top through the *acoustic window* of the bladder. By convention, the patient's head is to your left in viewing longitudinal sonograms. Immediately posterior to the bladder you see the pear-shaped uterus, its central cavity now a long lighter streak margined on both sides by the darker endometrium. The vagina angles upward and to your right.

214

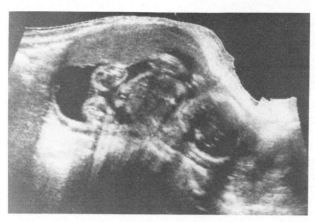

Figure 14-5. Longitudinal midline pelvic sonogram of pregnant patient.

A myoma would eccentrically thicken the wall of the uterus. A normal gestational sac would be seen distending it centrally. In Figure 14-5 you see a well-defined fetus in the third trimester in vertex presentation well up out of the pelvis, the beam of sound having entered through the abdominal wall. You can see the fetal head as a ring of white. Two legs and an upper arm can also be seen. The cresentic shadow of the placenta lies anteriorly near the abdominal wall (no placenta previa!).

Static sonograms like these at right-angled planes are in everyday use. Other ultrasonographic techniques record, instead of a stored or fixed image (like a radiograph), a continuous or dynamic image (like fluoroscopy). You will have heard of "real-time" scanning in which one or more transducers are used to image moving structures like the fetal heart. You can think of "real-time" sonography as similar to fluoroscopy, with the dynamic moving image on the screen being a tomogram. This has become an excellent survey method as well for quick screening of an area to be investigated, the usual static sonograms or high-quality real-time images then

being made at indicated locations.

Because of interference from bone, ultrasonography has little to offer in the imaging of the head, computerized tomography having taken over that sphere of medical investigation (except in the newborn where the fontanelle or suture opening can be used as a window). Similarly in the chest, because of the bony thorax and the air in the lungs, not much use can be made of sonography.

It is in the abdomen that sonography finds its principal use. There you will find it has so many applications you will need to be aware of that I must detail some of them for you. The pelvis is by no means the only usefully studied area, and with two careful mental observations you will easily learn and retain the rules relating to the upper abdomen as well: (1) always remember that bone, air, and barium block sound (bone and barium absorb it, having a very high density, and air transmits it only poorly); (2) realize that ultrasonography gives you structural data by telling you which are cystic and which solid masses, but that it cannot make tissue diagnoses.

215

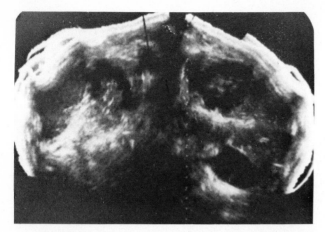

Figure 14-6. Normal prone transverse sonogram of the upper abdomen.

In the upper abdomen the study of the kidney is rendered difficult by the gas in stomach and intestine, so the patient lies prone. The transducer is moved across the costovertebral angle, projecting sound through the muscles of the back. Here in Figure 14-6 is a transverse sonogram of a patient lying prone. The beam has entered through his back and the kidneys are seen as two doughnut-shaped shadows. Renal parenchyma has a low acoustic impedance and is relatively sonolucent, and the central cluster of echoes you see represent sound reflected from the collecting system, renal sinus fat, and vessels.

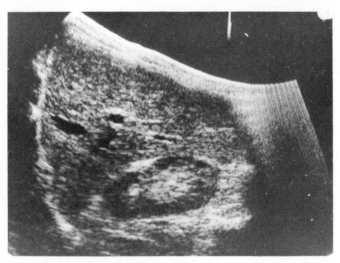

Figure 14-7. Normal longitudinal parasagittal sonogram 6 centimeters to the right of the midline. Patient's head is to your left.

In Figure 14-7 you have a longitudinal scan made in a parasagittal plane 6 centimeters to the right of the midline. The patient is supine, and the beam has entered anteriorly through the relatively homogeneous low-density liver in order to deliver enough sound to define the kidney clearly. Again you see the normal kidney as a ring of parenchyma, relatively sonolucent or *anechoic* (giving rise to few echoes), while the collecting system supplies a burst of returning echoes from its complex of interfaces. Notice that here there are two entirely anechoic structures in the liver, the right portal vein and the right hepatic vein.

216

Now compare Figure 14-8 and study the difference between this kidney and the one in Figure 14-7. Here there is a anechoic area in the center of the kidney, which is provided by a fluid-filled kidney pelvis. This patient had hydronephrosis, a condition easily diagnosed by ultrasound. We will further discuss the uses of sonography in the study of the kidney in Chapter 15.

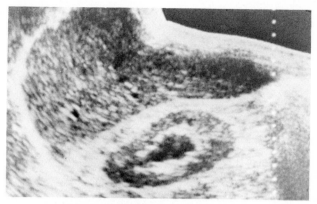

Figure 14-8. Longitudinal sonogram, plane comparable with that in Figure 14-7. This patient had hydronephrosis. (See text.)

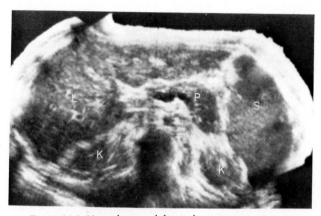

Figure 14-9. Normal upper abdominal transverse sonogram.

Figure 14-9 shows you a transverse sonogram in a supine patient made of the upper abdomen at a level 8 centimeters above the umbilicus, that is, high enough to avoid most of the problem of intestinal gas interference. On sonograms the exact plane is always recorded, transverse abdominal scans being said to be so many centimeters U+ (above) or U− (below) the umbilicus. Sagittal sonograms are defined in numbers of centimeters the plane of study lies to the right or left of the midline (sagittal) plane.

In Figure 14-9 you can define the liver (L), its left lobe stretching across toward the enlarged spleen, S (the patient clinically had splenomegaly). The tail of the pancreas (P) is seen just medial to the spleen, and the kidneys (K) posteriorly on either side of the forward-projecting spine.

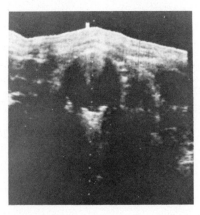

Figure 14-10 shows you a transverse sonogram made at the level of the umbilicus in a patient with a pulsating abdominal mass which proved to be a 5-centimeter aortic aneurysm. Figure 14-11 is the same patient's longitudinal sonogram. The head of the patient is to your left, remember, and the anechoic black abdominal aorta can be seen connecting with the large aneurysm. The transducer has been lifted from the skin surface (white blip) to indicate the location of the umbilicus.

Figure 14-10. Transverse sonogram in a supine patient at the level of the umbilicus shows an aortic aneurysm.

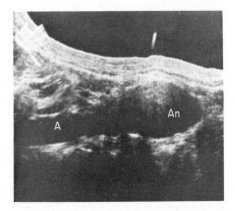

Figure 14-11. Longitudinal sonogram in the same patient. Note long anechoic aorta (A) and aneurysm (An). White blip is made by the operator to locate the umbilicus.

218

The gallbladder, often visualized with difficulty radiologically once it has become diseased, is easily imaged at sonography, since it is seen as a fluid-containing "cystic" structure close to or within the substance of the liver. Figure 14-12 shows you a transverse sonogram at U + 6 (6 centimeters above the umbilicus), which shows the gallbladder partly filled with sludge, a clearly seen level existing in this supine patient where the echo-producing solid particles have sunk to the bottom of a fluid-filled viscus. Figure 14-13 is the R6 longitudinal sonogram (parasagittal plane 6 centimeters to the right of the midline) on the same patient, showing the same findings, as you would expect.

Gallstones, whether visibly calcified on the plain film or not, are easily imaged sonographically, being denser (with a greater acoustic impedance) than bile, of course. In recent years this has become the method of choice in the diagnosis of gallstones, although cholecystography still finds a use in many patients adjunctively.

In Figure 14-14 you have a longitudinal sonogram showing a solitary gallstone lying on the posterior wall of the gallbladder. This case demonstrates another important facet of sonographic interpretation. Notice that the gallstone, perpendicular to the transducer, has no reflected echoes from structures directly behind it. It appears to cast a shadow, and this phenomenon has been aptly termed "shadowing." Note that a variety of echoes are returned from tissues behind the gallbladder wall on both sides of the stone.

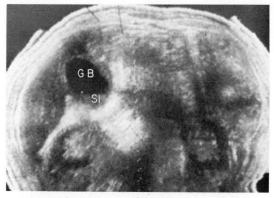

Figure 14-12. Transverse upper abdominal sonogram showing gallbladder (*GB*) with fluid level between bile and sludge (*Sl*) in dependent portion.

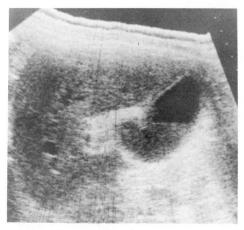

Figure 14-13. Longitudinal sonogram, same patient.

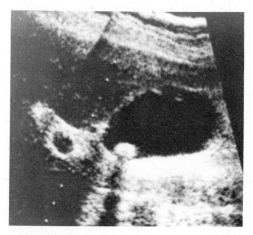

Figure 14-14. Longitudinal sonogram showing solitary gallstone in the gallbladder.

219

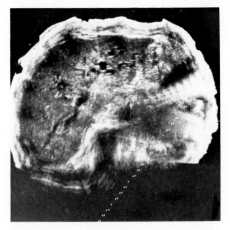

Figure 14-15. Transverse sonogram across upper abdomen in a patient with jaundice, showing dilated bile ducts in the liver.

Ultrasonography has also found one of its most dramatic uses as a screening procedure in patients with jaundice, by visualizing easily the dilated biliary tree within the liver in those with obstructive jaundice. Figures 14-15 and 14-16 show transverse and longitudinal sonograms on a patient with obstructive jaundice, and it is easy to see the cross-sectioned dilated sonolucent bile ducts inside the liver in both figures. In Chapter 15 you will find a somewhat more detailed discussion of the imaging workup of the jaundiced patient, with a fuller explanation of the various procedures available. One final caution: ultrasonography, unlike CT, is extremely "operator dependent" and is, in fact an art. Know your sonographer and find out how good he really is. His expertise technically, his familiarity with anatomy, and his judgment are vital to the success of his work. (It should be noted that this is true with compound-B scanning but less so in real-time scanning.)

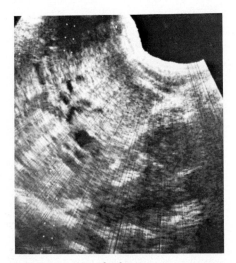

Figure 14-16. Longitudinal sonogram, same patient.

Breathing-Space Exercise

Now that you have been introduced to ultrasound, why don't you try your hand at reasoning out the answers to the following very practical questions? (Answers upside down).

(1)   Would you expect sonography to be as helpful in the diagnosis of aneurysm of the thoracic aorta as it is in aneurysm occurring below the diaphragm?

(2)   Why do you think ultrasound is often useful as a screening first procedure in patients with a question of obstructive nephropathy? Renal failure?

(3)   You know that sonography is useful in an obstetrical patient who is "too large for her dates." What possibilities must you consider in the patient who is "too small for her dates," and in which do you think ultrasound might help?

Answers

(1)   No, because both air and bone prevent proper sound transmission, and there is a lot of both bone and air in the thorax. Aneurysm of the aorta can easily be diagnosed by ultrasound *below* the diaphragm (provided there is not too much air in the gut).

(2)   Because it is easy to recognize the dilated collecting system inside the sonographic image of the kidney, either unilaterally or bilaterally. Other imaging facilities will then have to help you decide why there is obstruction. As to renal failure patients, sonography will exclude failure due to obstructive nephropathy and can also determine whether the kidney parenchyma has altered dimensions or texture.

(3)   Some possibilities for patient who is "too small for her dates":

(a) Inaccurate menstrual history	(ultrasound helpful)
(b) Fetal demise	(realtime = no cardiac motion)
(c) Missed abortion	(ultrasound = ? no fetus in utero)
(d) IUGR (intrauterine growth retardation)	(ultrasound does not tally with dates)
(e) Oligohydramnios	(ultrasound clear-cut)
(f) Ectopic pregnancy	(any kind of adnexal mass by ultrasound)

221

Computerized Tomography

As you discovered in Chapter 2, a computerized tomogram provides you with a schema of *density* values for a particular slice of your patient which you will learn to study with the regional cross-section anatomy in mind. An awareness of the relative attenuation of different tissues and organs and their interfaces with fat planes in particular, helps you as you look at CT scans. As you do so, you will be better able to understand anatomic relationships and proportions by knowing that those on CT scans are *living* dimensions rather than the necessarily distorted ones in the desiccated cadaver. There are also physiological implications in some of the observations you will make in serial CT scans. For example, in scans made across the upper abdomen the inferior vena cava can be seen to distend to twice its normal size during the Val Salva maneuver (in which the patient bears down against a closed glottis, as in pronouncing a forced "G" or "K").

Principles

To review briefly, in computerized tomography a thin collimated beam of x-rays passes through the body slice under study as the x-ray tube moves in an arc around the edge of the slice of patient. Carefully aligned and directly opposite the x-ray tube are placed special electronic detectors, a hundred times more sensitive than x-ray film, which convert the exiting x-rays on the other edge of the slice into amplified electrical pulses. These pulses vary in intensity in proportion to the degree of attenuation of the x-ray beam as it passes through the diagonal line of unit cubes of tissue in the mosaic of cubes composing that slice.

As fast as it is received, this information is stored in the computer, which then calculates the average x-ray absorption of each unit cube. This average figure is expressed in Hounsfield units on a scale in which water is arbitrarily assigned the figure of zero, everything denser than water having a plus number (up to +500 for bone), and everything less dense than water having a minus number (down to −500 for air.)

The attenuation value for each one of the unit cubes of tissue is converted into a dot on a TV monitor screen at its precise location in the cross-sectional slice, with the brightness or grayness of the dot proportional to the amount of x-ray absorption that cube was responsible for. The mosaic of dots thus represents the exact mosaic of cubes in terms of both location and density. The schema or density map so produced looks like a cross section of the body; of course, the smaller the units (pixels, as the units of the image are called) and the larger the number of them in the mosaic (matrix), the sharper the picture.

It is convention to view such tomograms from the patient's feet, so that his left side is on the viewer's right. Permanent images are obtained by photographing the screen. The x-ray dose per slice varies from one to four rads depending on machine design and is comparable to the exposure from conventional x-ray studies of the area.

Technique of scanning

Motion and high-density materials such as barium, a hip prosthesis, or surgical clips produce artifacts that degrade the image obtained. Older CT scanners required 2.5 minutes per slice, and patients had to be allowed to breathe quietly. The movement of abdominal organs during respiration is 1 to 2 centimeters, enough to distort smaller structures.

Newer models of scanners use only 1 to 10 seconds to complete a slice. Most patients can hold their breath for 5 seconds repeatedly, but of course many unconscious or very ill or dyspneic patients and small children requiring CT studies will be certain to produce motion degradation of the image. Mild sedation and reassurance beforehand by you as well as by the radiologist may help; but the *gantry*, or housing for the equipment, is huge and admittedly frightening to patients. It behooves you to inspect the CT room so that you can explain to your patient ahead of time that the procedure is as painless as having his picture taken, in spite of the look of the machine.

CT scans can be performed in the supine or prone position or with the patient lying on his side (decubitus). Usually, however, the patient is supine, as he is most comfortable and most relaxed in that position and can more readily keep still.

It is important for you to realize that computerized tomography most of the time should be considered an adjunctive study for special problems rather than a screening procedure. Other less expensive, less invasive procedures like plain films or ultrasound ought always to be used first if possible so that the CT study, when indicated, can be employed more precisely and more economically for the examination of the particular structure in question. One important exception is in head trauma, where one may go directly to CT without plain skull films in many patients. Because of the ionizing radiation involved, the female pelvis during the childbearing era must be examined most of the time by ultrasound rather than CT.

The use of contrast material for enhancement

Contrast media are almost routinely used during CT scanning for two basic reasons. (1) The GI tract can be tagged and thus distinguished from neighboring structures by having the patient swallow dilute opaque material. (Barium used in examination of the GI tract is too dense and produces artifacts.) (2) Intravenous administration of water-soluble contrast material will produce a temporary increase in the density of great vessels, of all capillary-perfused parenchyma, and, finally, of veins during CT scanning. This is called *enhancement* and is extremely useful. Dilated low-density branching channels within the homogeneous parenchyma of the liver, for example, on an initial scan without contrast could be either fluid-filled bile ducts or vessels. We can enhance the vascular bed with contrast medium, therefore, and if the observed channels are unchanged on a subsequent scan they are bile ducts, not vessels. Similarly, biliary or renal excreted contrast substances may be used, CT scanning being carried out both before and after the opaque is given so that the gallbladder, common bile duct, or kidney and ureters are seen as "dense" white areas of recognizable form and in the expected locations. On the other hand, *displacement* of these structures, although they are themselves not abnormal, will provide additional information with regard to soft-tissue masses being investigated.

As you have learned thus far, computerized tomography has important applications in the *chest*, where mediastinal masses can be more readily distinguished from normal structures than by plain tomograms and where small metastatic nodules, especially near the chest wall, can be recognized when they are not seen on routine chest films and are not detectable by any other means.

In Chapter 16 you will be learning the equally important applications in the *brain*, for CT has virtually revolutionized neuroradiology. However, for the moment I believe you will be able to learn to accept most easily the kind of information CT can provide by studying the normal scans of the *abdomen* in the rest of this chapter, identifying the structures as they appear in successive slices. Chapter 15 will organize and tally for you the indications for various special procedures, including CT, and the choice of procedures appropriate to a variety of common medical problems.

Body computerized tomography carried out in the abdomen is usually made transaxially at intervals of 2 centimeters, although each CT scanning study must be custom-tailored to the particular patient's problem. Of course, such serial slices give you composite information from which you can reconstruct the size and shape of any organ.

Begin by identifying the liver in Figure 14-17A. Note that as you look up from the patient's feet the liver is on your left and anterior. Ignore everything else and follow the change in shape and size of the liver down through all six sections made at 1-centimeter intervals in this patient.

Note how the dense vertebra changes shape depending on whether the cut is through the transverse processes in D and E or above or below them. The spinal canal is of course visible.

Locate the aorta just anterior to the body of the vertebra and slightly to the left of the midline, with dense white areas in its periphery which are calcified plaques in its wall. This series of scans has been carried out after intravenous infusion of contrast material, so that perfused structures and vessels are slightly whiter (enhanced). Note the branching white vessels in A in the homogeneous parenchyma of the liver, which fade away in successive sections. The intravenous contrast material used is excreted by the kidneys, so you see the renal parenchyma and calices as whiter than other organs. Those branching linear structures leaving the hilum of the kidney are vessels.

The stomach in A contains fluid and probably lunch. No oral contrast material has been given to this patient. Note that the (perfused) wall of the stomach is denser than its fluid content, and as you look from scan to scan you cross section first the body and then the antrum of the stomach; even the pylorus and proximal to it a peristaltic wave are seen.

The big black low-density areas on either side of the vertebra and posterior to the liver and spleen in B contain nothing but retroperitoneal fat. Follow those areas downward from section to section and study the kidneys, noting the initial appearance of their upper poles in B and the doughnut-shaped parenchyma around the upper calices in C before the hilum has been reached. The two kidneys are at nearly the same level in this patient; normally the left kidney is higher. The two hila are sectioned in E, where the kidney is seen as a crescent of parenchyma curving around the anteriorly directed hila. There is a tiny retention cyst in the posterior parenchyma of the right kidney in F.

Now find the inferior vena cava in F, just anterior to the vertebra a little to the right of the midline. If you follow it upward you can see it in C and D clearly receiving the left renal vein, which normally crosses in front of the aorta from left to right at this level. We are just above the pancreas. Note that anterior to the left renal vein in D you can see the splenic vein joined by the gastric veins forming the portal vein. In sections A and B the vena cava moves nearer the hilum of the liver. The dragon-shaped mass of the pancreas is seen first in section E, its tail extending toward the hilum of the spleen. Because the tail turns upward, the pancreas looks shorter in section F. See if you can figure out the identity of the two white (?vascular) structures just medial and posterior to the head of the pancreas in E and F. (There are matching labeled diagrams on the next page spread in case you need to check your findings.)

Figure 14-17. Series of normal computerized tomograms of the upper abdomen.

The two white structures in E and F are the superior mesenteric artery and vein. The artery is the smaller of the two.

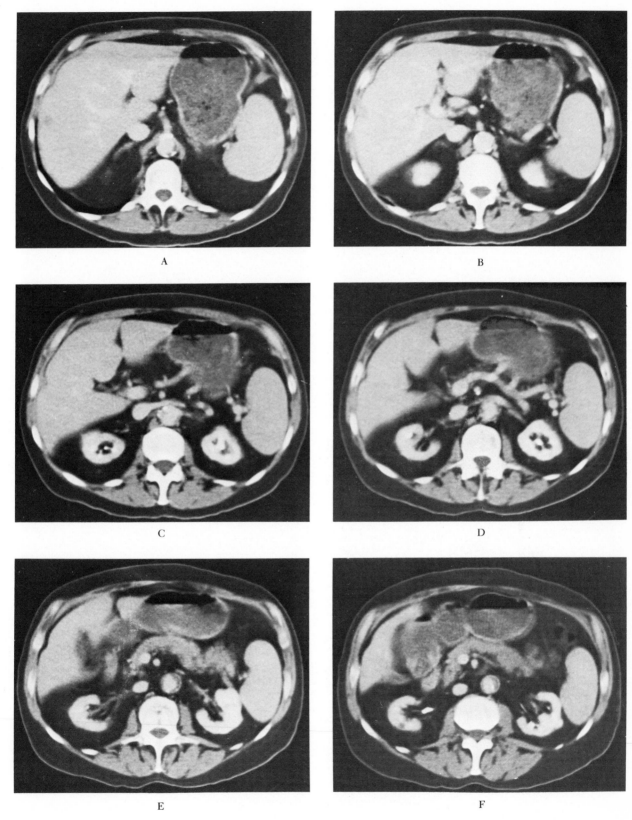

Diagrams to Match CT Scans in
Figure 14-17 (reprinted on opposite page)

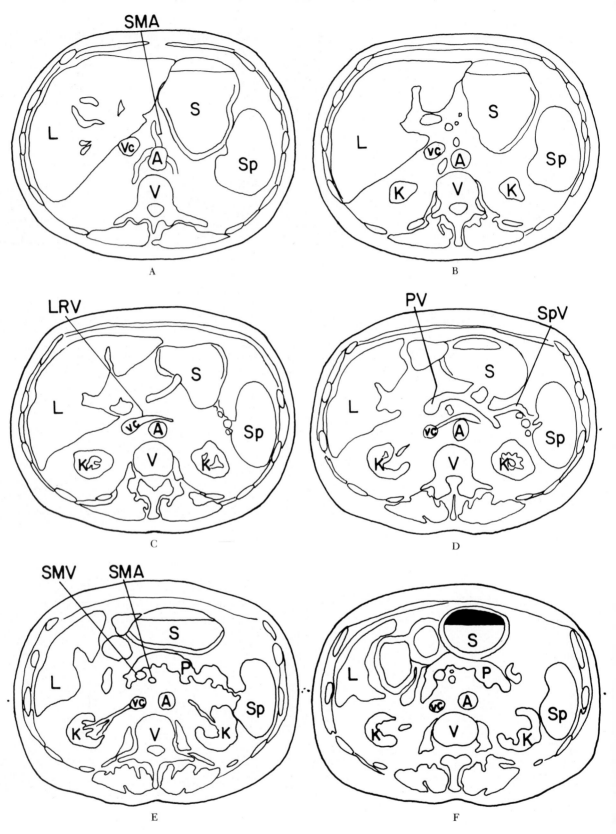

Figure 14-17 Reprinted

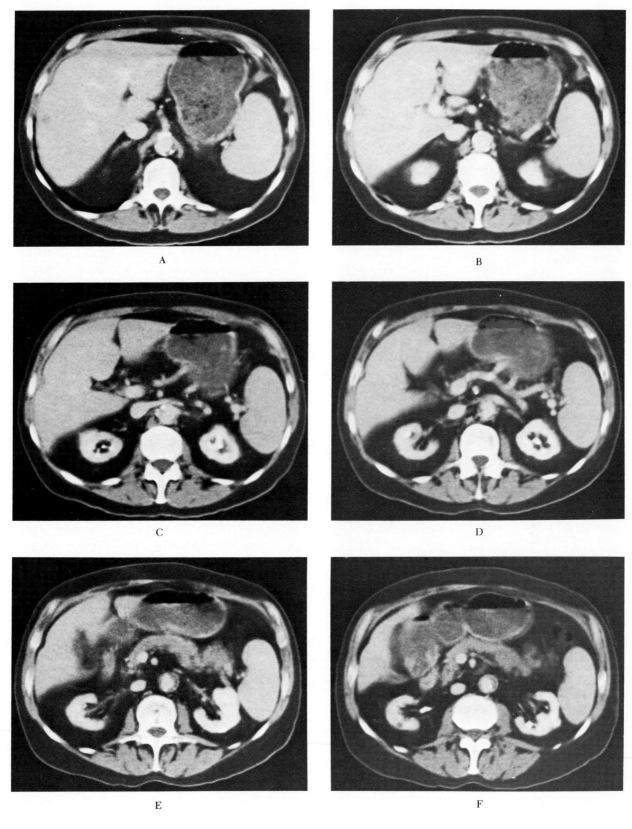

A

B

C

D

E

F

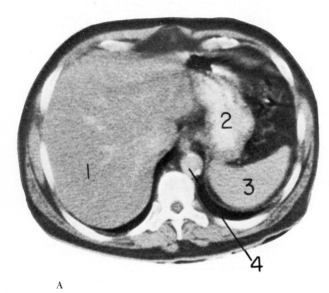

A

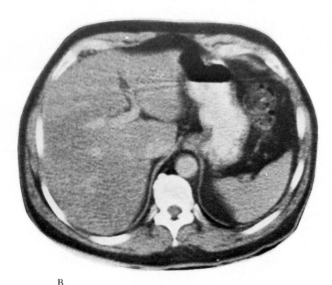

B

Now here is another series of normal CT scans for you to practice your skill on, studying all six cuts and identifying serially the liver, spleen, kidneys and their calices, aorta, vena cava, left renal vein, and pancreas.

Decide whether intravenous or gastrointestinal contrast medium has been given this patient by observing the density of kidney calices and stomach contents. Can you distinguish the head of the pancreas from the descending second portion of the duodenum in D? The superior mesenteric artery leaves the aorta anteriorly just above the point where the left renal vein crosses to the right. Can you find them both?

In this patient you can recognize the adrenal glands embedded in fat in sections C and D. The left adrenal looks like a flying bird and lies to the left of the aorta and posterior to the tail of the pancreas in this patient. The right is always seen just posterior to the vena cava as in C and D.

Still newer imaging techniques exist, proliferate, and are constantly compared, one with the other, in the current literature. I will be mentioning some of them at the very end of the last chapter.

Figure 14-18. Series of computerized tomograms on another patient. Use as an exercise to test your progress. You can check the numbers if you are in doubt as to the identity of any structures imaged.

(1) Liver
(2) Stomach with water-soluble contrast medium
(3) Spleen
(4) Aorta
(5) Kidneys
(6) Duodenum
(7) Head of pancreas
(8) Left adrenal
(9) Right adrenal
(10) Superior mesenteric artery
(11) Left renal vein
(12) Vena cava
(13) Diaphragmatic crura

228

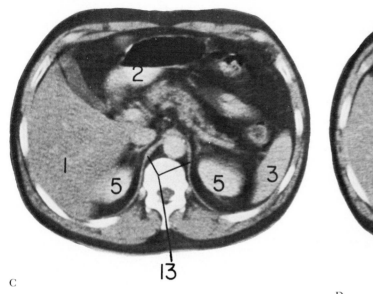

C

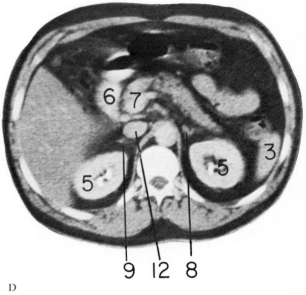

D

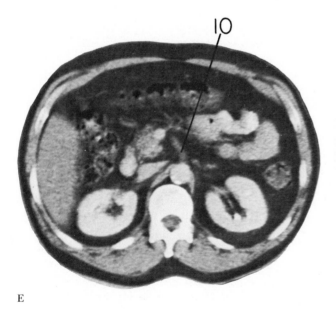

E

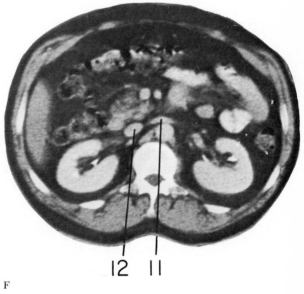

F

CHAPTER 15 Special Deductions Possible from Excretory and Secretory Contrast Studies: The Choice of Procedures

The Gallbladder

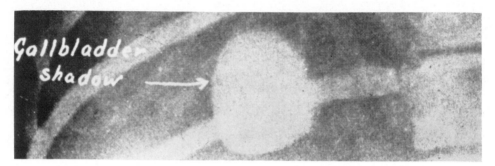

Figure 15-1. The first successful oral cholecystogram.

The discovery of *cholecystography* reads like a detective story, and the details of it are worth giving here because they illustrate so effectively the peculiar combination of intellectual alertness, hard work, and fortunate accident which so often produces a revolutionary new discovery.

When Warren Cole was in training as a surgical resident at the Barnes Hospital in St. Louis between 1921 and 1926, he decided, with Evarts Graham, to investigate the possibilities of producing a radiopaque drug which would be excreted in the bile. Abel and Rowntree, while searching for a cathartic which could be given hypodermically, had demonstrated that phenoltetrachlorphthalein was excreted almost entirely in the bile. A few years later Rous and McMaster had shown that the normal gallbladder concentrates bile eight to ten times by absorbing water from it. These facts, together with the knowledge that halogenated compounds are very radiopaque because of their high molecular weights, persuaded Cole and Graham that excretory roentgen visualization of the gallbladder might be feasible.

The first halogenated phthalein compound they were able to obtain from the Mallinckrodt Chemical Works was phenoltetrachlorphthalein. But the atomic weight of chlorine is only 35.5, compared with 80 for bromine and 127 for iodine. For this reason they planned early in their experiments to work with the soluble salts of bromine and iodine compounds. Accordingly, week after week they tried injecting into dogs and rabbits the sodium, calcium, and strontium salts of tetrabromophenolphthalein and tetraiodophenolphthalein.

They injected over 200 animals without obtaining a single shadow of the gallbladder. The animals were injected early in the morning and the radiographs made late in the afternoon, to allow time for the excretion and concentration of the opaque-loaded bile. Finally, a very dense shadow of what appeared to be the gallbladder *was* obtained in one dog, but the findings could not be repeated.

Discouraged, Cole was in the radiology department one afternoon studying that single positive examination (Figure 15-1) to be certain that the shadow could not represent a bone or something dense that the dog had swallowed. A radiologist saw the film and commented at once that it *had* to be the shadow of the gallbladder and that he believed it could only be a matter of time before the method would be used in humans.

With renewed conviction Cole then interviewed the attendant in the animal house, asking him whether anything different had been done for the dog in question on the day the posi-

230

tive test had been obtained. The caretaker denied that anything unusual had happened, but something about the manner of his reply prompted Cole to press him further, and he finally admitted reluctantly that he had forgotten to feed that dog at noon that day. Expecting a reprimand, the man was startled to have his hand shaken and his back slapped in a vigorous and grateful manner by Cole, who had realized at once that all the disappointing negative examinations were probably due to the fact that those gallbladders had emptied prematurely in response to the single daily feeding. *The dog who accidentally fasted all day had retained the concentrated opaque bile in his gallbladder until late afternoon when the films were made.* After this the studies progressed rapidly, and today, of course, the patient being prepared for oral cholecystography fasts overnight.

It would be unrealistic not to add to this miraculous story that years of investigative work subsequently went into the preparation of contrast substances that had minimal toxic side effects, could be given safely by vein or by mouth, and would produce roentgen shadows of the gallbladder more and more reliably. Today oral cholecystography is arranged in advance, the radiologist supplying the patient with the particular drug to be used, and the dose calculated according to body weight. The patient, fasting after a light supper, swallows the tablets of opaque drug the evening before the examination. Cleansing cathartics are not used because they interfere with the absorption of the contrast substance from the small bowel. Early in the morning the patient, still fasting, reports to the radiologist, and films are made in a prone oblique position (that is, with the gallbladder as close as possible to the film and not superimposed on the ribs).

The absence of a gallbladder shadow on the films obtained does not necessarily imply depressed function. A number of factors still influence the successful resolution of the test, just as

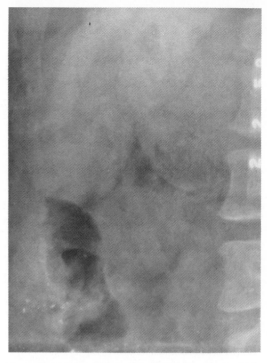

Figure 15-2. Faint shadow of the gallbladder obtained after a single dose of cholecystographic radiopaque medium. The gallbladder here lies just above the air in the right colon and superimposed on the tip of the eleventh rib.

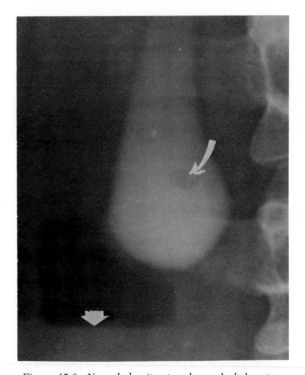

Figure 15-3. Normal density, two-day oral cholecystography. (Curved arrow indicates filling defect which does not fall to the fundus of the gallbladder in this erect film. Conclusion: tumor, not stone.)

231

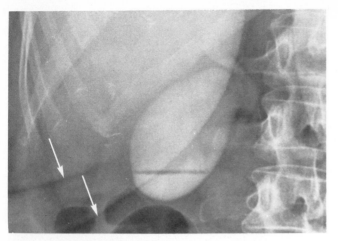

Figure 15-4. Oral cholecystogram with satisfactory visualization of the gallbladder, *which showed no abnormality and no filling defects in the usual prone films.* Here in a standing film, small cholesterin stones float as a lucent layer tangentially seen, finding their own level. (Arrows indicate soft-tissue shadows of breast and abdominal fatty fold.)

they did in Cole's original experiments. The patient may not, after all, have taken the tablets as he was instructed to do. If he took them he may not actually have fasted. If he indeed refrained from food, he may have had some nausea or diarrhea in reaction to the drug, preventing its retention in the small bowel long enough to allow for absorption. For these reasons the fallibility of the test is checked customarily today in negative cases by reexamination a day later. The patient adheres to a very light diet overnight, takes a *second measured dose* (*not* a double dose, which can be dangerous), and the following morning a second set of films is obtained.

A patient suspected of chronic gallbladder disease for some time may have been on a low-fat regimen for months and will begin the period of the cholecystographic examination with a gallbladder already filled with inspissated bile. It may even be necessary to maintain such a patient on a high-fat diet for a time in order to empty the organ of old bile before cholecystography is attempted.

Failure to visualize the gallbladder after properly performed oral cholecystography on two successive days may mean, then, that one of several different pathologic conditions is present. It *may* mean that liver function is depressed and the drug is not being excreted. (Cholecystography is contraindicated in frankly jaundiced patients, and above a serum bilirubin of 3 mg/100 ml it is usually considered that the test will be unsatisfactory.) *Or* the absence of a gallbladder shadow may mean that faulty absorption in the small bowel has interfered with the arrival of the opaque substance in the bloodstream.

Or there may be any of several sorts of obstruction present. Obstruction may be *gastrointestinal* (pyloric or duodenal), so that small-bowel absorption is delayed or interfered with. Or it may be *biliary*, in which bile does not reach the gallbladder to be concentrated (and visible—bile as first excreted is too dilute for resolution on the radiograph). Obstruction of the cystic duct, for example by a stone, will prevent bile from entering the gallbladder and there will be no visualization. Obstruction of the common bile duct (as by a stone lodged at the ampulla or an intraductal tumor) or compression from without (as in pancreatic carcinoma) will cause jaundice and consequent failure to visualize even a normal gallbladder.

Finally, chronic cholecystitis may cause nonvisualization because functioning of the organ is affected. It is important to remember that even when the gallbladder *is* successfully visualized, disease of that structure may be present. The gallbladders of patients with chronic cholecystitis are often successfully visualized for years before cholecystectomy is done, although the shadow obtained is faint and may show filling defects which represent calculi. In sum, then, *after properly performed oral cholecystography (with a repeat dose) nonvisualization of the gallbladder must be taken very seriously, but the problem may not be in the gallbladder itself. Even when there is visualization, mild chronic cholecystitis may be present.*

In patients in whom it is important to visualize the bile ducts, *intravenous cholangiography* may be carried out. The opaques used for intravenous cholangiography are more likely to cause reactions than those used in oral cholecystography, and the two procedures are not at all interchangeable. In fact, the gallbladder is poorly seen during intravenous cholangiography, while the ducts are usually not seen in oral cholecystograms. Intravenous cholangiography should be planned only after consultation with a radiologist and is used much less often than the oral method of study. It can only be performed in the x-ray department, as plain tomography is required, and it cannot be carried out successfully on a patient with a bilirubin above 2 milligrams.

Oral cholecystography therefore may give you information about function, but in most patients with suspected biliary disease the *newer imaging modalities* have now contributed such important additional diagnostic help that you will use them more regularly.

In a patient with upper abdominal pain whom you suspect of having *acute cholecystitis*, today you would employ isotope studies initially (PI-PIDA) and not attempt to visualize the gallbladder by cholecystography. In acute cholecysititis the cholecystographic contrast substance is reabsorbed at once through the hyperemic diseased gallbladder wall, and often also the cystic duct is obstructed, so that nonvisualization is the rule. However, in acute cholecystitis HIDA or PIPIDA scanning can usually show that the gallbladder does not visualize, indicating obstruction of the cystic duct. This can also be confirmed by ultrasonography which, in the hands of an experienced operator, may show stones and a thickened gallbladder wall.

In suspected *chronic cholecystitis* the two-dose oral cholecystogram is certainly indicated, but with poor visualization one often cannot settle the question of stones. Ultrasonography, so helpful in determining the presence or absence of stones in both the gallbladder and the common duct, tells you nothing about gallbladder function, on the other hand. The two procedures ought therefore to be used in tandem in this type of patient.

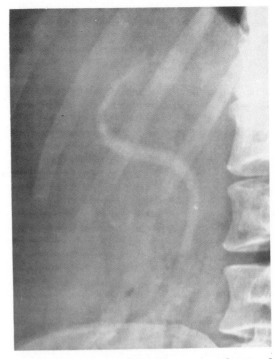

Figure 15-5. Intravenous cholangiogram, a visualization of the common bile duct in a patient whose gallbladder has been removed. Contrast substance administered intravenously.

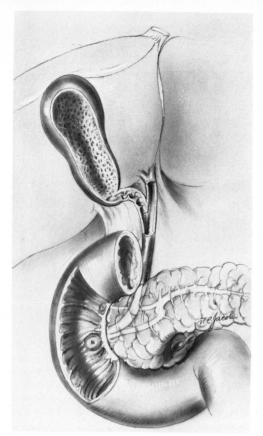

Figure 15-6. The biliary tree and pancreas. (Gallbladder reflected upward.)

The Biliary Tree and Pancreas

Great advances in the study of patients with obstructive jaundice have been made since the development of sonography and computerized tomography. In a patient with chemistries indicating a probability that jaundice is obstructive, the first approach should be sonography, which reliably indicates dilated biliary radicles in the liver, as you have seen in Chapter 14. CT also demonstrates dilated biliary channels, but should not be used until sonography has been tried, and then only because air in the gut may make the sonographic study impossible.

As soon as the presence of dilated ducts in the liver is established, *percutaneous transhepatic cholangiography* (PTC) is the next procedure in order. This is carried out by cannulating the dilated biliary tree via a fine needle introduced directly into the liver through the skin. As soon as bile is returned, one can be sure the needle tip is in one of the bile ducts; a water-soluble contrast medium is injected, filling the biliary tree down to the point of obstruction.

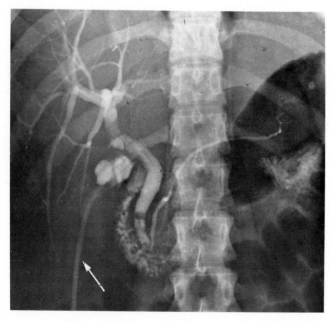

Figure 15-7. Operative cholangiogram, a procedure which has been used following cholecystectomy to visualize the biliary tree and determine whether there is free emptying of bile into the small bowel. Arrow indicates the catheter through which the contrast substance is being injected. It is attached to a T-tube placed within the common duct. There is some reflux into the bed of the gallbladder. The tree of hepatic radicles is visible as well as the common duct, and there is reflux filling of the pancreatic duct behind the dark, air-filled stomach. The duodenal loop is beginning to fill. Round radiolucencies in the lower part of the common duct could represent retained calculi.

234

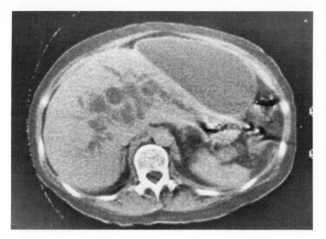 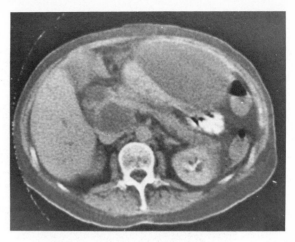

Figure 15-8 (above left) and Figure 15-9 (above right). Two CT scans of the upper abdomen on a patient with obstructive jaundice. (See text.) Figure 15-10 (right). Same patient. Percutaneous transhepatic cholangiography showing stones in the lower common bile duct.

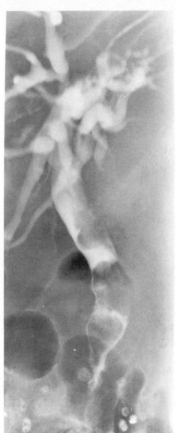

In Figures 15-8 and 15-9 you see CT studies carried out on a female patient of 65 who had been hospitalized for evaluation of jaundice and a history of bouts of abdominal pain over the previous 20 years. Ultrasonography (not illustrated here) indicated dilated bile ducts as well as the presence of pancreatic cysts. CT scans were made for the greater precision of information offered. Note the dilated biliary radicles in Figure 15-8 and the pancreatic pseudocysts in Figure 15-9, a lower cut. The patient's long history of pain suggested either cholecystitis with the passage of gallstones or pancreatitis or both. (She was not an alcoholic.) Her development of obstructive jaundice was worrisome and could have been due to stones in the common bile duct or to the development of carcinoma in the head of the pancreas.

The next step in this patient was, logically, a percutaneous transhepatic cholangiogram, which you see in Figure 15-10. There are several large filling defects seen in the dilated common bile duct. At surgery several large stones were removed successfully and the pancreatic pseudocyst arising from the tail of the pancreas was drained externally.

235

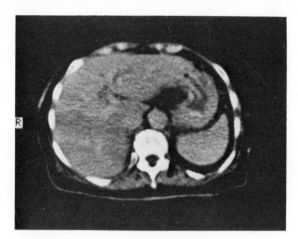

Figure 15-11

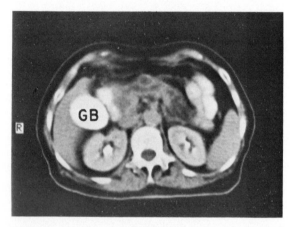

Figure 15-12. Made after P.T.C.; contrast has now filled gall bladder.

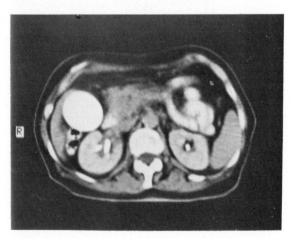

Figure 15-13

In the patient in Figure 15-11, who also had obstructive jaundice, dilated bile ducts are seen demonstrated by CT (sonography having proved not feasible because of ileus). In Figure 15-12, a cut made slightly lower down, there is contrast material in the gallbladder and also in the duodenum. One can identify an enlarged pancreatic head, especially taking together the two adjoining cuts in Figures 15-12 and 15-13. In this same patient a PTC (Figure 15-14) shows an abrupt, blunt, cutoff at the lower end of the dilated common bile duct and no filling defects. At surgery the suspected carcinoma of the head of the pancreas was confirmed. Now look back at the head of the pancreas in the other patient in Figure 15-9: it too is enlarged, but clearly by a *low-density* pseudocyst, not a solid mass.

Study of the inferior segment of the common bile duct below the point of obstruction can be carried out by direct injection of contrast medium through the ampulla of Vater. This is accomplished by fluoroscopically maneuvered fiberoptic cannulation of the ampulla and is called *endoscopic retrograde cholangiopancreatography* (ERCP). The pancreatic duct is usually also visualized.

In pancreatitis a large lumpy pancreas is seen by both sonography and CT, and pseudocysts are readily indicated by both procedures. *Selective arteriography* also has its place in study of the pancreas, but none of the imaging methods discussed has succeeded in producing reliable diagnostic information in pancreatic carcinoma. These various imaging studies cannot be thought of as competitive with one another, but should be used in an intelligently integrated manner.

236

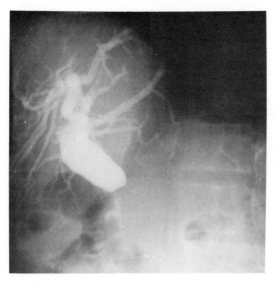

Figure 15-14. Percutaneous transhepatic cholangiogram (PTC) in patient shown on opposite page. (See text.)

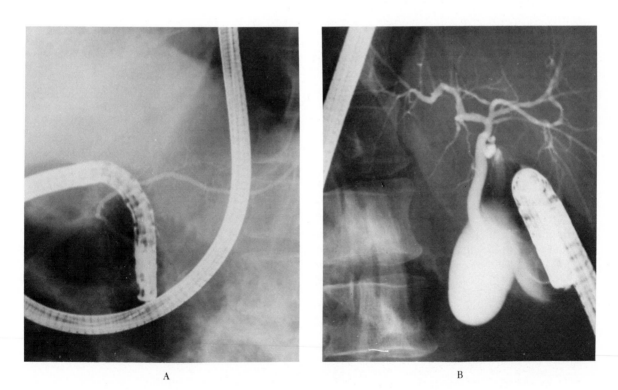

A

B

Figure 15-15. Endoscopic retrograde cholangiopancreatography (ERCP). A: The pancreatic duct visualized. B: The common bile duct visualized.

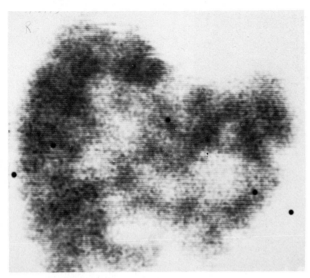

Figure 15-16. Isotope liver scan showing metastases from colon carcinoma.

The Spleen

The spleen can be studied by sonography, CT, isotopes, and angiography; cysts or subcapsular hematoma following trauma can both be readily diagnosed.

The Adrenal Glands

The adrenal glands are very successfully studied by CT, which has evolved as the method of choice in approaching adrenal mass problems. As you have seen, the normal adrenals can readily be imaged provided the patient has an adequate supply of fat around them. Location of both endocrine and nonendocrine tumors of the adrenals can be made with reasonable certainty if they are larger than 1 centimeter.

Evaluation of the Liver

The initial radiologic evaluation of the liver should begin with *radionuclide isotope scanning* (with technetium sulfacolloid). As you have seen, ultrasonography is able to demonstrate dilated bile ducts and hepatic cysts. CT confirms these findings in the patient in whom sonography has been difficult or impossible because of air in the gut. Intrahepatic masses can be studied by CT with and without enhancement after their presence has been indicated by isotope scans. Hepatic abscesses can be demonstrated as fluid-filled (low-density) areas in the liver parenchyma by either CT or sonography, and drained externally under control offered by either modality. Angiography, once widely used for liver problems, is now employed less routinely, as it offers only data on the vascular bed.

The Retroperitoneal Nodes

CT has become the method of choice in studying the retroperitoneal nodes in metastatic cancer or lymphoma. CT can determine the size of nodes very accurately, but cannot determine their microscopic involvement, of course. Nodes more than 1.5 centimeters in size are said to be enlarged. In "staging" Hodgkin's lymphoma, therefore, the CT scan should be made first. If it shows enlarged nodes, a lymphangiogram need not be carried out. This is a very uncomfortable procedure for the patient, but it does show involvement of normal-sized nodes. In staging one determines the extent of the disease in order to plan the treatment.

The Aorta and Vena Cava

Investigation of the aorta in determining the presence of aneurysm should begin with sonography, but when this becomes impossible because of the interference of intestinal gas, CT can be used. Angiography must follow in order to determine the size of the remaining lumen and the relation of the aneurysm to the aortic branches, particularly the renal arteries.

Thrombosis in the inferior vena cava is detected readily by sonography and CT has been employed, although *inferior vena cavography* with angiographic contrast material is still the best approach.

The Pelvis

Although CT may be used very successfully in men to determine the spread of bladder and prostate cancers, especially extension beyond the wall of the bladder, it is not a modality that can be used in females (because it employs ionizing radiation) except in pelvic malignancies, where CT gives valuable information to the radiotherapist. In most diagnostic pelvic problems in the female, sonography is the method of choice.

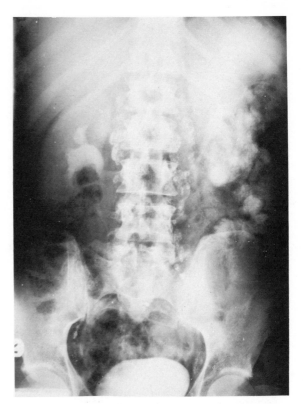

Figure 15-17. Patient with Hodgkin's disease. Both lymphangiography and intravenous urography have been carried out.

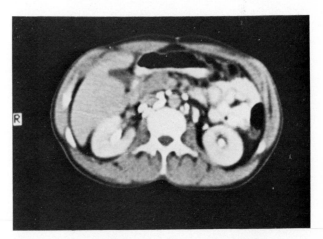

Figure 15-18. Same patient. CT scan, done after lymphangiogram, shows dense, enlarged periaortic lymph nodes. (Both oral and intravenous contrast medium have been given.)

239

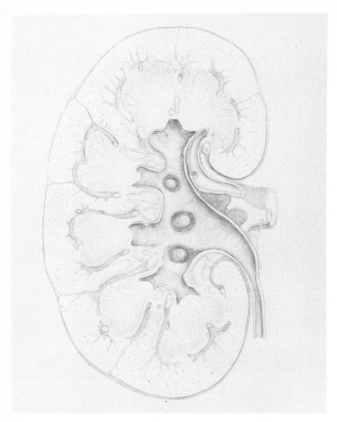

Figure 15-19. The anatomy of the kidney in coronal section.

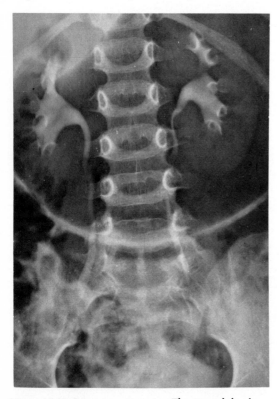

Figure 15-20. Intravenous urogram. The stomach has been distended with air to displace confusing bowel shadows.

The Kidney

Techniques available for study

Intravenous urography. The discovery in the late 1920s of radiopaque chemicals that are selectively excreted by the kidney revolutionized urologic diagnosis, and over the years it has become possible to study radiographically a great many conditions formerly diagnosed only at surgery. With few exceptions, the study of kidney disease should begin with the excretory study.

However, the intravenous urogram is to be considered a morphologic study rather than a functional study, for one cannot equate the density of contrast substance with overall kidney function. Kidney function is a highly complex matter and consists of many interrelated processes: glomerular filtration, tubular excretion, and reabsorption of water, electrolytes, and other substances. The density of contrast substance in the draining structures and parenchyma of the kidney must be interpreted in the light of any variation in the *fluid flow through the kidney* as well as fluctuations in renal physiology.

The drugs most widely used are excreted by the kidney almost entirely in the glomerular filtrate. This means that within less than a minute after intravenous injection enough opaque substance is present in the glomeruli and tubules within the renal parenchyma to give an appreciable whitening to the kidney shadow on an abdominal film. This has been called the "nephrogram phase" of urography and is the proper time to observe the size and shape of the kidney. The rule in studying the morphology of the kidneys on plain films and nephrograms is that *the normal length of the kidney is 3.7 times the height of the second lumbar vertebra in that patient.*

240

The calices, pelves, ureters, and bladder are seen in sequence following the nephrogram. The draining structures may be seen to fill from two minutes after the injection at the earliest; the filling of these structures increases to a peak within a few more minutes and then gradually fades. The entire length of the ureters is not normally seen filled on any single film, since they are constantly being swept by peristaltic waves. After 20 to 30 minutes, normally, the collecting system will be seen too faintly for further study, and all the visible opaque will be collected in the urinary bladder. Of course the kidneys continue to excrete the remaining opaque until the bloodstream is cleared.

The density of the opaque material seen in the collecting system will be decreased if there is low ureteral obstruction and the ureters are already filled with nonopaque urine at the start of the examination. The contrast substance will also be delayed in its time of appearance. In the presence of ureteral obstruction the faint excretion of opaque medium will be seen only after a lapse of time, and the study accordingly must be carried on much longer than the time conventionally devoted to intravenous urography. Much information is available from such late films made after several hours.

The *conventional intravenous urogram* commences with a preliminary plain film, which is always examined by the radiologist before the injection of contrast material, screening for calcification or stones which might be obscured by the contrast. (Ninety percent of kidney stones are radiopaque and dense enough to be seen on the plain film.) Then films are made at intervals, each being reviewed by the radiologist until he is satisfied that the examination has been completed for that patient. Thus every intravenous urogram is essentially a custom-tailored study. If there seems to be delay in excretion, the study will be prolonged. If the abnormality revealed on the first films suggests the need, additional special views may be obtained while the contrast material is still present.

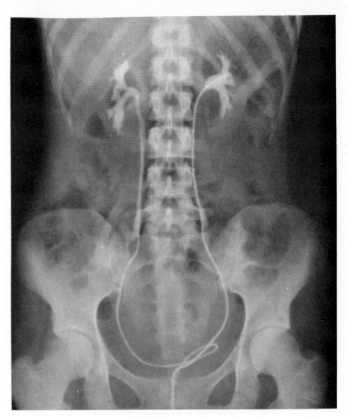

Figure 15-21. Retrograde pyelogram. Note catheters introduced into the ureters via a cystoscope, which has been removed.

Pyelography (either *retrograde*, in which visualization of the urinary collecting system is achieved via a cystoscope, ureteral catherization, and injection of contrast medium, or *antegrade*, via percutaneous puncture of the collecting system) can be done, but is less and less frequently used since it cannot be considered a nontraumatic procedure and affords no information with regard to the parenchyma of the kidney itself.

Sonography is extremely useful and widely employed in the evaluation of kidney disease, and has become the method of choice in screening for obstructive nephropathy (especially in renal failure) and in differentiating kidney cyst from solid tumor.

Computerized tomography and *angiography* are also employed in indicated situations, and *renally excreted isotopes* remain the best approach to assaying renal function.

241

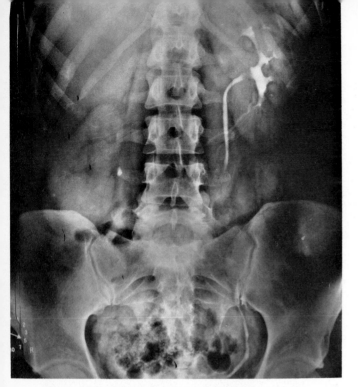

Figure 15-22. Patient who presented with hematuria had a history of ureteral calculi and now has acute right urinary tract obstruction.

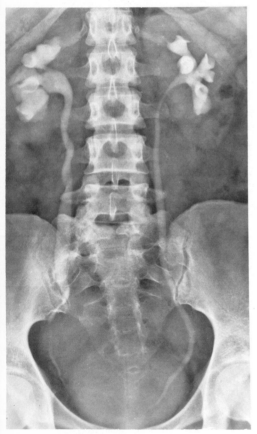

Figure 15-23. Early hydronephrosis due to pelvic masses.

Obstruction

Fluid flow out of the kidney may be prevented in numerous ways but the commonest is certainly *ureteral calculus*. Since 90 percent of renal calculi are radiopaque, the chance of recognizing the presence of one on the initial plain film of an intravenous urogram is excellent, and the study for stone should begin there. With one ureter obstructed by stone and non–opaque-containing urine backed up above it, a delay in the appearance of contrast medium in that kidney is to be expected; sometimes several hours are needed before the nephrogram finally appears. This has been called the "late white kidney" of acute renal obstruction. Ultimately opacification of the ureter down to the point of the obstruction will occur as excreted opaque mixes with retained urine. The obstructed kidney can also be readily screened by ultrasound, since the fluid-filled calices on that side will produce an echo-free center for that kidney on the sonogram.

It is surprising that any function remains in a chronically obstructed kidney; in advanced hydronephrosis the kidney will be converted into a thin-walled sac with only a slender rim of renal parenchyma remaining. The capacity of such damaged kidneys still to excrete urine containing the opaque medium and to concentrate it by reabsorption of water may be clearly demonstrated by making films over a prolonged period of time.

Figure 15-24 is a late film during urography which shows bilateral obstruction in an infant with a low congenital defect in drainage of both ureters. A sonogram would show bilateral dilated (echo-free) pelves, of course. Figures 15-25A and B show early and late urograms in another child with chronic unilateral high obstruction on the left at the ureteropelvic junction. In both children the cortex of the hydronephrotic kidney was a thin shell. After surgery to correct an obstructing aberrant artery, the second child's left kidney regained a normal appearance.

Obstruction to outflow of urine from the kidney is of course only one way in which the fluid flow through the kidney may be decreased. Interference to the blood supply to the kidney also decreases fluid flow through that kidney, and if this occurs on one side, the other kidney takes over the workload and excretes a much larger amount of urine than normal.

The obvious example is complete obstruction of a renal artery with total infarction of one kidney. This does occur, and an excretory urogram will show no opaque medium whatever on the ischemic side. Lesser degrees of interference with the arterial supply result in proportion to the degree of obstruction, and urine flow is slower, the urine remaining longer in the tubules before reaching the renal pelvis. This allows more time for water reabsorption, so that a smaller amount of more concentrated urine is to be seen in the draining structures of a kidney whose arterial supply has been partially cut off.

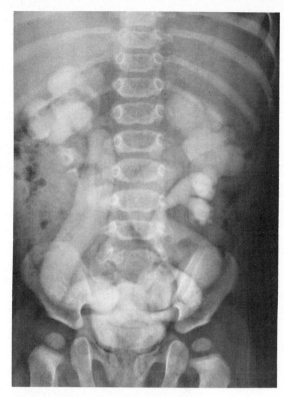

Figure 15-24. Advanced hydronephrosis in a child with congenitally defective drainage.

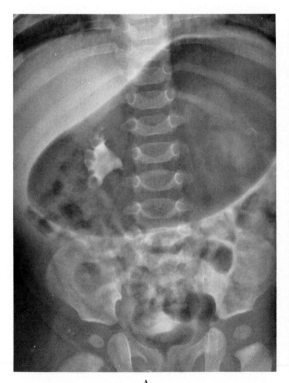

A

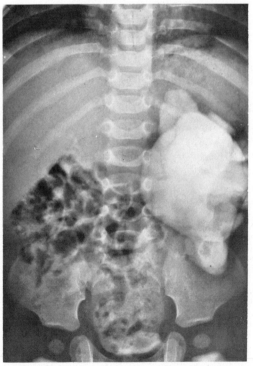

B

Figure 15-25. Intravenous urography, early (A) and four hours later (B), in a child with a palpable left abdominal mass which proved to be hydronephrosis due to obstruction just below the ureteropelvic junction.

243

In sum, then, *in studying plain films and intravenous urograms* you must carefully assay the size and shape of the two kidneys, the outline of parenchyma for each and its homogeneity, the appearance of the collecting structures and their rate of filling and emptying. *Failure of the kidney to visualize* should make you ask whether there is evidence for—

(1) No blood getting into the kidney (renal artery compromised)
(2) No blood getting out (renal vein thrombosis)
(3) Blocked drainage (such as a ureteral stone), or
(4) Destruction of the nephron system.

There are several ways in which the arterial supply to the kidney can be compromised other than by embolus. Rarely, the lumen may be reduced by extrinsic pressure. More often, intimal proliferation or sclerotic placques narrow the lumen. The restriction of arterial supply may affect the main renal artery or any of its branches, the entire kidney becoming ischemic —or only a part of it. The entire excretory capacity may be proportionally reduced—or only a small part of it.

Ischemia of renal tissue with increased excretion of renin has been shown to be etiologically related to the occurrence of some forms of hypertension. When such a condition can be demonstrated by renal arteriography and bilateral renal vein renin assay in persons who retain good function in the other kidney, hypertension may sometimes be cured or ameliorated by nephrectomy or reconstructive arterial surgery. This is true mainly in young hypertensives with renal artery constriction, and in their salvage the radiologist/angiographer certainly plays an important role.

The actual place for radiologic procedures in the workup of the patient with hypertension is important for every physician to understand clearly, since most of the hypertensive patients he will see in a lifetime of practice will have essential hypertension and normal IV urograms. Only very rarely will he see a patient with renovascular hypertension, and then he will have to eliminate other forms of hypertension before ordering selective angiography. Moreover, most of the other causes for hypertension are not diagnosed radiologically. Coarctation of the aorta *should* be recognized from unequal limb pressures on physical exam, and endocrine-related adrenal hypertension is a biochemical diagnosis. Although adrenal masses can be studied by CT and adrenal venography, those procedures are carried out subsequent to the laboratory evidence.

Certainly the physician ought not to make a routine of ordering urography on his middle-aged female patients with hypertension of some duration who respond well to antihypertensive medication. In the rare patient who is young and has suddenly become hypertensive, in whom coarctation and adrenal abnormality have been excluded so that renovascular hypertension is a strong possibility, it is renal arteriography the patient needs. Time and money are wasted in doing urography on that patient, especially when you consider that an IV urogram is a by-product of the angiogram, anyway. In such patients, after careful evaluation an alternative to surgical revision may be one form of *interventional radiology* (percutaneous transluminal angioplasty). In that nonoperative procedure the radiologist expands the stenosed vessel by pressure from within via a special catheter under fluoroscopic guidance. There is often a dramatic return to the normotensive state.

244

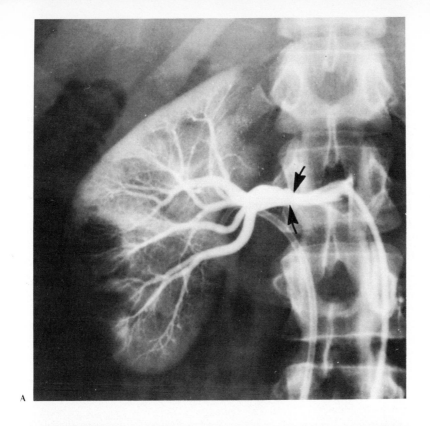

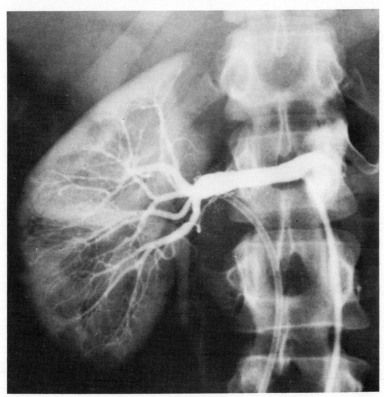

Figure 15-26. Interventional radiology in treating hypertension in renal artery stenosis. A (above): Selective renal angiogram in a young woman, 20, with severe hypertension thought due to renal ischemia (all other causes excluded). Arrow indicates area of stenosis of the renal artery. B (below): Repeat study, after balloon angioplasty, shows restoration of lumen caliber. Patient normotensive, off all medication.

Infection

The physician ought not to request intravenous urography on adult patients with urinary tract infections. Of course, the indications for urography in all patients with flank pain suggesting stone and those with hematuria are perfectly clear, but in the adult patient with only urinary tract infection no abnormal urographic findings can be expected and the examination is futile. Children with pus in their urine always need urography, on the other hand.

Most kidneys chronically infected from childhood do show important morphologic changes, demonstrable either on urography with tomograms or with CT. These consist of an overall decrease in size of the affected kidney and/or localized thinning of the parenchyma where pitting and scarring are to be seen on the surface of the surgical specimen. When you examine a plain film, always make a habit of estimating kidney size and shape and trace its normal smooth, plump outline.

Perinephric abscesses are easy to diagnose by both ultrasound and CT, and one of these procedures should be carried out as soon as the diagnosis has been suggested clinically.

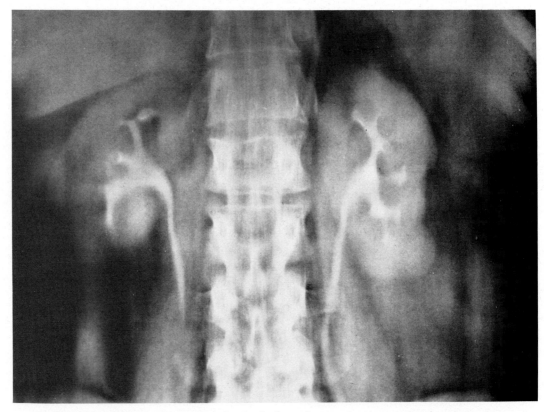

Figure 15-27. Tomogram during urography clearly shows the irregular scarring of pyelonephritis. Note that both kidneys are small. (Rule: normal length of the kidney should be 3.7 times the height of the patient's second lumbar vertebral body.) There is also a striking irregular scar indenting the parenchyma of the lateral margin of the left kidney.

Renal masses

Because the kidney secretes fluid, it is subject to the development of retention cysts of various kinds. Although these do not fill with excreted opaque because they are walled-off collections of fluid, their presence in the kidney distorts the parenchyma and the draining structures on urography in a characteristic fashion. Even more precise is the recognition of cystic renal masses by either sonography or CT. A renal mass discovered clinically or by urography should be studied at once, with sonography as the less invasive procedure, CT being used only when sonography is impossible. Polycystic kidneys have so classic and pathognomonic an appearance on both sonogram and CT scan that those procedures are used for screening in families of patients with polycystic disease.

In the patient with no hematuria, determination by sonography that a renal mass is cystic (with good through transmission, a sharp far wall, and no interior echoes) is usually sufficient evidence to terminate the study. Few cysts require treatment. Cyst puncture can be carried out for confirmation; obtaining a clear aspirate proves the diagnosis. However, the patient with hematuria must have additional diagnostic procedures (CT, aspiration, angiography) before the diagnosis of simple cyst can be accepted.

If, on the other hand, sonography indicates a renal mass not classically a cyst (for example, poor through transmission, an indefinite margin, or interior echoes), the patient is a surgical candidate and renal angiography is usually done in order to inform the surgeon as to the vascular anatomy of that kidney.

In masses which seem cystic at sonography but have thick walls on CT, one must suspect a tumor that is partially necrotic. Puncture can be carried out for tissue diagnosis, and if the fluid is bloody or dark the patient ought to be explored, since tumors are known occasionally to arise in the wall of a benign cyst, and cytologic study of aspirated fluid does give some false negative results.

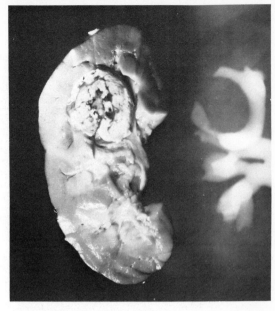

Figure 15-28. Sectioned specimen and radiograph of the same specimen injected with a radiopaque material before sectioning, to show the caliceal deformity produced by such a tumor mass. Small hypernephroma. Sonography, CT, and arteriography would all give important additional information.

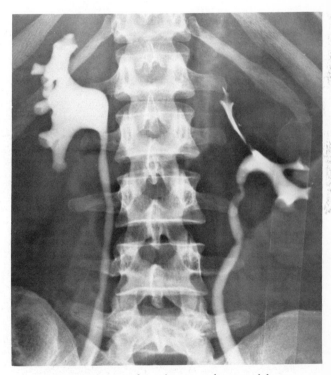

Figure 15-29. Retrograde pyelogram, catheters withdrawn. Note stretching distortion of the upper and middle calices on the left around a "mass," which proved at sonography to be a cyst.

247

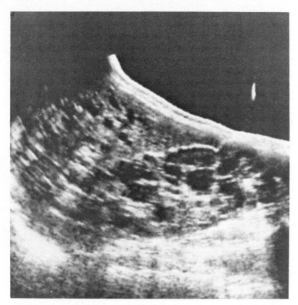

Figure 15-30. Supine longitudinal sonogram on a patient with cystic disease of both kidneys and liver. (White blip made to show location of umbilicus.)

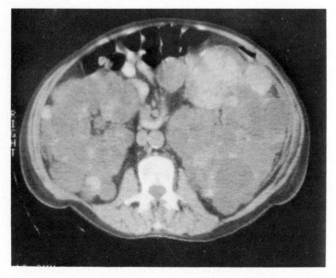

Figure 15-31. CT scan in a patient with polycystic kidneys.

Figure 15-32. Workup of a patient with renal mass: cyst. The patient, age 58, had a large palpable mass on the right, thought at first to be the liver. However, her hematuria justified an excretory urogram early in her workup and, as you see in A, the right renal draining structures are distorted and pushed upward in the abdomen by a large renal mass. Ultrasonography, the correct next procedure (B) shows a large sonolucent mass with excellent through transmission, clearly a cyst. Cyst puncture showed perfectly clear fluid. No further workup was necessary, but a CT scan was done (C) and shows the right kidney parenchyma stretched around the cyst, whose attenuation coefficient was that of water.

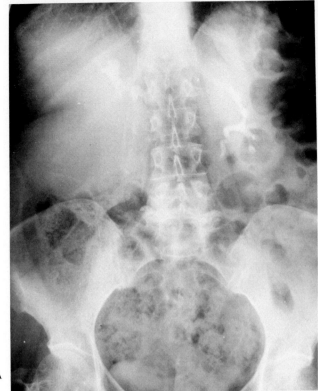

A

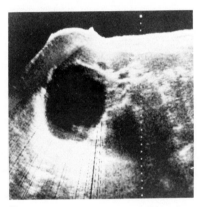

B

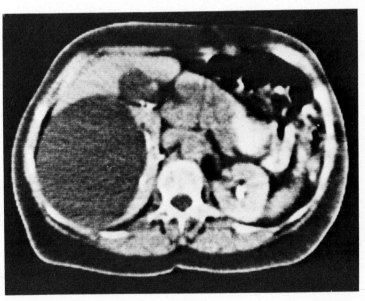

C

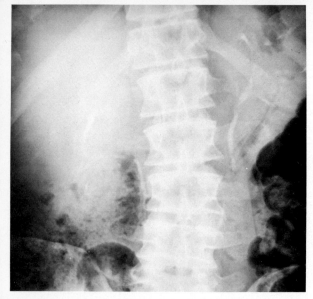

A

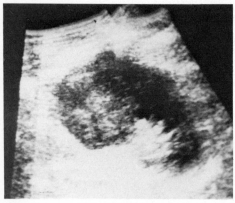

B

Figure 15-33. Workup of a patient with renal mass: tumor. Patient, a man of 51, had painless hematuria and was discovered to have a large right abdominal mass which, as you see in A (his IV urogram), distorted the right renal collecting structures. Next step, sonography (B), shows a large renal mass with many echoes, probably tumor. CT scan (C) shows a large intrarenal mass of mixed attenuation, parts of which may be cystic but which appears to conform to the impression of tumor. Therefore, to help the surgeon, angiography is in order (D) and shows clear-cut evidence of a large, partly necrotic tumor which distorts the vascular tree. There are pooling and tumor vessels. Surgery: clear cell carcinoma.

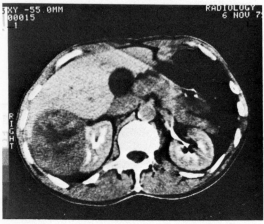

C

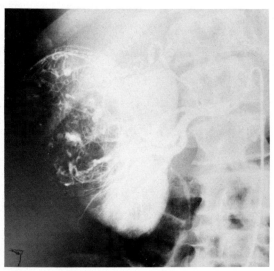

D

250

Trauma

Renal trauma may be suspected in a patient with hematuria after any kind of accident. The trauma may be slight (contused kidney, self-curing) or catastrophic (fractured kidney, torn major vessels requiring immediate surgery). Quite severe degrees of trauma in between these extremes often heal themselves without repair surgery, and while any patient with hematuria after trauma needs an excretory urogram to evaluate the situation and to make sure that he has both kidneys, in many the *treatment* is watchful support.

The Lower Urogenital Tract

All patients with hematuria and any with bladder symptoms require direct observation by cystoscopy, not just urography. Many types of lower urinary tract pathology are unclear or missed on urography and must be viewed directly to be recognized. Bladder morphology and outlet obstruction can be studied by *cystography* (radiographs after urethral instillation of opaque) and by *cystourethrography* (Figure 15-34).

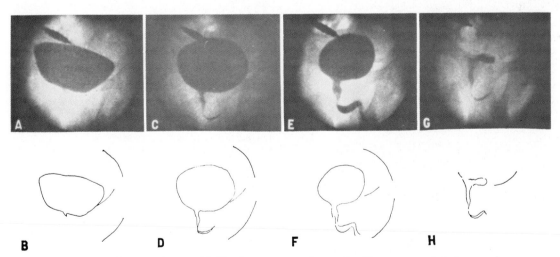

Figure 15-34. The normal urinary bladder during cystourethrography. Here you see a technique employing cinefluorography, in which rapid photography of an intensified fluoroscopic image of the bladder enables one to record and study its manner of contraction. The bladder contracts differently in patients with neurogenic (upper and lower motor neuron) disturbances of micturition.

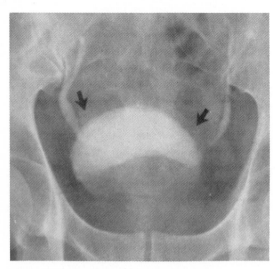

Figure 15-35. The opaque-filled urinary bladder (cystogram) in a patient with prostatic hypertrophy. The filling defect elevating the floor of the bladder is the enlarged prostate gland. Arrows indicate thickened bladder wall.

Unknown

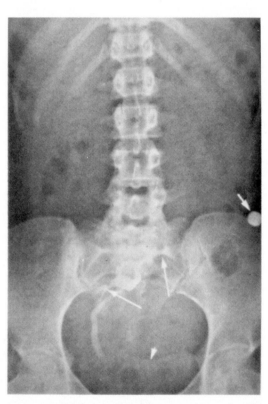

Figure 15-37 (*Unknown 15-1*). This patient was referred to radiology for intravenous urography because she had had blunt trauma to the back while playing volleyball and developed hematuria. Decide: (1) whether with this history *you* would have referred her for intravenous urography; (2) what all the arrows are indicating; and (3) your provisional diagnosis.

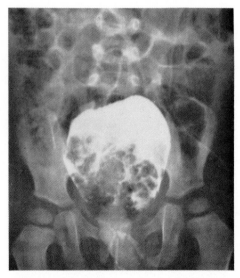

Figure 15-36. Cystogram shows many radiolucencies outlined by the opaque material within the bladder. These represented malignant tumor nodules.

Contrast Reactions

Oral Opaques

Barium is inert and passes through the intact GI tract with perfect safety. Water soluble opaques occasionally used in the GI tract are hypertonic and may be dangerous in debilitated or dehydrated patients or infants because of the massive shifts of fluid that may result.

Intravenous Opaques

Radiographic opaques used intravenously and excreted by the liver or kidney very occasionally produce undesirable reactions, and all physicians should be aware that intravenous administration of contrast substances may result in such episodes while the patient is being examined.

Reactions may be quite mild with pallor, sweating, a feeling of warmth, nausea, vomiting, and anxiety, and the injection should be stopped at once. These probably occur in about 5 percent of all such studies.

Reactions may also, very rarely, be severe; fatalities (generally due to cardiovascular collapse in anaphylactoid reactions) are reported to occur about once in 14,000 cases. For this reason no such studies should be carried out without an emergency cardiopulmonary support system being available.

CHAPTER 16   Skull and Bones

Bones are much more interesting than most people think them during the years in medical school. It is probable that no segment of medical information *could* maintain an aura of fascination against tedium like that felt while memorizing the origins and insertions of muscles. Perhaps the memory of that tiresome and difficult task continues long afterward to cloud the subject of bone at a time of learning when the metabolic disease processes in which bone shares as an organ are being studied. The student cannot afford today to neglect the bones and their function and change, their growth and ultimate microscopic structure. He must be able to imagine what is going on in the bony skeleton in the immobilized patient with a healing fracture, and

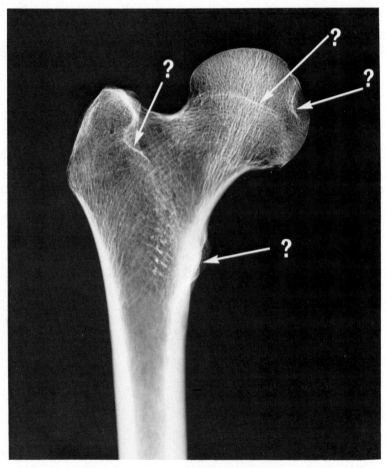

Figure 16-1. Can you explain precisely why the details of the radiographic shadows marked with arrows should have been produced by the anatomic structures they represent? (Rhetorical query; not an unknown.)

not just at the site of the fracture but throughout the body as a result of enforced inactivity. The physician must be able to predict to what extent invasion of his patient's bones by metastatic tumor, for example, will alter blood chemistry. He must understand the formation of kidney stones in hyperparathyroid patients who develop extensive bone destruction and a significant increase in calcium excretion.

The possibilities for diagnosis available through radiography of the bones were partly anticipated by Roentgen himself in the first months after the discovery of the new ray. The technical improvements early in this century made possible a much greater sharpness of detail. A finer focal spot, which could be kept cool, enabled the technician to define the shadows of individual trabeculae in spongy bone. At the same time, finer granules of chemical in the gelatin base improved the photographic properties of radiographic film. More recently, magnification studies produced by placing the film farther from the patient's body also allow for resolution of individual trabeculae.

Today bone is studied by x-ray at a gross level, as in routine medical radiography and also at a microscopic level, finely ground sections of compact bone less than 2 microns in thickness being radiographed in close contact with high-quality, fine-grained film. *Microradiography* in comparative studies of bone in health and disease is rapidly becoming one of the most informative investigative tools in medical research, and collateral autoradiographic studies with radioisotopes embellish that information by adding a time record of tagged change, as you will see later in this chapter.

Begin by understanding at a gross level the radiographic reasons for the appearance of the details questioned in Figures 16-1 and 16-2. If this chapter is to be successful at all, it must eradicate completely any lingering feeling of ennui you may have when you think of bones. Radiology can show you better than any other discipline this quite magical part of medical learning.

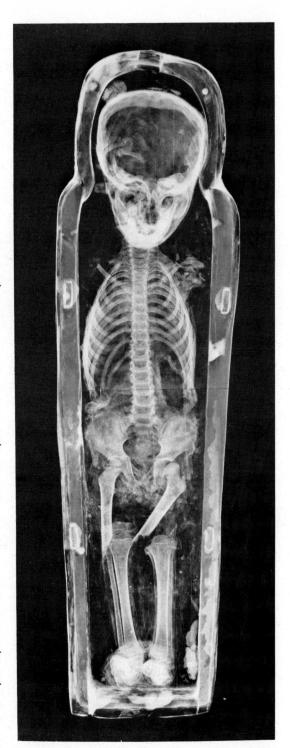

Figure 16-2 (*Unknown 16-1*). Radiograph of a child's mummy, undisturbed since about 100 B.C. What can you determine about the remains? How do you know it is a child? How would experts determine his age in years at the time he died? In precisely what ways is his sketeton abnormal?

255

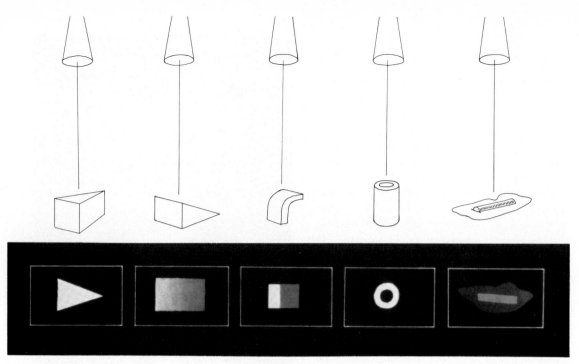

Figure 16-3. (See text.)

Carry forward, now, the general principles about radiographic shadows which you learned from rose petals in the first chapter, and apply them to the folds and variations in thickness of the compact cortex which invests the great tubular bones. Examine the several hypothetical examples in Figure 16-3 and the approximate radiographic images below them.

Assuming uniform composition for all five "objects" (which actually you can assume only up to a point for compact bone), the wedge casts a different shadow according to the direction in which the ray traverses it by a simple rule of summation, of thickness. The curved sheet of bone obeys the same principles which applied to the curved rose petal. The cylinder seen end-on becomes a circle in the radiograph, and if it were radiographed from the side would produce two parallel lines of tangentially projected "cortex," just as you see it in the lower part of Figure 16-4C. Finally, the sheet of bone with a thicker ridge across it will radiograph as a gray area with a streak of white.

It is just as important to think three-dimensionally about the radiograph of a single bone as about the whole chest, for you must add together the shadows cast by all its parts. The shadow of the femoral shaft which you see in the radiograph in Figure 16-4C includes not only the denser shadows of the lateral and medial cortex which has been x-rayed in tangent, but also sheets of gray representing the anterior and posterior cortex which has been projected en face. You will have identified the fovea capitis in Figure 16-1, but did you account for the white streak which limits it laterally as the cortical bone at the base of the hollow, caught tangentially in this projection? Note that in the lateral projection (Figure 16-4D) the inferior cortex of the lesser trochanter is similarly caught in tangent. You know from 16-4C that the cortex of the bone thickens quite suddenly below that point. For this reason the lesser trochanter appears in D as a more radiolucent area above a generally denser one and is separated from it by an even denser white horizontal line, which is its own inferior cortex in tangent.

To the folds and thickness of the compact bone, finally, must be "added" the shadow of the trabecular bone inside. As you have seen in Figure 16-1, the trabeculae themselves vary in distribution and thickness within a piece of spongy bone.

256

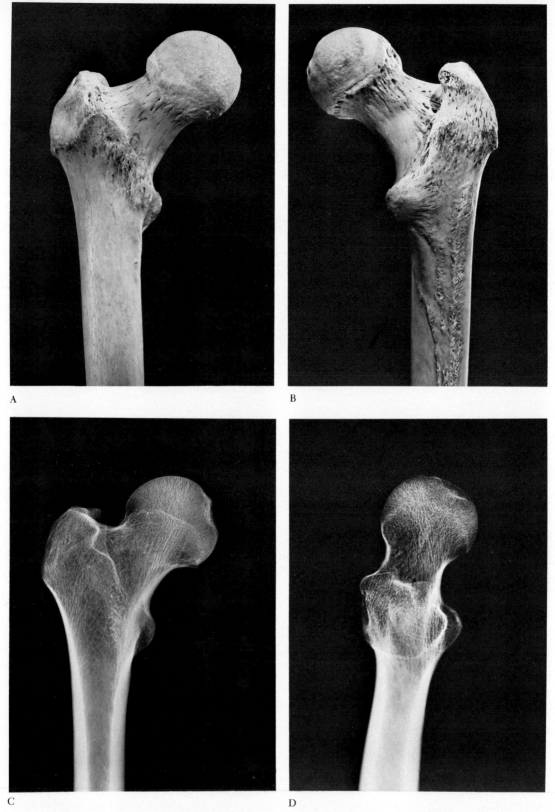

A

B

C

D

Figure 16-4. Anterior and posterior photographic views of the upper femur (A and B) to help to account for the details of shadows seen in the radiograph (C). A lateral radiograph (D) made at right angles to C provides different shadows because the projection is different, although the same anatomic structure can be identified.

257

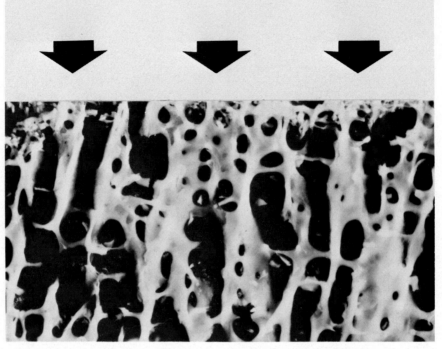

Figure 16-5. Microphotograph showing trabecular arrangement developed with weight bearing (arrows).

Notice that the trabeculae in the upper femur are arranged in a series of arching parallel struts which closely follow the line of stress developed within this part of the bone in man, who stands erect and carries the weight of his trunk upon the two femoral heads (Figure 16-4C). The arrangement of these struts to bear weight differs from that of the similar spongy bone within the upper femurs of quadrupeds, and it is interesting to reflect how those trabeculae must have adapted themselves first in *Pithecanthropus erectus*.

Figure 16-5 is a microphotograph of the trabeculae in a coronal 3-millimeter slice of bone from the upper tibia and shows adaptation to weight bearing delivered from above. Note the major struts of bone joined and reinforced by minor horizontal ones, which are much more slender. In other areas, of course, spongy bone is more uniform in structure, the trabeculae assuming the form of curved sheets with communicating spaces between them all more or less the same size and radiographing as you would expect, without conspicuous strands of white like those in the upper femur.

When you look at films of bones, therefore, think of the folds and variations in thickness of the investing cortex and then consciously add an inspection of the pattern of the trabeculae inside. For the gross level at which you view routine medical radiographs, remember that optical limitations permit you to resolve shadows of only the larger trabeculae. The myriads of finer ones are not seen as defined white shadows, but contribute a diffuse overall whiteness to the shadow of the bone you are inspecting.

In radiographs in which there was even the slightest motion during the exposure, you will find that you cannot see any trabeculae at all. You will probably not see them either in films which have been made of an extremity in plaster. Learn to look for the trabecular pattern, but to discount its absence in types of examinations in which such a degree of detail was not technically possible.

Learning to think from the gross level of detail in bone films down to the microscopic level and then reversing that process is, in general, the orientation of this chapter.

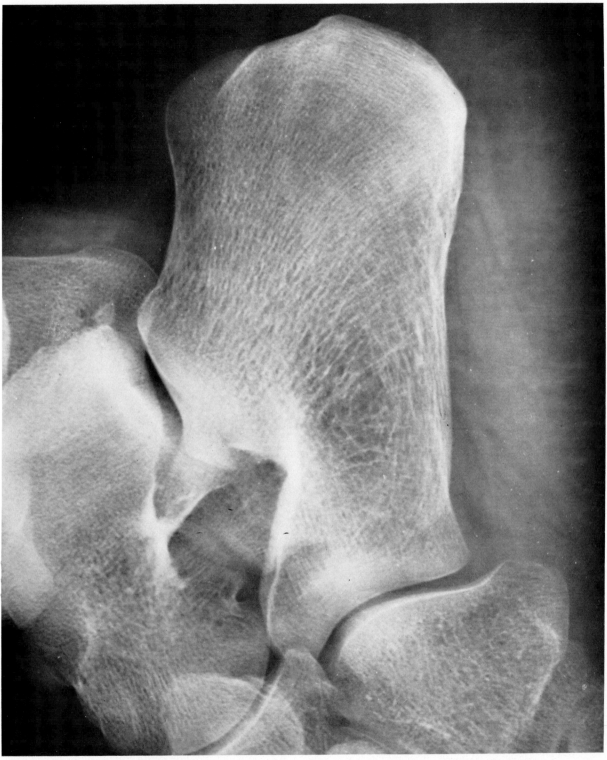

Figure 16-6. Magnification study. Lateral projection of the foot. (Sole of the foot parallel with side margin of the page.) Note the trabeculae, which arch backward and downward from the calcaneotalar joint toward the weight-bearing point under the heel.

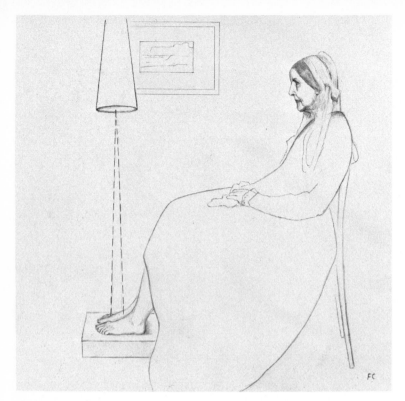

Figure 16-7

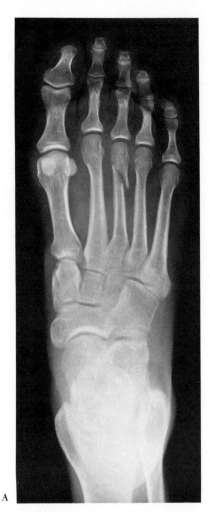

A

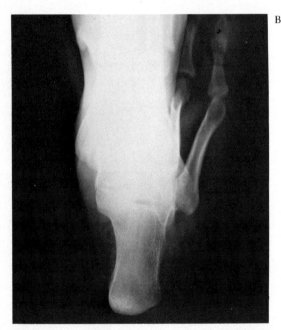

B

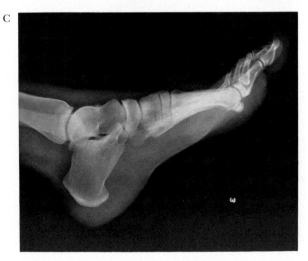

C

Figure 16-8. Three different views of the foot. How would you rearrange Mother Whistler to obtain B and C? (See text.) (*Unknown 2:* Has she anything abnormal?)

260

The various projections in which films of the bones are made are largely a matter of convention based upon standard investigations determining which ones combine to produce most information. You will become accustomed to the AP and lateral views, which are routine. Additional views often have to be designed in order to show to the best advantage a particular lesion in a particular patient.

Figure 16-8A is the conventional AP view of the foot, made as in Figure 16-7; note that the lower parts of the tibia and fibula are superimposed upon the proximal part of the foot. The added density causes the loss of all detail *at the technical exposure suited to so thin a part as the toes.* Some information about the talus and calcaneus, the ankle joint, and the lower leg is derived from the lateral view (C), and if additional AP information is needed about the calcaneus, for example, it can be obtained with view B, made by directing the beam downward from above and behind the heel.

With exposure factors calculated for greater penetration and by use of the Bucky diaphragm on thicker bony parts, it is usually possible to produce a film with the cortical details of superimposed bones, appearing as though seen through one another. Thus it is often necessary to subtract intellectually the overlapping folds of the cortex of one bone in order to trace the cortex and structure of another which is superimposed upon it in the conventional views.

Familiarity with the anatomic details of the bones is of great help in interpreting radiographs, and by the same token it is possible to learn and review anatomy by "accounting for" the details of the roentgen image. Compare, for example, the difference in the radiograph of the *hip* which will be produced when the lower extremity is externally rotated, with the appearance which you would find in a film made with the leg rotated internally as far as possible. You will find that in looking at films of bones there are certain key points which, once learned, identify for you the projection you are seeing. In ordering films of bones you should always indicate the location of pain and the provisional diagnosis.

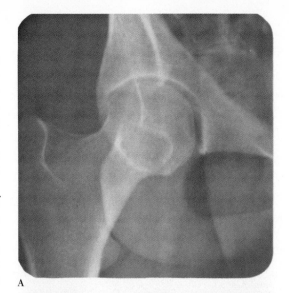

A

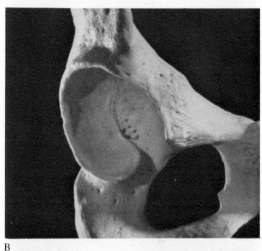

B

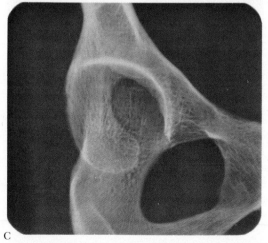

C

Figure 16-9. The shadow of the acetabulum superimposed on that of the upper femur. A: Radiograph of patient. B: Photograph of specimen. C: Radiograph of specimen (without femur).

261

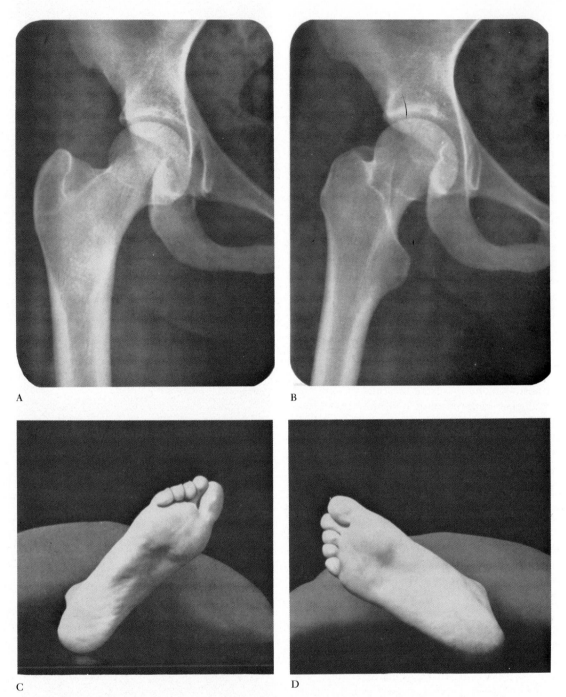

Figure 16-10. Radiographs of the hip made with the lower extremity internally and externally rotated as per text. Note the changes in the appearance of the trochanters. Compare with the appearance of the hip when radiographed straight AP (Figure 16-4C). The lesser trochanter can thus become an index to the degree of rotation present when the radiograph was made.

Fractures appear on radiographs as dark streaks across the white of the bone, of course because there the continuity of both compact and spongy bone is interrupted, soft tissues and hemorrhage usually separating the fractured fragments slightly. If the fracture is a simple one, a single dark line will be present. If a comminuted fracture occurs with several separate fracture planes communicating, then several lines should be present (Figure 16-11). Sometimes the obvious presence of several fragments indicates that the fracture is comminuted, although only one major fracture line can be seen because the additional planes of fracture are so oblique to the direction of the beam used that overlap of bony margins prevents your "seeing through" the planes of the extra fractures. In Figure 16-11 two fracture planes can be seen and one more supposed: that for the fracture of the greater trochanter. Remember that such communicating planes of fracture may curve, so that only part of the bony separation is ever appreciated in a single projection. Remember too that while interruption of the continuity of the cortical compact bone is the clearest indication of a fracture, the spongy bone is also fractured, and depending on the direction and character of the trauma, the surfaces of spongy bones may become impacted. When this happens the fractured trabecular surfaces are jammed into one another and the trabeculae become enmeshed, so that there are innumerable fragments of bone lying closer together than is normal. As you could predict, a radiograph made with the beam parallel to the plane of fracture and impaction will produce an area of increased whiteness because of the greater density existing there.

The radiolucent cartilaginous disc of the epiphyseal plate in immature bones may lie in the plane of the beam of x-rays and so also appear on the film as a linear dark area crossing the bone. It is usually easy to distinguish from a fracture line, however, because it is not an abrupt break in the cortex but smoothly bounded on the epiphyseal side of the radiolucent area by a white line, the denser bony disc of the epiphyseal plate where little or no growth is occuring.

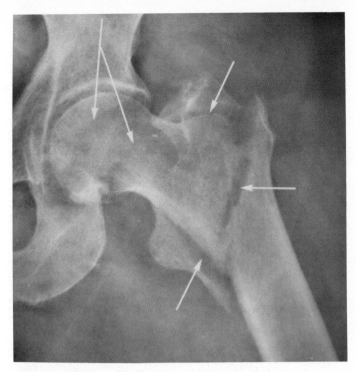

Figure 16-11. Intertrochanteric comminuted fracture of the left femur. Longer arrows indicate the overlapping margins of the anterior and posterior rims of the acetabulum. Shorter arrows indicate three communicating fracture planes, one through the femur at the intertrochanteric line, one through the base of the lesser trochanter, and a third (not clearly seen) through the greater trochanter, its outer cortex showing loss of continuity.

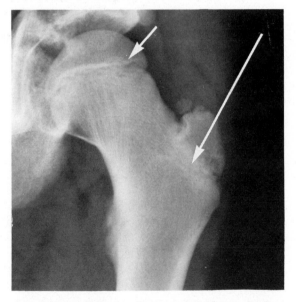

Figure 16-12. Child's hip showing growth plates to be distinguished from fractures. The epiphysis for the femoral head appears before 8 months and fuses at about 18 years; the one for the greater trochanter appears at around 2 years and fuses at about 16 years.

263

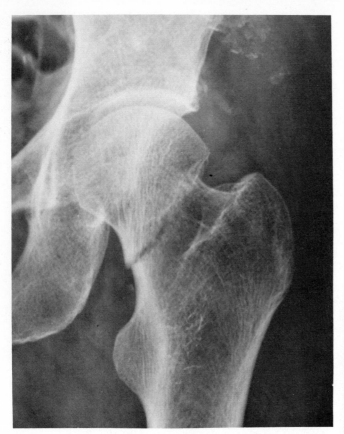

Figure 16-13

of the other metatarsophalangeal joints in the same foot, a procedure you will find convenient in looking at radiographs of joints and bones. In degenerative joint disease only traces of the interposed cartilage remain, spurs of bone form at the joint margins, and the overall density of the adjoining bone is increased. Note that there are also fragmentation and hypertrophy of the sesamoid bones found normally about this joint (compare Figure 16-8A).

Figure 16-15 is an example of similar changes about the hip joint.

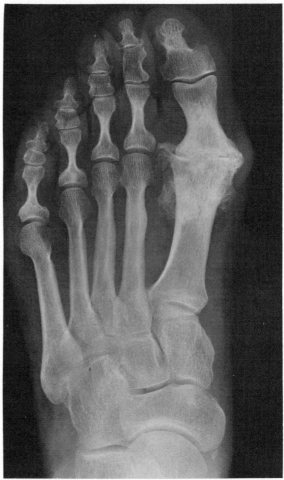

Figure 16-14

You will be able to make a diagnosis of the type of fracture in Figure 16-13. At the same time note the roentgen characteristics of the normal hip joint with its dense white acetabular roof seen in tangent and the radiolucent area just below it which represents the cartilaginous layers lining the acetabulum and investing the femoral head. Compare the thickness of cortex of the head of the femur with that of the acetabulum and of the femoral shaft lower down. Dislocations of joints are often combined with fractures.

When chronic injury to a joint impairs its integrity, the width of the radiolucent zone (which includes both the joint space itself and the two thicknesses of radiolucent articular cartilage) decreases, while mechanisms of reaction and protection produce increased amounts of dense bone on both sides of the joint. The result is what you see in Figures 16-14 and 16-15, both very common. Figure 16-14 is an example of degenerative arthritis of the first metatarsophalangeal joint with soft-tissue swelling (bunion). Here you can use for a normal comparison any

264

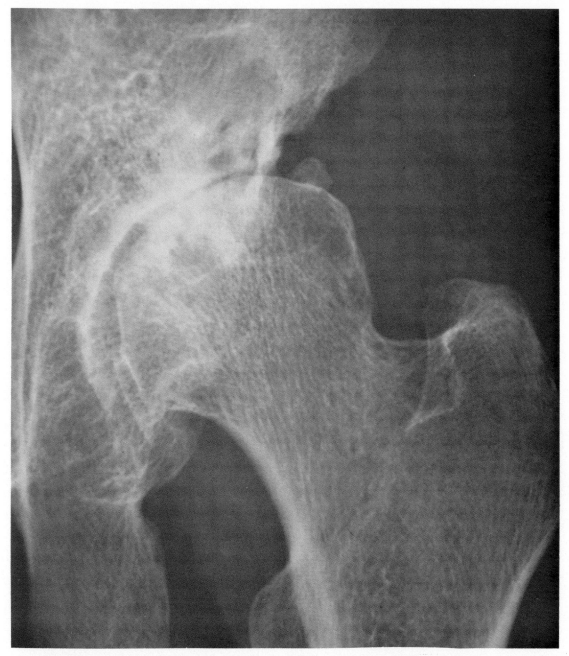

Figure 16-15. Degenerative joint disease of the hip. Note narrowing of the joint space and reactive density of new bone on both sides of the joint, commonly referred to as *malum coxae senile* and understandably frequent in older people after a lifetime of weight bearing. In arthritis which develops in a joint following inflammatory disease, on the other hand, complete obliteration of the joint may occur and the radiolucent joint space may entirely disappear.

Fracture Clinic

The illustrations on the next four pages constitute an exercise in fracture diagnosis, framed as unknowns because they are more interesting so. *Not every film contains a fracture, however, as would be the case in the same group of patients if you were seeing them at random in the emergency ward.* All these patients have been injured.

> The roentgen findings you are looking for are—
> Breaks in the continuity of cortex
> Radiolucent fracture lines
> Overlap where the added density of cortical bone seen through cortical bone creates a white area
> Fragments of bone without explanation even in the absence of a visible fracture
> Denser areas where impaction of spongy bone has occurred, which must be seen in two views
> Flocculent density in soft tissues in healing fractures (callus), visible only after it calcifies.

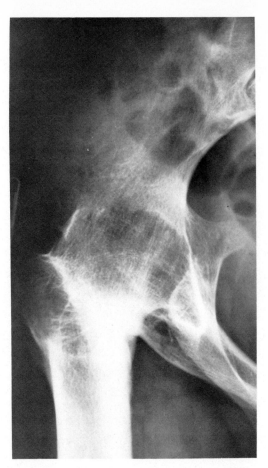

Figure 16-16 (Unknown 16-3)

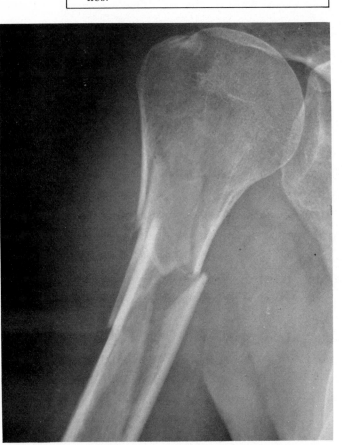

Figure 16-17 (*Unknown 16-4*)

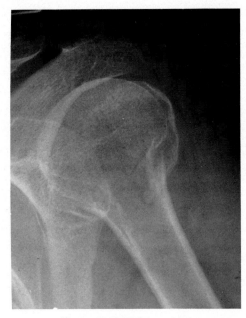

Figure 16-18 (*Unknown 16-5*)

266

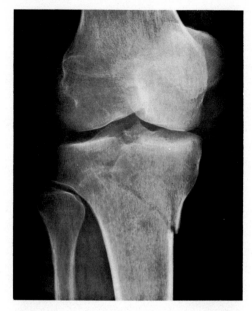

Figure 16-19 (*Unknown 16-6*). Oblique view of the knee following injury.

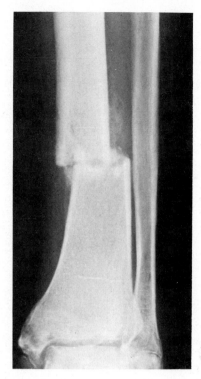

Figure 16-20 (*Unknown 16-7*). Fresh or old fracture?

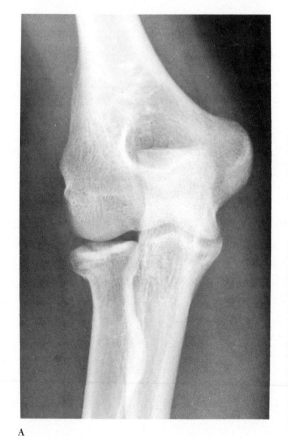

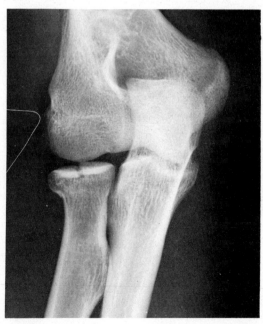

A

B

Figure 16-21 (*Unknown 16-8*)

267

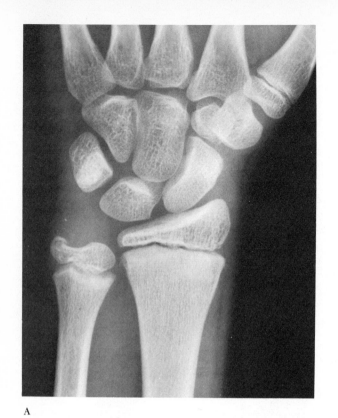

A

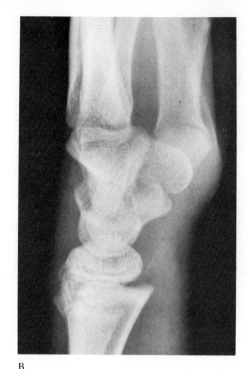

B

Figure 16-22 (*Unknown 16-9*)

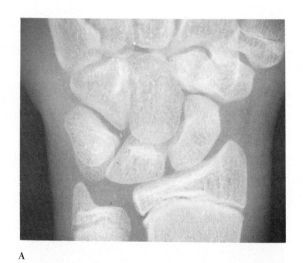

A

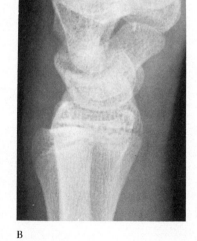

B

Figure 16-23 (*Unknown 16-10*)

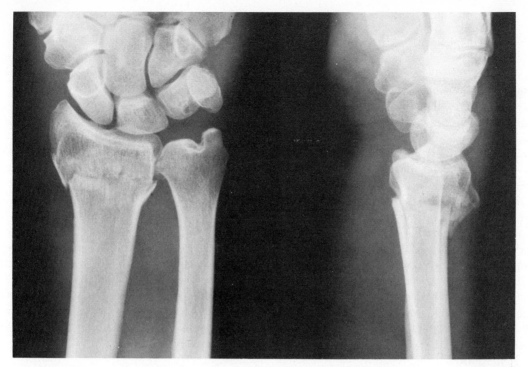

Figure 16-24 (*Unknown 16-11*). Lower forearm and wrist of an adult after a fall on the outstretched hand. What is different about this fracture from the ones you have been looking at? Identify the carpal bones in the two views.

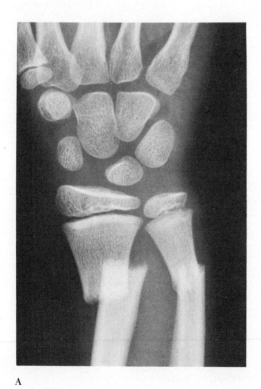

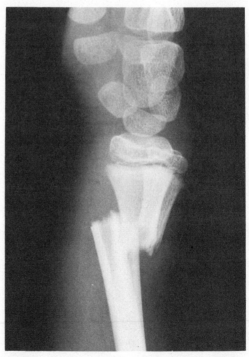

A

B

Figure 16-25 (*Unknown 16-12*). Diagnose and plan management. Patient fell out of an apricot tree.

269

When a fracture appears to have occurred through bone which was already abnormal and may therefore have been abnormally fragile, it is called a *pathologic fracture*. Figures 16-26 and 16-27 are examples.

In Figure 16-26 a cylindrical cuff of bony cortex has been eroded by pressure from within, although you observe the thinning best where you see cortex in tangent medially and laterally. Across the thinned segment of bone at the level of the arrows a jagged fracture has occurred and is seen on the lateral surface as a distinct interruption of the cortex. Note that the bone appears to be expanded by the pressure, a common finding in benign intraosseous tumors and cysts which increase in size so gradually that new bone can be laid down under the periosteum in a protective response to the weakened structure as the erosion occurs from within. This is an example of a *unicameral bone cyst*, common in children and occurring, as you see it

here, at the metaphyseal end of the shaft close to the epiphyseal growth plate. Tumor, too, erodes bone and produces a radiolucent area wherever bone has been destroyed.

Figure 16-27 is the upper femur of a patient with Paget's disease, and a transverse fracture has occurred across the shaft several centimeters below the lesser trochanter. Although it characteristically thickens bone, Paget's disease also weakens its structure and the bone withstands stresses and strains less well than normal sound tubular long bone does. As additional evidence of weakness of the bone, note that this fracture has occurred straight across, whereas it is more usual for sound tubular bone in midshaft to fracture irregularly in ragged points and with comminution. Compare the appearance of the cortex in the fractures of previously sound tubular bone you have just seen (or have seen in your own fracture patients) with this very abnormal bone structure.

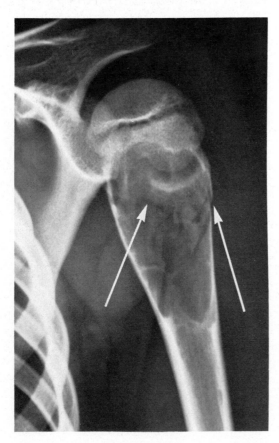

Figure 16-26

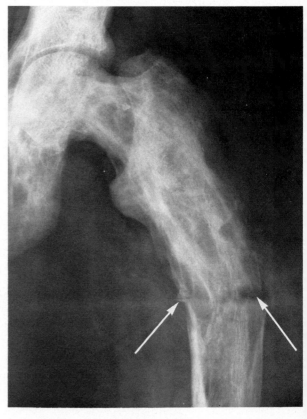

Figure 16-27

270

What types of pathologic bony change, then, can be appreciated at the visual level afforded by conventional roentgen techniques in which the film is placed close to the patient and the bone in question appears approximately life size? There follow examples of various changes matched against specimen photographs of the bones in question.

Figure 16-28. Upper pair: *Giant cell tumor* of the proximal end of the radius. There is destruction of the cortex for several centimeters down the shaft, but of varying degree. The tumor has not destroyed all the spongy bone within the head of the radius close to the joint surface.

Lower pair: *Sarcoma* of the tibia. Here the rate of growth has certainly been faster, and the entire medial cortex was destroyed before a fracture of the bone occurred. The ragged appearance of the destructive border is much more in keeping with the progress of a malignant tumor than the smooth erosion allowing time for expansion of the entire bone in Figure 16-26.

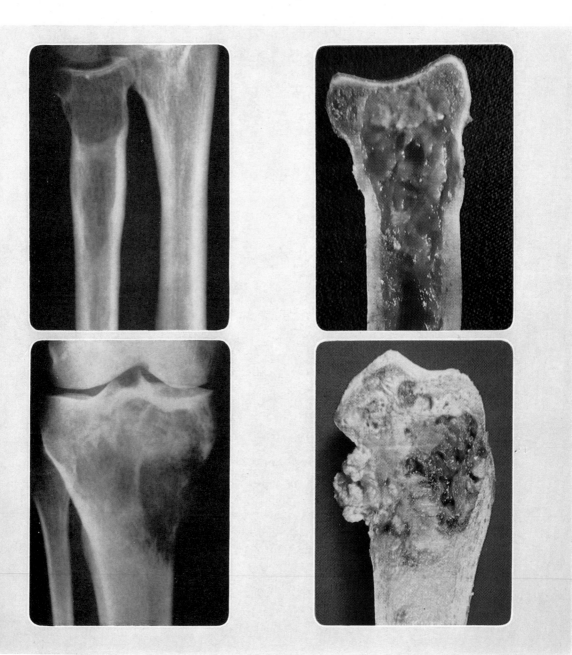

Figure 16-29. The cortex markedly thickened by addition of new bone from beneath the periosteum in a boy with *osteoid osteoma*. Note that you can follow the old cortex from below upward in the radiograph to an area about 4 centimeters in length where it has been largely destroyed. At the center of this segment of destroyed cortex and at a point which is also opposite the thickest part of the newly superimposed cortical bone, there is an oval area of radiolucency. This represented the nidus of the osteoid osteoma, seen as a reddish pulpy projection from the wedge of bone removed at surgery.

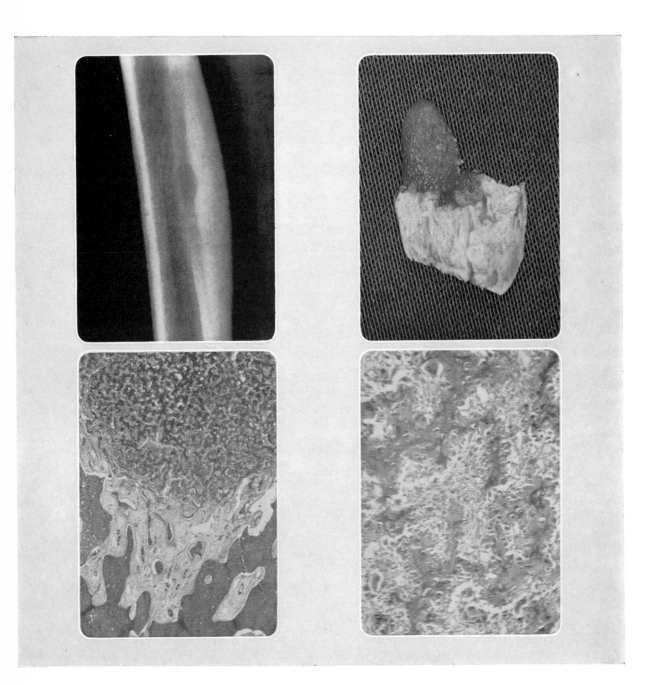

Figure 16-30. Two patients with *chondrosarcoma*, a relatively slow-growing malignant bone tumor which characteristically shows calcification within the tumor. The two illustrations on the left are from one patient. They show the effect on the upper femur of a chondrosarcoma which is growing principally *outside* the bone. The illustrations on the right are from a patient whose tumor began *inside* the bone and grew slowly enough to expand it. Compare the cortex in the two cases.

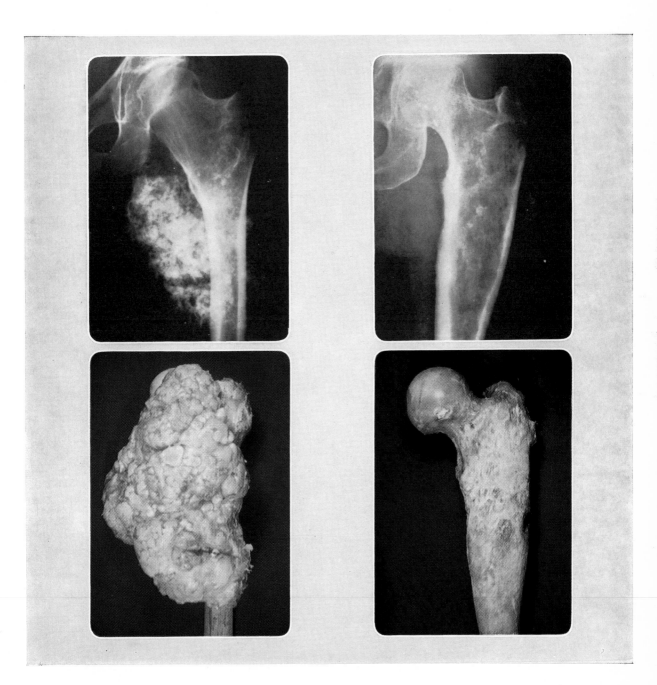

Figure 16-31. This is the lower femur from a child who died at age 4 of *leukemia*. While you see here only the radiograph of the specimen, the same destructive changes would probably have been appreciable in films made shortly before death. Note the numerous radiolucent defects caused by growing lymphomatous tumor in which the thickness of the cortex is generally decreased and also perforated in many areas. Take note, while you are about it, that the cartilaginous part of the growing epiphysis surrounding its bony center is "visible" in the radiograph of the specimen because air surrounds it, whereas in a radiograph of the patient it is not seen because soft tissues and cartilage have about the same radiodensity. Destruction at the metaphysis close to the growth plate is common in leukemia, and almost all faults, vitamin deficiencies, injuries like lead poisioning, and many other pediatric problems may be diagnosed from films of the long bones.

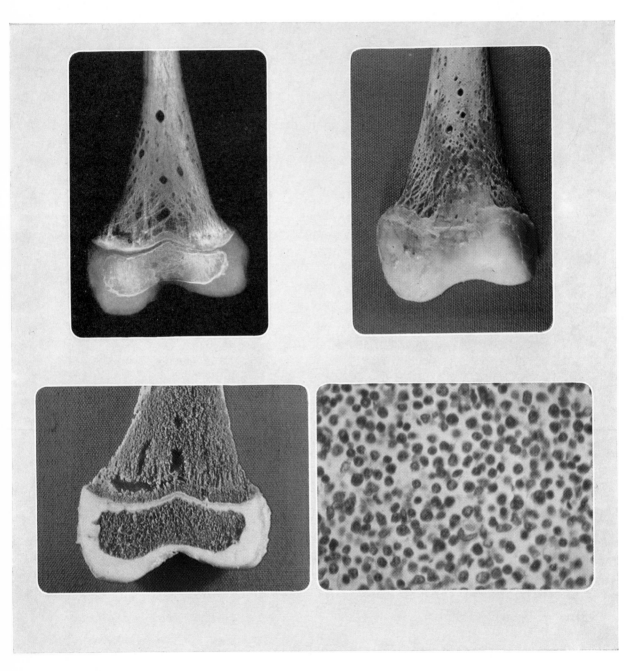

Figure 16-32. Bone destruction in the skull, the result of diffuse involvement of the diploe and perforation of the inner and outer tables in a patient who died of *multiple myeloma*. Above, photograph and radiograph of the specimen top of the calvarium. Punctate areas of radiolucency like this will be seen antemortem on skull films made in the AP and lateral projections, for example, in patients with myeloma or metastatic malignancy. Below, a specimen of rib from the same patient. While these are classic bone lesions in myeloma, you will need to remember that they occur late in the disease. The diagnosis should be made biochemically at a much earlier stage, when the bone films will probably be negative.

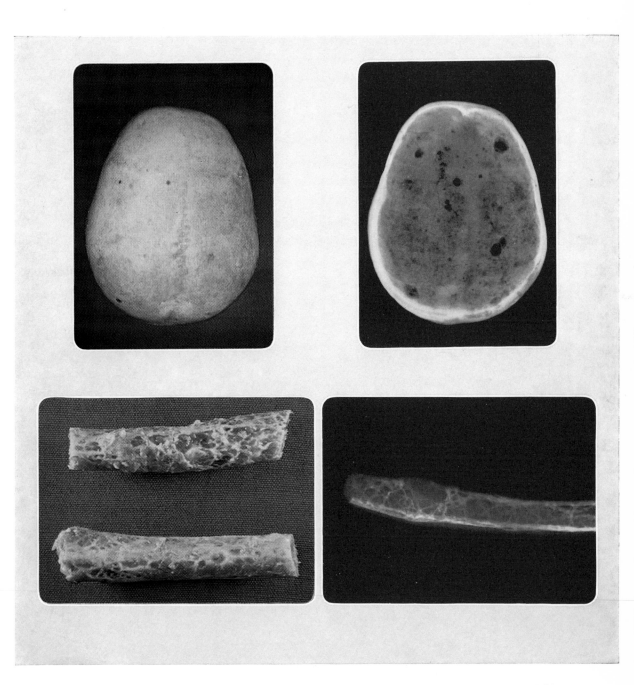

Figure 16-33. Localized destruction of the calvarium in an area involved by a large focus of *metastatic neuroblastoma* in a young child. Tumor projects upward from the external surface of the skull in the photograph. Note that in the radiographed specimen slice of calvarium the destruction of bone is actually less extensive than one believes on first inspection of the photographs. In radiographs made of the live patient with this type of diploic destruction, spotty loss of density in the diploe and loss of continuity or thickness of the tangentially seen cortical tables may be expected.

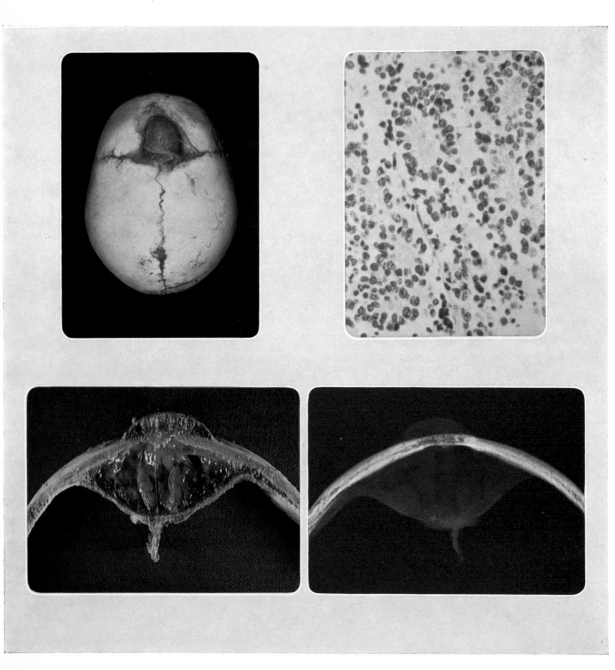

276

Figure 16-34. Excrescences of new bone arising from the outer surface of the cortex will appear as you see demonstrated here in a patient with *calvarial hemangioma*. The first illustration is a special tangential view with the technical factors of the exposure decreased for details of the protuberant bone only; note that the skull itself has not been penetrated. Compare this with the radiograph of the specimen and with photographs of the whole fresh specimen and of a slice of that specimen after maceration. The latter can be matched in precise detail against the radiograph of the specimen.

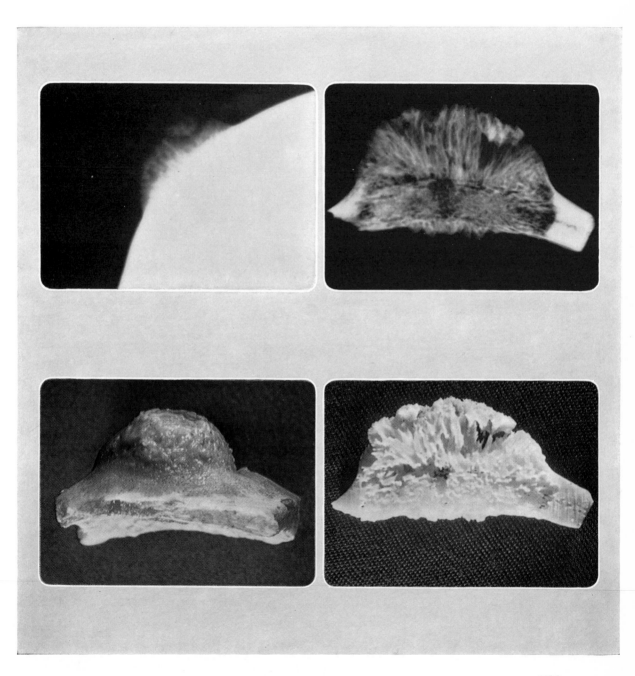

Figure 16-35. Diffuse destruction of spongy bone by tumor usually allows preservation of the shape of the bone for a time, with ultimate collapse when the supporting function of the cortical shell is impaired by erosion and multiple fragmentations. Here, in a patient with diffuse *myelomatosis* involving the marrow spaces in the spongy bone filling the vertebrae, extensive destruction of the bony trabeculae of cancellous bone and later of the cortical boxy envelope has resulted in varying degrees of vertebral collapse. Note the reciprocal "expansion" of the intervertebral discs, which are inclined to assume a more spherical shape if destruction of bone above and below allow it.

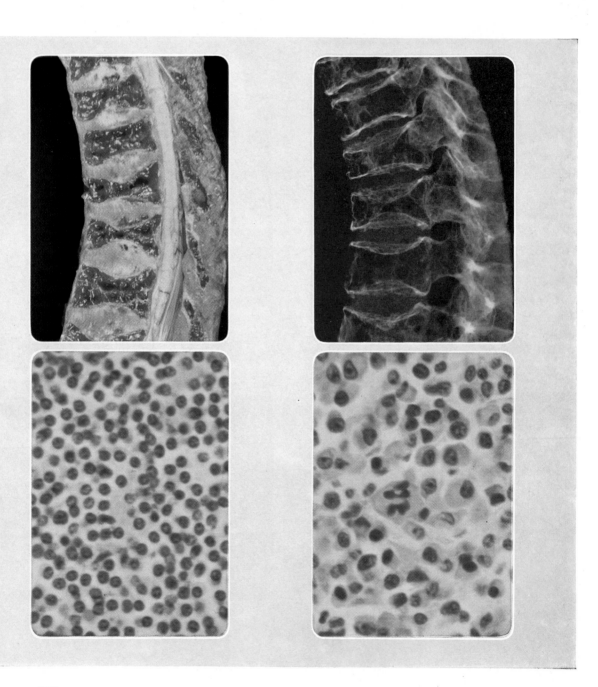

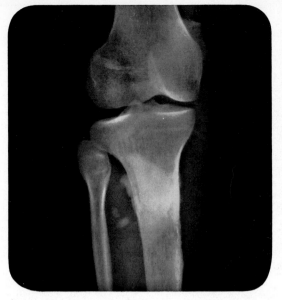
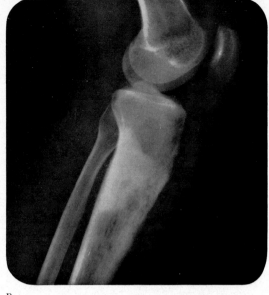

A   B

Figure 16-36. When, on the other hand, a tumor invading the marrow spaces between trabeculae of spongy bone characteristically produces dense new bone, as does this *osteosarcoma* of the tibia, an area of *increased* density will be visualized in the radiograph. In two views at 90 degrees it clearly occupies the central part of the bone. There is also some spotty cortical destruction here, and dense new tumor bone is seen in the soft-tissue part of the tumor lateral to the tibia.

In sum, then, conventional roentgen studies of bones will often be able to visualize localized or diffuse *increase* in bone thickness and will also be able to show evidence of localized or diffuse *decrease* in bone mass, either of compact bone or spongy trabeculae, or both. Sometimes the particular location and character of the bone change offer evidence to the experienced viewer which permits him to all but label the disease entity. Sometimes there is nothing characteristic about the changes present, and they can only be described and the possibilities named which fit in with the clinical story.

To give you an example, the *diffuse bone loss* which occurs in the early course of many cases of multiple myeloma cannot be distinguished radiologically by anyone from a *similar decrease in bone mass* which occurs commonly in patients of the same age group for a variety of metabolic reasons and is named *osteoporosis*. Once the bone shadows of the myeloma patient do begin to show spotty areas of trabecular and cortical destruction (as in Figure 16-35), a much more positive roentgen interpretation is possible in light of the clinical picture. Early in the course of either myeloma or osteoporosis, the microscopic change in the bone is similar, since it is indeed a diffuse thinning of all bone, though for very different reasons.

Osteoporosis is a term which has been decried by many, but it is not actually a bad description of what occurs, for bony trabecular plates do become "porous" when they are perforated by holes. The "sponge" produced is a finer one, then, with relatively more marrow spaces and relatively less bone. In the same fashion the juxtamedullary part of the compact bone is tunneled into and converted to spongy bone in a patient with developing osteoporosis, so that the much denser compact bony layer under the periosteum is narrowed. Seen in tangent in the radiograph, the cortex appears thinned.

The borderline of the normal in judging the thickness of either compact bone cortex or individually seen trabeculae is not easy to define clearly. It is not easy for either the radiologist or the pathologist when they are considering the problem of a particular patient, because so many factors determine bone thickness. Genetic heritage, habitual activity, nutrition, and age all influence bone mass, so that a range of differing thicknesses may be normal for each of a group of patients. You can better appreciate this problem in orientation if you now review briefly the microscopic structure of compact bone.

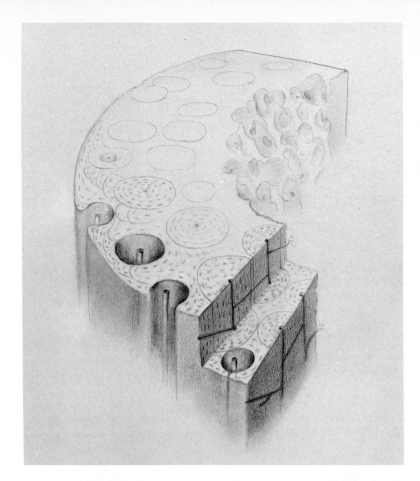

Figure 16-37. The structure of compact bone. This diagram has been adapted from Ham and shows both horizontal and vertical cut faces of the femoral shaft at a level where cortex begins to be lined with trabecular bone. The diagram has been simplified for clarity; note in the microradiographs (Figures 16-38 and 16-39) that normally in an adult there are many more osteones in the full thickness of femoral cortex.

Focus down intellectually upon a cross section of the full thickness of the cortex of the femoral shaft you were looking at in Figure 16-1 and you will be seeing the structure diagrammed above in Figure 16-37. The cross-cut face reveals numerous sectioned *osteones* (or haversian systems) with their central vessels. The vertical cut enables you to recall that the basic functioning adult bone unit is a cylinder of very minute dimensions. These cylinders, the osteones, are connected with one another via their branching central arteries, and compose, in effect, a breccia of units mortared together to form a mass. They are of a high order phylogenetically and do not exist in the bones of many lower animals. Structurally they produce a type of bone (and there are several types, remember) which is of excellent resilience and beautifully designed for adaptation in response to changing needs. Such a composite of arterially connected units begins to be laid down in the bones of the human infant, replacing a far less well designed type of immature bone, phylogenetically much earlier in type and resembling a woven fabric rather

than a masonry wall. Even in the infant osteones are found to be concentrated in regions of particular stress such as important tendon insertions. Eventually in the adult most compact bone is composed of osteones mortared together by lamellar bone matrix, as you can see in Figure 16-38, a microradiograph of a thin-ground cross section of the shaft of a long bone which might have been sliced off the face of the diagramed bone wedge in Figure 16-37.

The osteones in such microradiographs are seen as rings of varying density about dark central holes which once contained arteries. Osteones vary in radiodensity because they are of different ages and therefore contain somewhat different amounts of mineral apatite; mineral is precipitated very rapidly into the organic collagen bone matrix when it is first laid down, and after that more slowly over a period of several years.

The useful life expectancy of an individual osteone is around seven years, at the end of which time it is removed by erosion from within until an empty cylinder exists where it once was tra-

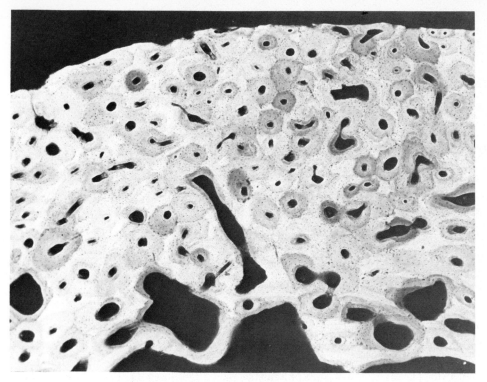

Figure 16-38. Microradiograph of a transverse section of normal femoral cortex. The specimen was not prepared by sectioning decalcified bone, but was sawed off and then ground down to a thickness of a few microns in a fresh state retaining its natural calcium content. The radiograph was made with the specimen closely in contact with a photographic film, so than an x-ray shadowgram of the variations in radiodensity of a histologic section of bone is produced.

versed by the central artery and lined by sheets of mesenchymal cells. These differentiate into osteoblasts and lay down new layers of bone matrix concentrically, one within another, until the central artery is again surrounded by a new osteone. The osteoblasts become engulfed in the bone matrix they elaborate (after which they are called osteocytes), continuing to function via minute canaliculi which radiate from their surfaces in all directions like the spines of a burr. These communicate with the canaliculi of other osteocytes nearby so that bone is able to be transfused with fluid and electrolytes, functioning throughout life as an organ no less important than the liver or kidney. Because the osteoblasts become engulfed in concentric cylindrical layers of matrix, they will appear in cross section as arranged in concentric circles about the artery, just as you see them in the diagram and in the microradiograph. You would *expect* the cells to be radiolucent compared with the mineralized matrix around them and could predict that in the microradiograph they would appear as minute black dots. Note that some of the osteone

circles in the microradiograph are very dark; these are the younger ones, less completely mineralized than their white, denser, older neighbors.

If the patient in Figure 16-38 had recently been given an injection of tagged (artificially rendered radioactive) calcium, the younger osteones which you have identified would now contain much larger amounts of that calcium load, since they are mineralizing at a more rapid rate than their seniors. An *autoradiograph*, made by placing a fine-grained photographic film in close contact with a section of bone like the one which was x-rayed to produce Figure 16-38, would show darker spots in the precise locations of the younger osteones because radioactivity of the calcium isotope produces silver precipitation in the film. When microradiographs, autoradiographs, special stain studies, and photographs made with polarized light *of the same bone section are matched in register*, an invaluable means of studying bone pathophysiology emerges.

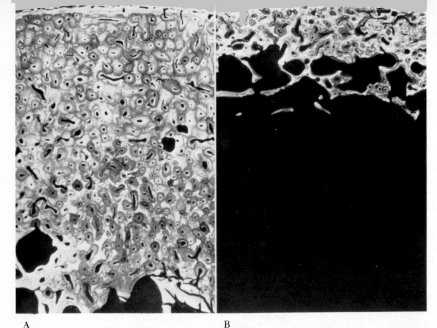

Figure 16-39. Microradiographs of normal cortex (A) and the cortex in postmenopausal osteoporosis (B), taken from precisely the same location on the lateral surface of the femur. The periosteal surface is at the top and the medullary surface below (see text).

A   B

By means of such studies the rate at which osteones form and are mineralized, removed, and restored can be recorded for healthy as well as abnormal bone. The gross appearance of a bone is so suggestive of permanence and durability that it is difficult to accept intellectually the degree to which bones are being constantly changed and remodeled throughout life and the extent to which they do reflect and share in virtually every disease condition. In learning to comprehend these changes, it is essential to think clearly of the "flow" prevailing normally in the bones at various periods of life. The infant and young child grow in many ways and at different speeds from year to year, and their growth bonewise has been charted and documented extensively. However, most of us fail to comprehend fully that bone laid down in one site this year will begin next month to be removed, to accommodate for developing changes.

Take any given tendon insertion site as an example. During childhood growth spurts, when the long bones are increasing in length very rapidly, an important muscle tendon inserted at one point soon functions at a disadvantage unless it is moved again close to the joint it subtends. The adductor muscles, arising from the pubis and inserting into the femur posteriorly along its entire length, powerfully adduct the thigh. However, the adductor longus inserts into the linea aspera on the posterior surface of the bone in about midshaft, a location in which little or no change is occurring, while the adduc-

tor magnus inserts further down into a more limited area by a heavy aponeurosis and just above the margin of the epiphyseal growth plate. Here new bone is forming and extending the length of the femur at a very rapid rate indeed. If the tendon insertion of the adductor magnus remained attached at one point, it would soon be inserting farther up the femur and would adduct the thigh much less efficiently.

The concentration of osteones located along the linea aspera in early childhood and at all tendon sites allows for a mechanism of adaptation. By destruction and reconstruction of osteones at slightly different locations, it is possible to maintain in an area optimal for function the heavy cortex into which tendon fibers insert. Thus the bones, like every other tissue, adapt and change with growth until maturity. Through the prime years doubtless many individual osteones manage to live out their seven-odd years of usefulness in the same location, but others are removed before that time in order to accommodate to changes pertinent to the habits or activity or health of the individual. If a carpenter gives up his trade and learns another more sedentary one, the heavy concentrations of osteones under the tendon insertions in his dominant arm will gradually be decreased. The young mental patient who recovers after several years of depression and inactivity and takes up the latest dance step must throughout his body increase the rate of bone building.

With the advent of postmaturity and the waning years, however, the process of bone replacement flags. The normal stimuli to the maintenance of healthy bone begin to diminish. Activity decreases. The rocking chair takes the place of squash. The appetite declines, and less adequate supplies of proteins, vitamins, and minerals essential to proper bone building are available. Hormonal stimuli to bone maintenance gradually abate with advancing years in both men and women, although these changes, occurring earlier in women, have time to produce in them the atrophy of bone known as postmenopausal osteoporosis, which might best be thought of as the *net decrease in bone mass prevalent in old age.*

In Figure 16-39 you can judge for yourself the lengths to which this decrease in bone mass may be carried. The cortex of the elderly woman in B has gradually been decreased to one-fourth the normally maintained cortex in A. In serial bone studies taken at different ages this process may be observed to occur in two ways coincident in time. Individual osteones which are removed fail to be replaced adequately and the cortex takes on the appearance of a Swiss cheese. At the same time the juxtamedullary part of the cortex is gradually converted into spongy bone, the innermost trabeculae being replaced least well and finally disappearing altogether.

Cancellous bone located in the ends of long bones and filling the bodies of the vertebrae, for example, also shares in this attritional process in aging individuals. The high-magnification photographs in Figure 16-40 will give you an unforgettable concept of net decrease and increase in bone mass of cancellous bone, which is composed not of osteones but of sheets of lamellar bone and which is laid down or removed by the surface activity of osteoblasts and osteoclasts.

When you consider that bone mass may be decreased either by failure to replace it when it is removed in the course of normal bone maintenance (osteoporosis), or by some extraordinary process of bone destruction, you will understand that the radiographs of bones in these very different conditions may indeed be indistinguishable. The acceleration of bone destruction occasioned metabolically in hyperparathyroidism is an excellent working example to contrast

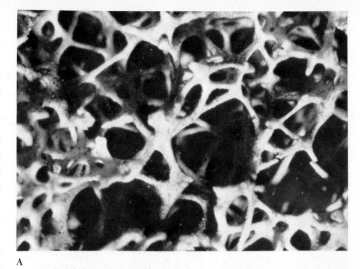

A

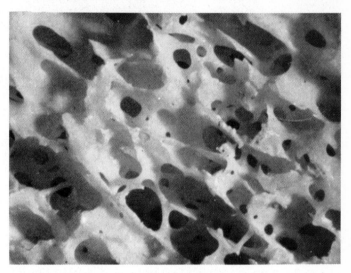

B

Figure 16-40. Cancellous bone, porotic (A) and sclerotic (B). The normal is somewhere in between.

with the much more gradual loss which occurs in osteoporosis. Both result ultimately in a pronounced decrease in bone mass, but in hyperparathyroidism the decrease occurs relatively rapidly and by a process still incompletely understood in which innumerable osteoclasts appear to destroy bone actively. This occurs in every part of the bone—on the vast total surface of the trabeculae, within the cortex, and also under the periosteum—whereas no change at all occurs in osteoporosis. The total decrease in bone mass is appreciable in bone radiographs, of course, as decreased radiodensity, but in hyperparathyroidism the distinctive subperiosteal destruction of bone may also be seen tangentially on films of the best quality, constituting a dependable diagnostic finding.

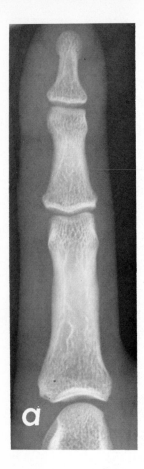
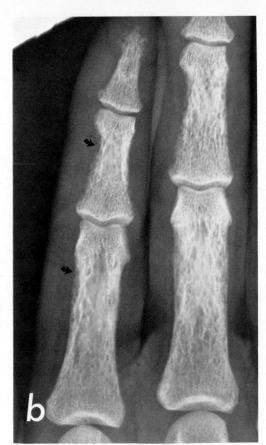
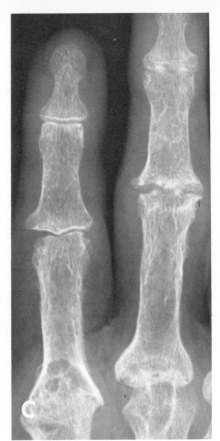

Figure 16-41

Variations in the appearance of cortical and cancellous bone which can be recognized from radiographs may be gauged from the six magnification studies of fingers on this page and the next. The engravings you see here were reduced by about half from the original magnification prints, and you are therefore seeing the details as though you looked at a routine radiograph of the hand through a low-power magnifying glass.

The finger in *a* is a normal one from a young man. The relative thickness of compact bone in midshaft in the proximal phalanx as well as the size of the individual trabeculae and the marrow space intervals between them are to be compared with the abnormal bones in the other five illustrations.

In *b* you will recognize the bone destruction occurring subperiosteally in hyperparathyroidism, not to be seen in any other bone disease and therefore distinctive. For this reason films of the hands are often requested in patients suspected of having hyperparathyroidism. Note the erosion of the terminal tuft of the distal phalanx

as well as the appearance of destruction in the areas of compact bone, thinning the cortex.

In *c*, the fingers of an elderly man whose activity had been limited for a prolonged period of time by generalized rheumatoid arthritis, the destructive joint changes are the finding which first strikes you. But look also at the cortex and note how thinned it is even in midshaft well away from the joints. In *any* severe generalized illness in which activity is sharply reduced, the development of osteoporosis is inevitable. Failure of bone replacement, of course, takes a long time to produce a significant net change in the entire bone mass, so that osteoporosis is to be anticipated in an illness of long duration. However, in very sudden and almost total interruption of activity such as that which occurs in the patient with poliomyelitis or one who is virtually immobilized in plaster following a severe accident, important changes in calcium metabolism that are largely the result of decreased bone building may have to be watched for, and ultimately osteoporosis develops to a point where it becomes appreciable radiographically. Thus the

284

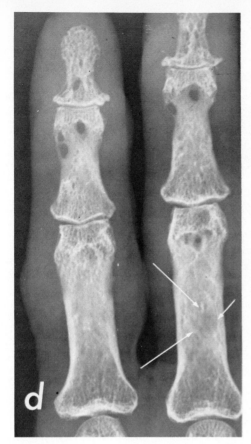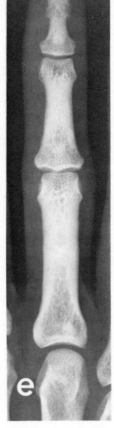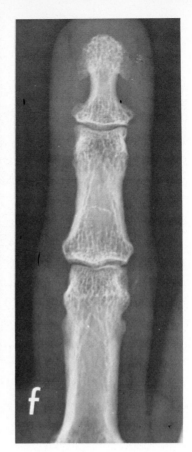

Figure 16-41 (continued)

radiographic picture in many bone diseases is complicated by the *additional* development of osteoporosis superimposed on other findings.

In *d* sharply margined areas of bone destruction are seen scattered throughout the bones, the result of pressure from granulomatous foci in a patient with sarcoidosis. Note that when these involve principally the compact bone they are much easier to recognize. When mainly trabecular bone is being destroyed, as frequently happens in widespread metastatic malignancy, a good deal more bone must be missing before one can see the change radiographically. Something of this sort is going on here in the vaguely lucent area between the arrows. The reason is of course that such areas of loss are masked by superimposed bone. Thus, in a lateral radiograph of the spine, areas of trabecular bone destruction up to 1 centimeter in diameter in the vertebral bodies will not be visible even in retrospect when their presence has been confirmed at autopsy. It is for this reason that bone isotope scans with m99 technetium are used for screening for metastases to bone, since that method

gives much earlier evidence for them than plain films.

The patient in *e* had osteopetrosis, or marble bones, an inherited fault in which the maintenance and reconstruction of bone seems to be impaired so that bone accumulates, the cortex is thick, and marrow cavities may be obliterated. All bones are affected, and patients who are severely afflicted in early infancy die apparently as a result of failing hematopoiesis. The net bone mass is strikingly increased.

In *f* form is faulty. This finger would be recognized by experts as having the typical alteration of form seen in acromegaly. Compare the widely flanged tuft of the terminal phalanx with the others on these two pages. The bones as a whole are broad, and the bases of the phalanges splayed. Note the distinctive soft-tissue changes as well. The classic acromegalic history of increasing sizes for shoes and gloves is as much due to increase in the soft tissues as to increase in the size of the bones. Roentgen findings of this sort may suggest a diagnosis not suspected clinically or confirm one which is.

285

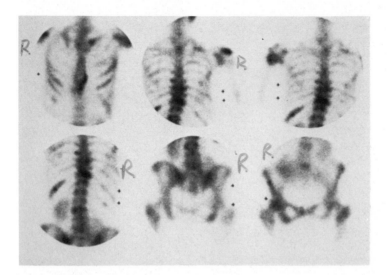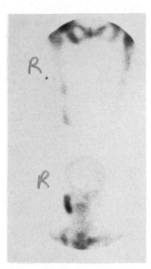

Figure 16-42. Series of technetium bone scans in a patient with breast carcinoma shows uptake of the isotope as dark patches. Note asymmetry of distribution of metastases (lower left rib, right side of mandible, right shoulder). Some of these scans were made AP, some PA.

Additional diagnostic techniques include isotope bone scans and computerized tomography; ultrasound, however, has no place in bone work because it is absorbed almost entirely when it encounters bone. CT is increasingly used in extremity work to provide a second (cross-sectional) plane of data as an adjunct to conventional films. It is also helpful in locating obscure fractures in areas difficult to radiograph, such as the spine and the base of the skull.

Technetium m99 labeled phosphorus bone scans will provide information about areas in bone in which there is rapid turnover and increased vascularity much earlier than conventional radiographs of the best quality can detect any changes at all. However, the bone scan evidence is very nonspecific, since uptake will be observed in such diverse conditions as tumor, osteomyelitis, and arthritis!

The correct current use should be as an early screening procedure in patients clinically suspected of any of these conditions. Thus a child suspected of osteomyelitis from pain and fever localized to a bone clinically will show isotope evidence up to two weeks sooner than bone destruction can be visualized on ordinary radiographs. This makes early therapy possible. Similarly, a patient with a known primary malignancy of a type which usually metastasizes to bone can be screened for bone spread as a guide to appropriate therapy before ablative surgery is contemplated.

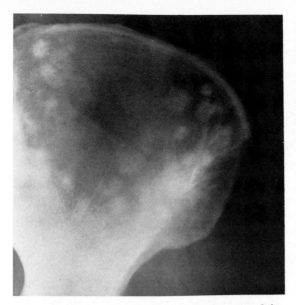

Figure 16-43. Osteoblastic metastases in the wing of the ilium. Such *increased* density is caused by new bone formation locally. Malignant metastases from carcinoma of the *prostate* most frequently produce osteoblastic foci in bone.

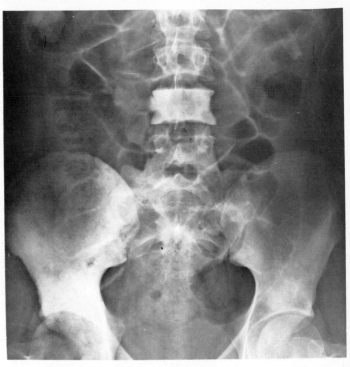

Figure 16-44. Asymmetrical blastic metastases in prostatic carcinoma. Note that here the increased bone density is diffuse rather than spotty.

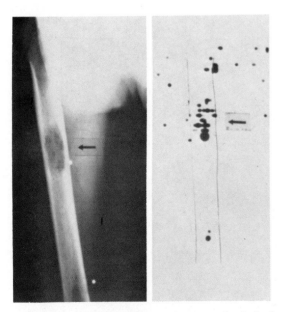

Figure 16-45. Solitary osteolytic metastasis in the shaft of the femur matched against a photoscan of the area after an injection of a radioisotope admirably suited to such studies because of its high rate of uptake in tumors and its rapid decay. Scans are also useful in determining metastatic disease which is not yet detectable in radiographs.

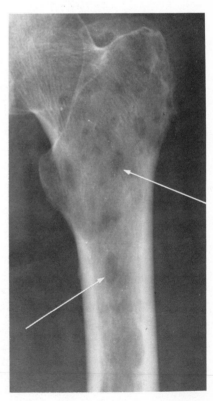

Figure 16-46. Osteolytic metastases in the upper femur. *Decreased* density due to destruction by growing tumor is usual in metastases from *kidney, lung,* and *thyroid.*

287

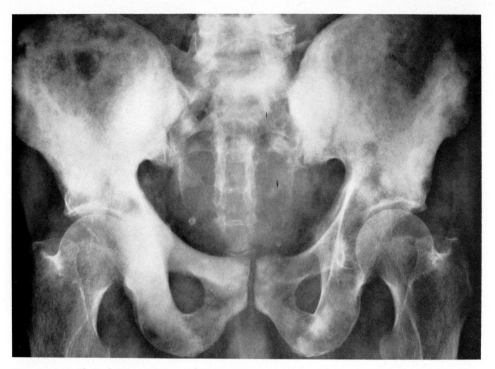

Figure 16-47. The pelvis in a patient with prostatic carcinoma. Asymmetrical dense white areas are involved by diffuse new-bone-forming metastatic disease. Note that the bone is not enlarged with thickened cortex as it is in the patient with Paget's disease below.

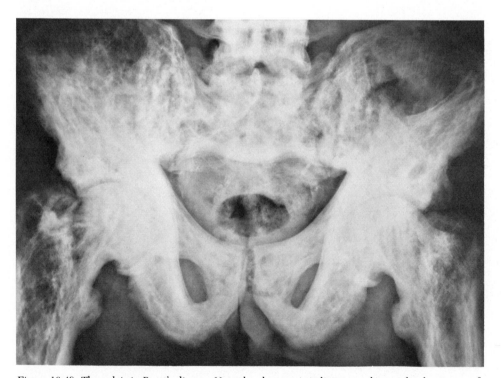

Figure 16-48. The pelvis in Paget's disease. Note the characteristic linear streaking and enlargement of bone, not present in Figure 16-47. This is an important distinction, since the two diseases are apt to be common in the same group of patients.

288

The Skull and Brain

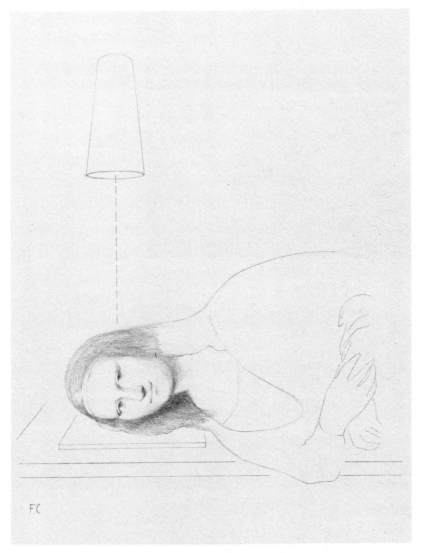

Figure 16-49

Radiography of the skull and brain is already an extensive branch of medical radiology about which many books have been written. The skull film must be viewed, like any other radiograph, while thinking in three dimensions, and the superimposed bony parts must be subtracted one from the other. The usual set of skull films comprises a series made AP, PA (in several degrees of sagittal flexion of the neck), lateral (each side in turn close to the plate), as well as one of the basilar projections in which the ray is directed so that it superimposes the complex basilar structures upon the less complex calvarial cap. The lateral view of the skull shows the two halves of the coronal suture superimposed. The two parts of the lambdoidal suture are seen. Sutures usually remain visible throughout life, distinguishable from fracture lines by their serpiginous character and white margins, while a fracture will be more linear, not at all marginated, and usually more radiolucent. Study the normal skull films on the next pages.

The Lateral View

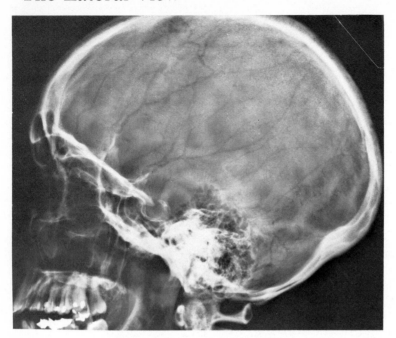

Figure 16-50. Normal lateral film.

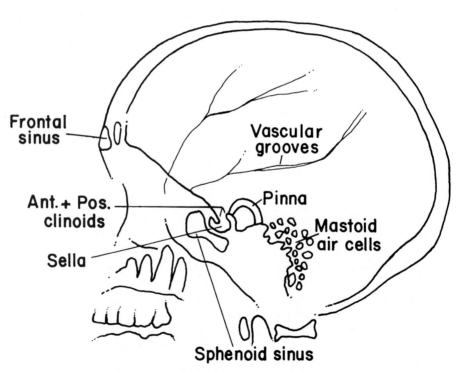

Figure 16-51. Labeled diagram to match Figure 16-50.

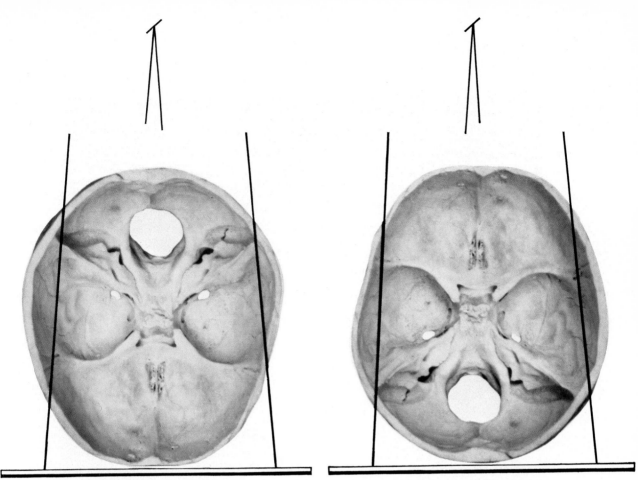

Figure 16-52. PA projection.

Figure 16-53. AP projection.

Skull films made PA and AP will look different to you, because in one the orbits are close to the film while in the other they are projected from far away and therefore show larger round circles of bone.

These photographs, made from above looking down into the unroofed skull, will help you to identify the anterior, middle, and posterior fossae, the sella, anterior and posterior clinoids, and the superimposed petrous tips in the lateral radiograph opposite.

The sagittal suture is not seen, of course, in the lateral view, but the coronal and lambdoidal are, one side superimposed on the other. Note that the face is "burned out" on the lateral film; facial fractures would be missed if you had ordered skull films instead of a facial series.

291

The PA View

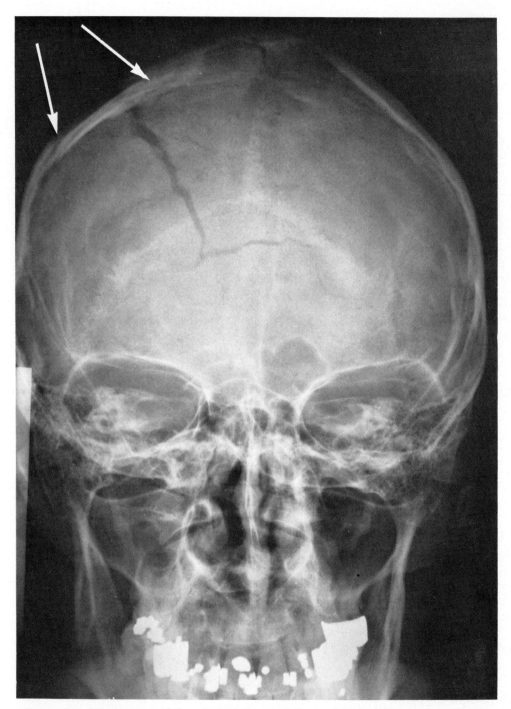

Figure 16-54. PA projection with fractures both linear and depressed. A plate of bone seen in tangent (between the arrows) is slightly depressed. This is not a simple linear fracture but a comminuted one, therefore. Note fillings in the teeth. Identify: odontoid seen through the nose, frontal sinuses, petrous tips with internal auditory canals seen through orbits.

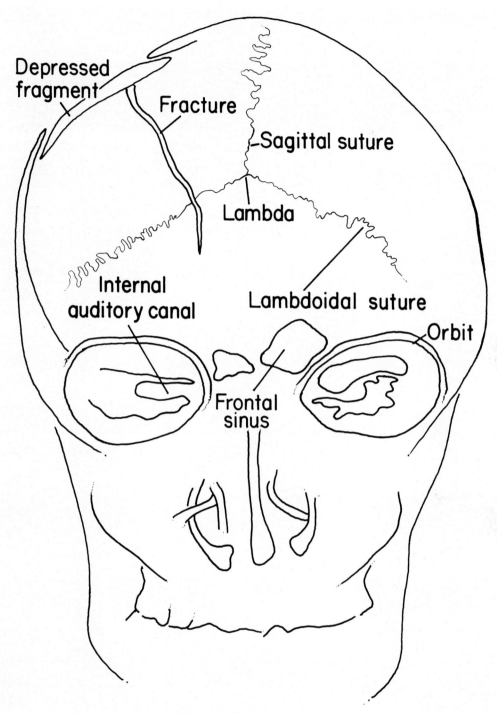

Figure 16-55. Labeled diagram to match Figure 16-54.

The Basilar View

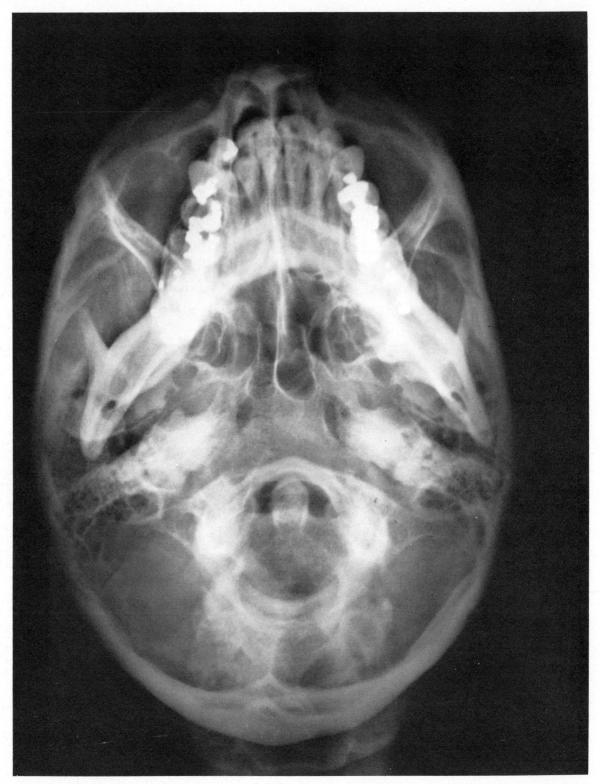

Figure 16-56. Inferior-superior or basilar view of the skull. Normal. Identify: mandible, foramen magnum, odontoid, petrous tips, foramen lacerum, foramen ovale, foramen spinosum, and sphenoid sinus.

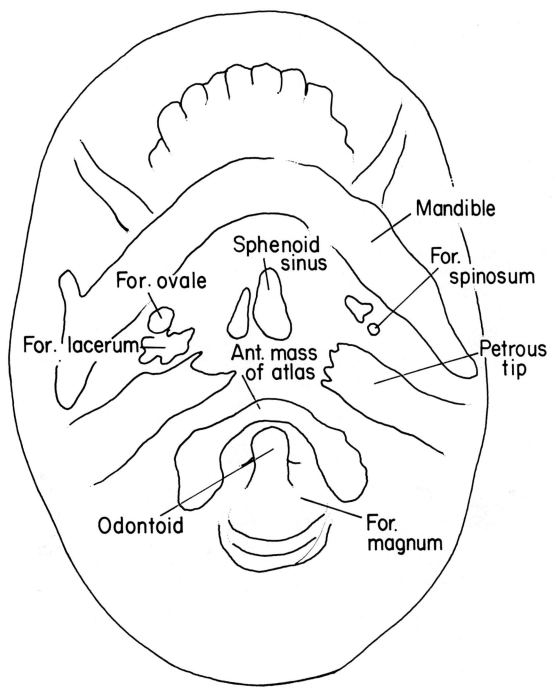

Figure 16-57. Labeled diagram to match Figure 16-56.

CT or Skull Films in Head Trauma?

You will find that today patients are having skull series made much less frequently than they used to do, and that being able, yourself, to study skull films without help from the radiologist is seldom necessary. This is true for two main reasons. First, one no longer screens for bone metastases by making a "skeletal survey" (which includes the skull); one employs a bone scan for the purpose of screening and then documents areas of increased uptake with radiographs (which *are* more specific).

Second, physicians are beginning to realize that it is an obsolete procedure to request skull films automatically on head trauma patients. It is vital to decide in such patients *whether there is significant (and much more important) neural injury.* The presence or absence of a linear skull fracture is incidental and can in any event be demonstrated later on, when the proper study by CT has been made and the patient's clinical condition permits. Of course when inspection shows evidence suggesting a *depressed* fracture, skull films may have to be made tangential to the plane of the depressed fragment as a guide to the neurosurgeon.

Computerized tomography has revolutionized neuroradiology, and well-educated general practitioners know that any patient with a history of loss of consciousness and neurological symptoms after head injury should go straight to the nearest CT room for study. It is not a question of radiation exposure (the exposure from CT is about equivalent to that for a skull series) but rather of efficiency in diagnosis that may be life saving. *CT is able to demonstrate early and minimal subdural hemorrhage, and precious time would be wasted filming the skull in the conventional way.* Well-conducted studies have shown that injury to the brain or tearing of intracranial vessels often occurs when no skull fracture is present.

A first-rate history and neurological examination, followed if negative by serial checks of the neurological status, should be the concern of those who provide primary care for head injury patients, and if aberrations are present, such as loss of consciousness, vomiting, or pupillary difference, the next step is an emergency CT study. If it is not available at your hospital, have your patient transferred to one where it is. The linear skull fracture, if present, requires no separate treatment and can be documented with films later if necessary. Remember this when you are pressured to order skull films by patients' families or their lawyers. *Tell them the brain comes first.*

In patients in whom the injuries are only facial, you should order *facial films*, not skull films. They are made quite differently. Facial fractures can be missed and are seldom seen well on routine skull films.

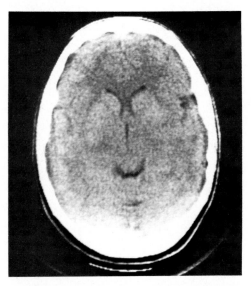

Figure 16-58. CT section showing normal midline and para midline structures (for example, anterior ventricles, third ventricle).

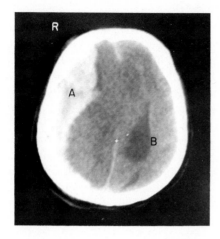

Figure 16-59. CT scan shows (A) enormous acute subdural hematoma after head trauma (the right ventricle is entirely obliterated); (B) dilated left ventricle secondary to shift of midline structures and obliteration of the third ventricle. (Surgery attempted but the patient died on the table.)

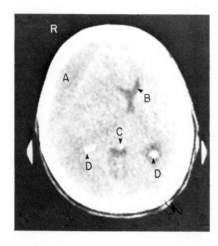

Figure 16-60. Another patient with large chronic subdural hematoma (A). Note shifted and compressed lateral ventricles (B); calcified pineal, also shifted to the left (C); calcified choroid plexus (D). At operation about 100 cubic centimeters of blood was removed. Patient did well postoperatively.

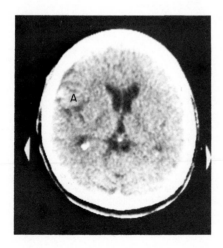

Figure 16-61. Same patient as in Figure 16-60 some time after the operation. CT scan shows midline structures returned to normal position. (A) indicates area of residual atrophy from chronic compression.

297

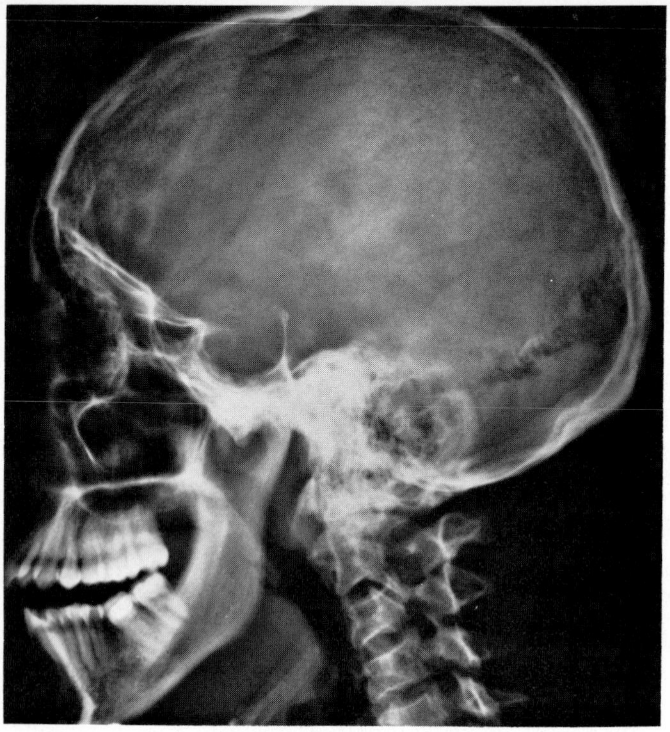

Figure 16-62. Pituitary tumor with enlarged sella. Note that the posterior clinoids are thinned and tilted backward.

Skull Films in the Nontraumatized Patient

In nontraumatized patients the skull series is often diagnostic, of course, and you will want to review those films with your radiologist, informing him with regard to the history and working clinical diagnosis. A variety of disease conditions cause more or less distinctive *intracranial calcification*, for example. These include slow-growing gliomas, arteriovenous malformations, meningioma, craniopharyngioma, old infection (abscess, tuberculoma, toxoplasmosis), and congenital aberrations like the Sturge-Weber syndrome. Cranial calcifications are also to be seen normally (pineal gland, choroid plexus, falx) and are unimportant.

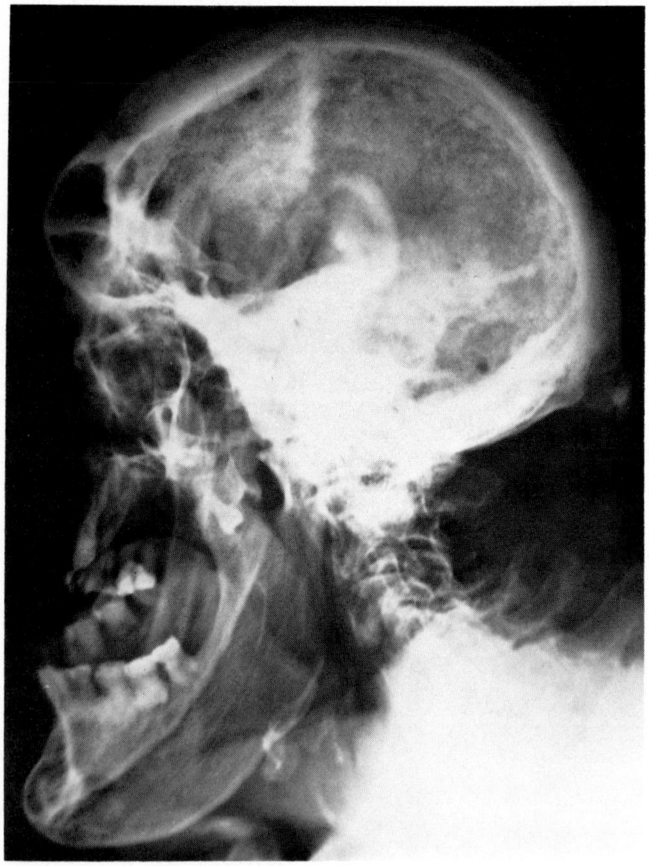

Figure 16-63 (left). Acromegaly with marked overgrowth of the mandible, but the sella turcica normal in size in this patient. More commonly the sella is enlarged.

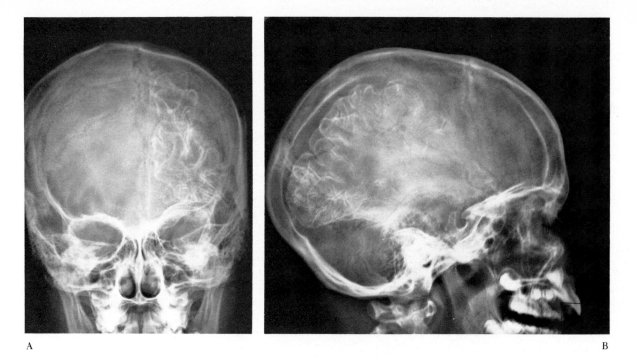

A   B

Figure 16-64. Intracranial calcifications of many kinds have been catalogued, some distinctive for the condition they occur in, others quite unspecific. Here wavy irregular calcifications in the parieto-occipital part of the brain have an appearance characteristic of that seen in Sturge-Weber syndrome (encephalotrigeminal angiomatosis). The fundamental lesion in this condition is an anomalous development of the blood vessels of the skin, meninges, and underlying brain, with the cutaneous angiomas, or "port-wine" marks occurring in the trigeminal distribution. Calcification has been attributed to disturbance of circulation through the angiomatous channels with focal infarctions. Note how calcification and smaller size of hemicalvarium containing it indicate cerebral hemiatrophy. Both would be evident on computerized tomography.

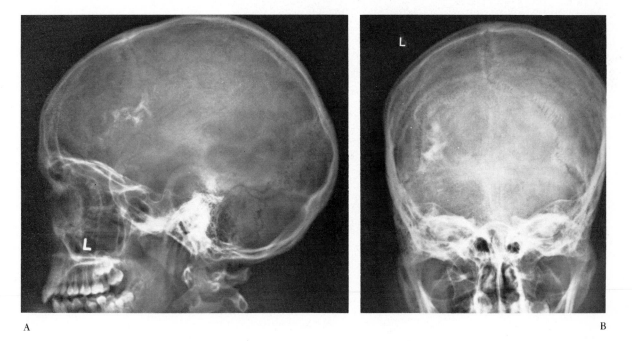

A   B

Figure 16-65. Can you locate this intracranial calcification?

299

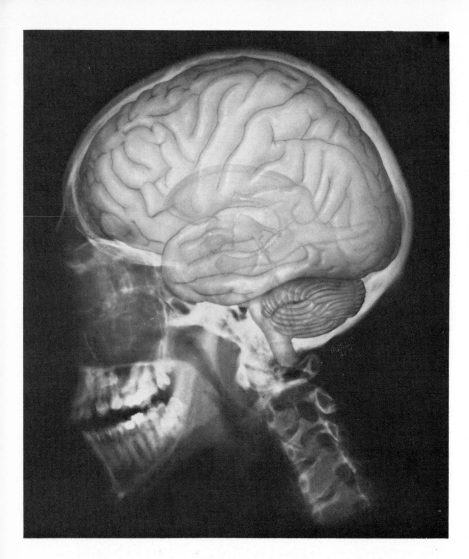

Figure 16-66A. Superimposition of the apparently transparent brain and its ventricular system on a lateral radiograph of the skull will help you to visualize the relationships and to think three-dimensionally about skull films and air studies. Identify the two lateral ventricles (superimposed in this projection), the third ventricle, the aqueduct, and the fourth ventricle. Note how the temporal horns of the lateral ventricles extend forward, appearing to cross the aqueduct, although intellectually you know the temporal lobes to be far lateral and the aqueduct midline.

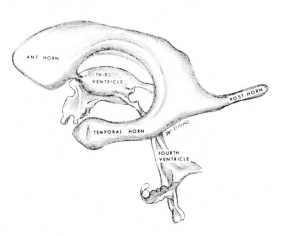

Figure 16-66B. Labeled diagram of the ventricular system.

The Brain

Before computerized tomography was evolved, several more invasive procedures were much used. *Pneumoencephalography* involves the introduction of air via spinal puncture, with subsequent filming of the head in several projections. The air, as a radiolucent contrast substance, fills the arachnoid spaces over the surface of the brain and the ventricular system. This procedure is quite uncomfortable to the patient and is seldom performed today, since almost all the same information can be obtained by CT with no discomfort or subsequent morbidity for the patient, and computerized tomography can be performed as an out-patient study.

Cerebral arteriography with injection of contrast substance into both right and left carotids and vertebral arteries (or any one of them) uses the displacement of the visualized arterial tree and the presence of abnormal vascularity to locate and define masses. Intravenous contrast enhancement is used during CT studies, just as it is elsewhere in the body, to emphasize the difference between well-vascularized and poorly-vascularized tissues, or to demonstrate breakdown in the blood-brain barrier. Cerebral arteriography per se is most commonly used today in the demonstration and localization of cerebral aneurysm.

Because computerized tomography is many times more sensitive to slight differences in the density of tissues, the anatomy of the brain and the ventricles is well outlined and even the difference between gray and white matter seen, rendering slight degrees of cortical atrophy visible.

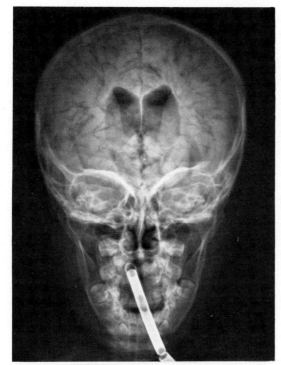

A

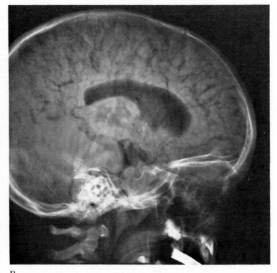

B

Figure 16-67. A: Pneumoencephalogram. Air is injected into the spinal canal and is seen here in the subarachnoid space over the brain and filling the ventricles. (Slight convolutional atrophy present.) B: Lateral view.

301

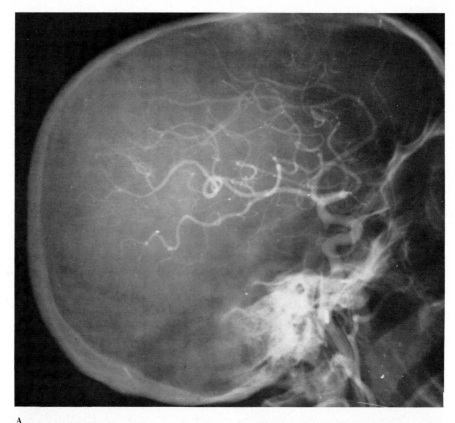

A

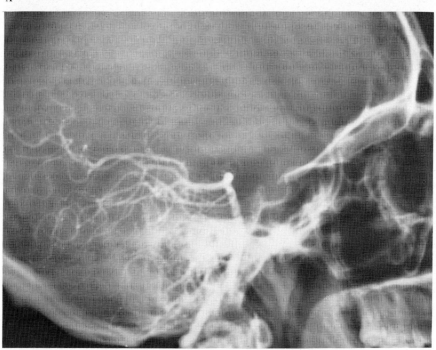

B

Figure 16-68. Cerebral arteriogram. A: Carotid artery injection. B: Vertebral artery injection.

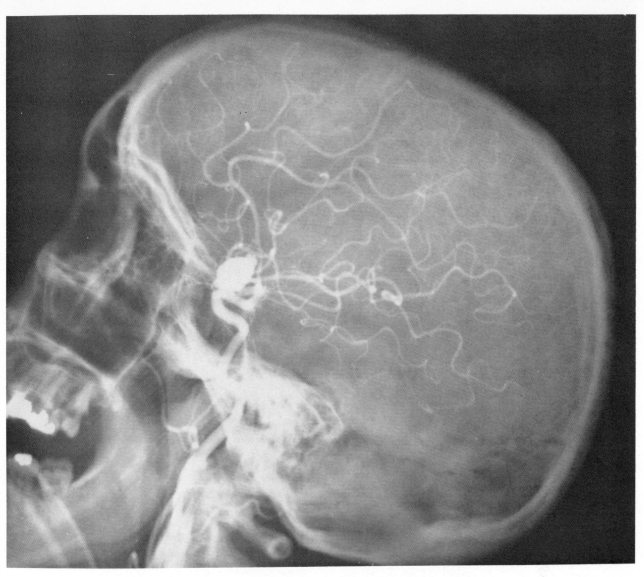

Figure 16-69. Cerebral arteriogram. Follow the course of the carotid artery upward to the cranial cavity. The pool of opaque material is in an aneurysm.

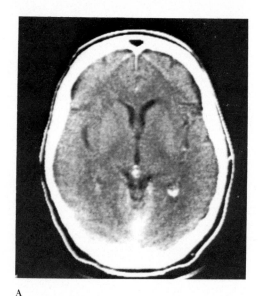
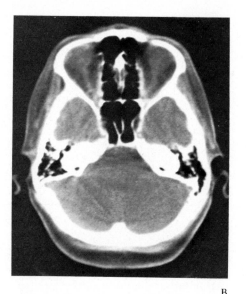

A   B

Figure 16-70. A: Normal CT scan. Note ventricles, calcified pineal gland behind the third ventricle, and calcified choroid plexus bilaterally. B: Lower scan through the base of the skull. Note petrous tips and mastoid air cells.

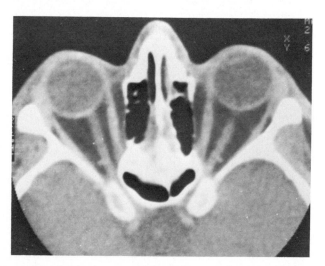

Figure 16-71. CT scan through the orbits. Note globe of the eye, lens, medial and lateral rectus muscles, and optic nerve embedded in the retro-orbital fat.

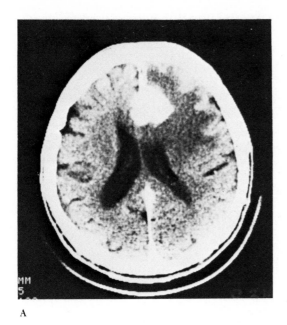

Figure 16-72. Falcine meningioma demonstrated on CT scan (A) and at cerebral angiography (B and C below)—early and late studies (subtraction technique) showing the late "stain" of retained contrast substance in the tumor.

A

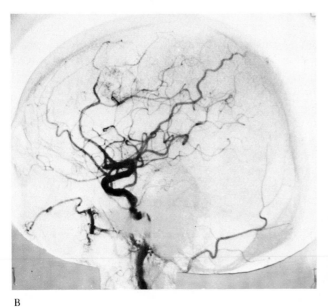

B

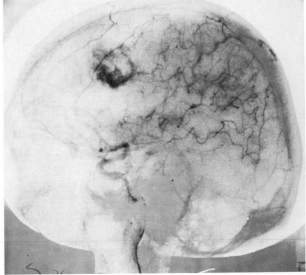

C

305

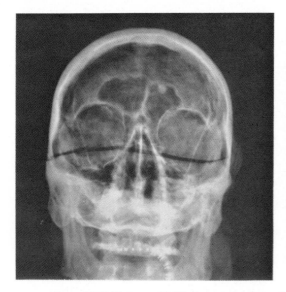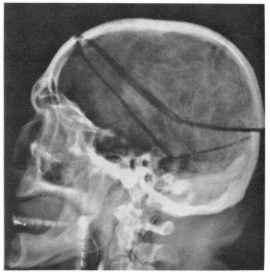

Figure 16-73 (*Unknown 16-13*). Try your hand at radiologic medicolegal detective work. These are radiographs made at the request of the coroner after the prosector had failed to establish the cause of death. The deceased had apparently been beaten to death in a drunken altercation. During the fight he had received multiple cuts from a soft-drink bottle and at autopsy numerous contusions were seen about the face, but there was no evidence of skull fracture or of intracranial hemorrhage. What cause of death, indicated by these films and noted by the radiologist, was confirmed by reexamination of the corpse?

The final unknown serves as a last reminder that roentgen shadows are essentially logical, and that from roentgen density as a clue to composition, and from form as a clue to structure, even unfamiliar objects may be recognized.

In the same fashion, disease processes whose roentgen appearance you have not yet seen will appeal to you as logical when you do see them, because you will think in terms of the pathologic change you know to have occurred. For instance, you will *expect* osteomyelitis to appear as an ill-defined, ragged area of destruction in bone visualized late in the illness, since dissolution of a rigid structure takes time to occur. It will not surprise you, therefore, that the patient with acute osteomyelitis must usually be treated presumptively before the roentgen findings are definite, and that for this reason bone scans are used early and treatment instituted: films are useful and important in following the course and progress of the disease rather than in affording a means of identifying it early.

Bone growth, too, is beautifully documented in serial films, like time-lapse studies of opening flowers. Vagaries of growth can be analyzed and comprehended through such serial studies. If you want to appreciate the fascinating patho-

logic implications evident from such studies, hunt out the film envelope of a patient in your hospital (there must be one!) who had achondroplasia, the familiar classic form of dwarfism, diagnosed in infancy and followed into adulthood. Compare his films with the pattern of growth in normal bones, measuring in the stunted femurs and square pelvis the failure of cartilage proliferation at the growth plates. Many such adventures in thinking await you in the next few years as you familiarize yourself with the roentgen appearance of normal and abnormal bones.

Future advances in neuroradiology may come with digital angiography and nuclear magnetic resonance. Digital angiography is a technique whereby the faint opacification of arteries after *intravenous* injection of contrast medium is accentuated by serial computerized subtraction. This produces an "arteriogram" without an arterial catheter or injection. Present resolution limits the study to the extracranial circulation, but advances are expected.

Nuclear magnetic resonance (NMR) scans are obtained by placing the patient in a magnetic field and exciting his protons with radiofrequency radiation. The number of protons varies in different tissues, and since the speed of relaxation of the hydrogen atom depends upon its chemical surroundings, different tissues can be distinguished from one another. Although at present experimental, NMR shows great promise, especially in the diagnosis of white-matter disease. It is likely that for the foreseeable future NMR and CT of the head will be useful as complementary procedures. Both are exciting advances for you to think about.

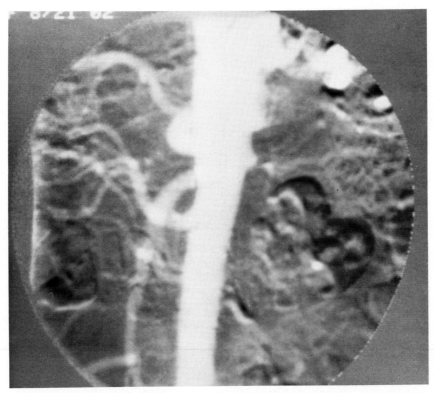

Figure 16-74. Digital video subtraction. *Intravenous* contrast medium with digital video subtraction technique in a young patient with hypertension successfully demonstrates absence of *arterial* perfusion of the left kidney.

Appendixes

Index

APPENDIX A Answers to Unknowns

Unknown 1-1 (Figure 1-14)

The pair of dice on the right have been loaded by boring holes into the substance of the die, filling with heavy metal, recapping, and repainting the dots. Bits of lead wire have been used. Of the loaded pair, the die on the left has been x-rayed with the loaded face down as it would tend to fall. The die on the right has been turned on its side and then x-rayed. Note that you are now looking through it from the side, so to speak. The loaded face is down and very dense. The upper part of the die has been evacuated and left empty, increasing its tendency to fall with the "2" facing up—or the "5," depending on which is chosen by the tamperer.

Unknown 1-2 (Figure 1-15)

No, not an egg with a nail in it. The oval object could not be an egg because its radiodensity falls away at the edge and is much greater and fairly uniform in the center. Therefore, this must be a solid oval body of considerable density and homogeneous composition, except for the nail, which actually was in the center of it. The dark streaks are air in the interfaces after it has been cracked open. The object was a mineral bolus found in the stomach of a horse. The nail, typical of those used for shoeing horses, had undoubtedly been swallowed many years ago and remained in the stomach. The "stone," a concretion like a gallstone, had been built up around it gradually.

Unknown 2-1 (Figure 2-22)

If you "saw" Figure 2-22 as a rather curvaceous posterior view, old habit tricked you! This is a radiograph of the last slice of the cadaver. The only bony structures in this slice are the posterior shell of ribs, the spinous processes of the vertebrae and the sacrum.

Unknown 2-2 (Figure 2-23)

Radiograph of a midline sagittal slice of a female cadaver. It can only be a midline slice: the uterus, sternum, and vertebrae are present, whereas the breasts, rib shadows, and pelvic bones are absent.

Unknown 3-1 (Figure 3-13)

The ribs are numbered correctly. Structures indicated by white arrows are cervical ribs arising from the last cervical vertebra.

Unknown 3-2 (Figure 3-14)

The eighth rib on the left is fractured close to its vertebral end. There is also a fracture of the lateral margin of the scapula.

Unknown 3-3 (Figure 3-15)

Fractured clavicle. Air from a break in the skin has infiltrated the soft tissues (subcutaneous emphysema).

Unknown 4-1 (no figure in text)

Search the patient's clothing for a straight pin; then order another chest film, specifying your reason for doing so. The technician will make sure that there is no straight pin *outside* the patient. The radiologist will determine whether there is one *inside*, altogether unlikely in this case, but a risk not to be taken preoperatively. Figure A-1 shows a chest film of a different patient in which a hat pin actually was in the left main bronchus. A photograph of the recovered hat pin has been superimposed on the radiograph. This patient, needless to say, was not talking comfortably. Foreign bodies are more commonly seen in the right main bronchus. Why?

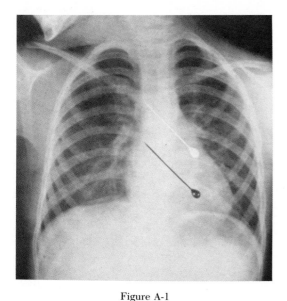

Figure A-1

Unknown 4-2 (Figure 4-22)

You see spotty densities well out in the lung parenchyma which do not taper like vessels. A small circular gray shadow with a darker interior suggests a cavity. Obviously, at age 23 inflammation of some kind is more likely than tumor or lung insult through employment, neither of which is very plausible from the story. Certainly tuberculosis, a strong possibility, must be ruled out by collateral laboratory procedures. If the chest film made three months before (or any other fairly recent film) can be obtained for comparison, it may be easier to judge the age of the process. You can discard consideration of an inflammation one day old and probably that of one week, since involvement of lung tissue enough to produce infiltrative densities, a cavity, and the story of weight loss indicate a somewhat older process. The best choice would be subacute inflammation one month old—although that is not entirely satisfactory either, since earlier changes *might* have been missed on the insurance film.

Unknown 4-3 (Figure 4-23)

The left shoulder girdle is missing, removed surgically because of a malignant bone tumor. Note that the medial part of the left clavicle is still present.

Unknown 4-4 (Figure 4-24)

The clavicles are normal. The scapulae, rotated well out, appear normal, their margins seen crossing the upper ribs near the lateral chest wall. The anterior ends of the two first ribs have a curious appearance due to calcification in the costochondral junction. You will see this often. Clavicles and ribs are symmetrical without distortion due to rotation. The hila and lung markings would pass for normal, with the exception of the lung parenchyma seen in the window formed between the posterior parts of the right fifth and sixth ribs and the anterior tips of the first and second ribs. Here you see some increased density, not present in the comparable interspace window on the left. In a far anterior body-section study (Figure A-2) this density is more clearly seen, placing it near the anterior tips of the first two ribs. It proved to be a malignant tumor arising in the pleura.

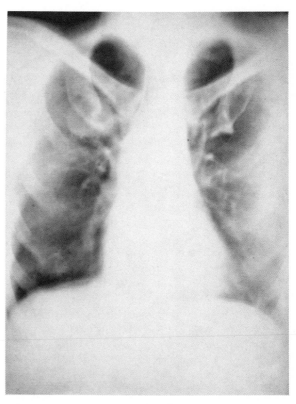

Figure A-2

311

Unknown 5-1 (Figure 5-13)

Pneumonia of the superior segment of the RLL. You would hear rales posteriorly. The heart border is clearly seen. Therefore the lung density must be behind the heart in the lower lobe.

Unknown 6-1 (Figure 6-7)

The diaphragm is elevated by large amounts of air below it in the peritoneal space (pneumoperitoneum), one method of putting the lung at rest in pulmonary tuberculosis. The diaphragmatic leaves are seen as thin sheets of muscle, the right at the level of the ninth rib and the left a little lower. Liver and spleen are displaced downward and medially. The patient was unable to pull his diaphragm down well in inspiration because of the air cushion below.

Unknown 6-2 (Figure 6-18)

The bones are normal, as are the soft tissues in this male patient. The heart and mediastinum appear to be slightly deviated to the left. The diaphragmatic shadows are at the level of the eleventh rib and appear normal. The left costophrenic sinus is normal; the right one is blunted and appears to contain a small amount of fluid, since there is a short fluid level there. There is a pneumothorax on the right, the lower and middle lobes being almost completely collapsed and very dense. The upper lobe is still partly expanded. There are mottled densities in the parenchyma of this lobe. The left lung field is abnormal, with an area of density in the middle of the sixth interspace measuring about 2 centimeters in its longest dimension. (All this you can say about this film without any clinical information and, you observe, without mentioning any diagnosis.)

If the above report were to reach you, the physician, and you were already pretty sure that your patient had tuberculosis, the points in this report would give you just what you wanted to know, namely, that there is a pneumothorax on the right, as you suspected from your physical examination, and that the disease is probably bilateral, which you may not have suspected. The radiologist would have been thinking the patient had tuberculosis, of course, and might add to his report in summary that the findings are most consistent with that disease, although both you and he know that these roentgen findings could possibly be caused by several other disease conditions. If the radiologist takes a shortcut here and in his summary simply says, "Bilateral tuberculosis with pneumothorax on the right," he is, admittedly, reading from his knowledge based on experience that no other disease is *very* likely to give just this picture. He also assumes that such a patient will not be treated for tuberculosis by you without bacteriologic confirmation.

Unknown 6-3 (Figure 6-19)

This fluid level could not be inside the thorax, since it extends beyond the rib cage. It is an air-fluid level inside a breast prosthesis in a mastectomy patient.

Unknown 7-1 (Figure 7-24)

There is consolidation of the right upper lobe (note air bronchogram) with some elevation of the minor fissure indicating a degree of atelectasis, not unusual in pneumonia. With the clinical story and these findings, one would treat as pneumonia.

Unknown 7-2 (Figure 7-25)

The absence of the left diaphragm should strike you. Considering the absence of the diaphragm and the apparent depression of the left hilum, there may be some shift of the mediastinum to the left. The lateral view shows only one diaphragmatic shadow, and taking the two views together, this indicates density at the base of the left hemithorax. Some pneumonic infiltrate, some atelectasis, some pleural fluid are all possible. When you are told that the patient had a three-year history of fever, wheezing, cough, and left chest pain, you are compelled to consider first the presence of chronic infection at the left base, possibly with some decrease in size of the left lower lobe to explain the depressed hilum. You cannot reasonably consider acute left lower lobe atelectasis with this history. The presence or absence of fluid could be established at fluoroscopy.

The film in Figure A-3 was made two years later. There is now obvious shift of the mediastinum to the left. At surgery this patient proved to have a benign tumor in the left lower lobe bronchus, and massive atelectasis was present.

Unknown 8-1 (Figure 8-22)

A soft-tissue mass containing dense calcium deposits would have been visualized by CT located close to the trachea and superior vena cava, corroborating the plain film and tomographic studies. Diagnosis: possible hamartoma, but probably old infection.

Unknown 8-2 (Figure 8-23)

The second scan shows several small soft-tissue nodules in the lung which were confirmed on chest films a month later when they had increased in size. The patient finally agreed to chemotherapy, which afforded him time to arrange his affairs.

Unknown 9-1 (no figure in text)

Bronchogenic carcinoma may first cause symptoms in a wide variety of ways. You probably have on your list all the following:

(1) Silent infiltration of the lung. Likely to be discovered only on routine physical examination or check chest film.

(2) Obstruction of a bronchus. May cause cough as the initial symptom, or occasionally hemoptysis. Radiograph may look entirely normal if the mass is small and close within the hilum. Will eventually appear on the radiograph as a

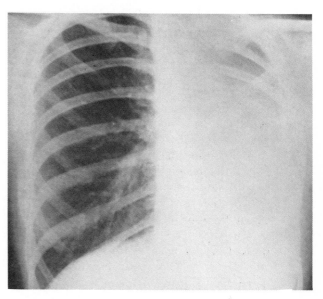

Figure A-3

mass of increased density within the lung or close to the hilum, and may appear at the time of the first examination as:

(3) Atelectasis of the segment of lung distal to the obstructed brochus.

(4) Atelectasis with pneumonia distal to the obstruction.

(5) Pneumonia, apparently a simple inflammation clinically, but which does not clear and improve on schedule with appropriate treatment. (You must be very suspicious of repeated episodes of atelectasis in the same lung segment and of recalcitrant pneumonic infiltrations in the lungs of patients in the cancer age group.)

(6) Bronchogenic carcinoma not infrequently metastasizes early to the pleura. The patient may therefore appear at your office for the first time complaining of symptoms and presenting signs of pleural effusion, without other complaints or findings.

(7) Bronchogenic carcinoma metastasizes to bone very commonly, and if such involvement occurs before other symptoms bring the patient to your office, he may be complaining of bone pain anywhere at all. You may see him because of a fracture which has occurred through bone invaded by tumor.

(8) Distant metastases to parenchymatous organs may occur early while bronchogenic car-

313

cinoma is still asymptomatic in the chest. Such a patient may therefore present himself for help with symptoms of a brain tumor or with almost total adrenal gland destruction, to mention only two possibilities. Radiographic study of his chest may reveal the shadow of the primary tumor, or if the tumor is small and has metastasized very early, the chest films may at first be entirely negative.

(9) Bronchogenic carcinoma may metastasize early to the lymph glands and bring the patient to you because of pressure from such glands on any of the mediastinal structures. Notable among these patterns of initial difficulty is one in which the trachea is surrounded and compressed by tumor nodes, resulting in dyspnea and wheezing. The vascular structures of the superior mediastinum may also be compressed, giving the symptoms of superior vena cava obstruction, for example.

(10) Bronchogenic carcinoma may invade the pericardium, presenting initial symptoms of pericardial effusion.

(P.S. There are still other possibilities!)

Unknown 10-1 (Figure 10-35)

The young man shows borderline cardiac enlargement to measurement, but the concave left border and general shape of his heart suggest left ventricular hypertrophy out of proportion to his age. The too-prominent aortic knob confirms this impression; it is not the aortic shadow you expect for a young man. This patient had malignant hypertension of some standing.

Unknown 10-2 (Figure 10-36)

Left ventricle, left atrium, and aorta are opacified. Opacification of the atrium implies insufficiency of the mitral valve. The atrium is obviously dilated.

Unknown 10-3 (Figure 10-37)

In myxedema the heart shadow is frequently enlarged and, pathologically, this is found to be due to a combination of dilatation of the chambers, some increased bulk of the heart muscle, and frequently pericardial effusion. A combination in this patient of a thickened, myxedematous myocardium and arteriosclerotic compromise of its blood supply might well contribute to the advent of failure. Here the angiocardiograms establish the extent to which the increased size of the heart shadow is due to the pericardial effusion and thick myocardium rather than to failure with dilatation. Echocardiography is in order.

Unknown 11-1 (Figure 11-51)

Cervical vertebra of a giraffe. It, too, has only seven.

Unknown 11-2 (Figure 11-52)

The upper half of the abdomen is blank and airless. There is no air in the stomach which can be clearly identified. The spleen is obviously enlarged and it lies close against the flank. There is no displacement of the colon away from the left flank stripe. Both kidneys appear to be depressed, as do all air-containing structures. This patient had Hodgkin's lymphoma with massive enlargement of both liver and spleen. That diagnosis could not be made from the film, of course, as there is nothing distinctive about the roentgen findings.

Unknown 11-3 (Figure 11-53)

The plain film shows a round, sharply demarcated area of radiolucency overlying the sacrum, and the barium study shows the sigmoid colon lifted up over this "mass" and apparently flattened against it posteriorly across the rectosigmoid junction. At surgery, as predicted by the radiologist, a 10-centimeter cystic mass was removed, which proved to be a dermoid cyst and to contain thick, grumous, fatty material. Note the calcium-dense shadow overlying the sacroiliac joint on the right, which was contained in the cyst and consisted of a rudimentary tooth. Teeth are often present in dermoid cysts, and the combination of a circumscribed radiolucent shadow with a density resembling a tooth is dependable roentgen evidence identifying the nature of such masses.

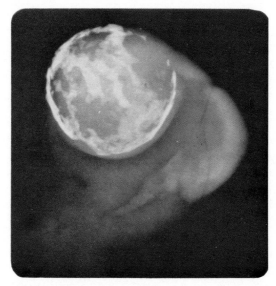

Figure A-4. Radiograph of the specimen (spleen with calcified cyst).

Unknown 11-4 (Figure 11-54)

The anterior surfaces of the bodies of the last two thoracic and the first lumbar vertebrae show marked erosion in the lateral view. The AP view shows erosion of the left lateral surface of L1, the most extensively involved of the three. The aorta below this level is strikingly calcified, but at the level of L1 it is deviated sharply anteriorly. The patient had a large aneurysm lying against T11, T12, and L1. Note well the calcified aorta seen through the bones on the AP view.

Unknown 11-5 (Figure 11-55)

Peripheral calcification in a splenic cyst located close to the diaphragm and indenting the stomach. The patient was Norwegian and had no symptoms and no important findings. The spleen and cyst were removed surgically, and in Figure A-4 you see a radiograph of the entire specimen. Microscopic examination showed no evidence of parasitic infection. The cyst contained clear fluid and may have resulted from trauma many years before.

Unknown 11-6 (Figure 11-56)

Dark subcutaneous fat can be seen outlining the elbow and flexed forearm and the buttocks. The crescentic gray shadow above the fetus is the placenta in its normal location high in the uterus. Compare the thickness of the uterine wall over the fetal rump.

Unknown 13-1 (Figure 13-10)

Four spot films of the antrum of the stomach and duodenum show a small round filling defect arising from the greater curvature about 3 centimeters from the pylorus. The defect is present on all films and represented a gastric polyp.

Unknown 13-2 (Figure 13-43)

Large scrotal hernia containing part of the barium-filled sigmoid, which extends well below the pelvic brim.

315

Unknown 15-1 (Figure 15-37)

(1) Yes, you would have sent the patient for excretory urography; any patient with hematuria after trauma needs that study.

(2) The shortest arrow points to the perivesical fat on the roof of the urinary bladder (seen tangentially). There is a soft-tissue mass above the bladder filling up the rest of the pelvic bowl. It was palpable on bimanual pelvic examination and proved to be a solitary pelvic kidney (two long arrows indicate the collecting system.) No kidney shadow could be seen on either side in the usual location on any of the patient's films.

The hematuria cleared without treatment, on rest and watchful support. Had the symptoms been more serious and life threatening, it would have been vital for the surgeon to know that she had only one kidney and where it was located! (The fourth arrow indicates a snap on the patient's gown. Anything *that* symmetrical is likely to be an artifact.)

Unknown 16-1 (Figure 16-2)

The legs have been broken in order to shorten the mummy, doubtless to make it fit into a burial case which the embalmer had on hand. The lower femurs have been removed, and the arms are also missing. The mummy probably dates from no later than 1000 B.C., because after that time much more packing was used in the preparation of embalmed bodies. Embalmers were often dishonest and left off parts of the bodies entrusted to them. Radiographs have shown that the "trunk" was sometimes filled with animal bones and trash and included only the human skull.

Unknown 16-2 (Figure 16-8)

Mother Whistler has a spiral fracture of her third metatarsal. Let no one say she did not put her foot down with Jimmy!

Unknown 16-3 (Figure 16-16)

Fused hip, of long standing, following tuberculous arthritis. The joint space and cartilage have disappeared. Note bony trabeculae crossing the region of the joint.

Unknown 16-4 (Figure 16-17)

Comminuted fracture of the humerus extends into the base of the greater tuberosity.

Unknown 16-5 (Figure 16-18)

Impacted fracture of the neck of the humerus.

Unknown 16-6 (Figure 16-19)

Fracture of the medial condyle of the tibia, the fracture line extending downward from the joint surface to the medial side of the tibia, with some depression of the fragment. The obliquity of the projection used here may be appreciated from the position of the patella.

Unknown 16-7 (Figure 16-20)

Radiograph of a fractured tibia several weeks after the injury, made the day the initial plaster cast was removed. Shadowy flocculent white material (callus) is taking on mineral, which tells you that this is not a fresh fracture.

Unknown 16-8 (Figure 16-21)

Fracture of the radial head is easier to see in B, an oblique view. Note offset of white bone at the fracture point in A.

Unknown 16-9 (Figure 16-22)

Fracture of the distal end of the radial metaphysis at the wrist with displacement of its epiphysis. Note white overlap of bone in AP view, always a clue to the presence of subtle fractures.

Unknown 16-10 (Figure 16-23)

No fracture is present. This is a normal immature wrist. Note that in children it is the convention to radiograph also the noninjured extremity as a mirror image for comparison with the injured part. You will always be able to distinguish a growth plate from a fracture because it is smoothly marginated by white lines.

Unknown 16-11 (Figure 16-24)

Impacted fracture of the radius 1.5 centimeters from the radiocarpal joint. The typical Colles' fracture adds a fracture of the styloid process of the ulna, not present here. If you subtract the slender shadow of the ulna from that of the radius in the lateral view, you will be able to appreciate the degree of impaction, fragmentation, and slight angulation of the distal fragment of the radius.

Unknown 16-12 (Figure 16-25)

Fracture of both bones of the forearm with overriding due to muscle pull which must be reduced, set end to end, and immobilized in good alignment in plaster. Trees are off limits for several months.

Unknown 16-13 (Figure 16-73)

Suffocation. The man is edentulous. A lower denture is in its normal place against the mandible, but the upper denture lies vertically behind the tongue. A large fragment of the soft-drink bottle was found lodged in the denture.

APPENDIX B Credits

Chapter 1

Figure 1-1. The late Dr. M. Sosman brought this from Australia.

Figure 1-3. From *Medical Record* 149, Feb. 15, 1896.

Figure 1-4. Courtesy Dr. W. Felts, Minneapolis, Minn.

Figure 1-5. From *Fundamentals of Radiography*, p. 25, published by Eastman Kodak Co., Rochester, N.Y.

Figure 1-8. Courtesy Dr. D. Eaglesham, Guelph, Ontario, Canada.

Figure 1-9. Courtesy Dr. E. Comstock, Wellesville, N.Y., and C. Bridgman, Rochester, N.Y.

Figure 1-10. Courtesy C. Bridgman, Rochester, N.Y., and S. Keck, New York, N.Y.

Figure 1-11. From *Fundamentals of Radiography*, p. 6, published by Eastman Kodak Co., Rochester, N.Y.

Figure 1-14. Courtesy C. Bridgman, Rochester, N.Y.

Chapter 2

Figure 2-1. Courtesy Dr. A. Richards and the publisher, *Medical Radiography and Photography* (hereafter *MR&P*) 32:28.

Figure 2-2B. Courtesy Drs. W. Macklin, Jr., H. Bosland, and A. McCarthy, and the publisher, *MR&P* 31:91.

Figure 2-4. Courtesy S. McPartland, Brooklyn, N.Y.

Figure 2-5. Courtesy C. Bridgman, E. Holly, Dr. M. Zariquiey, and the publisher, *MR&P* 32:49.

Figures 2-7, 8. Courtesy Dr. H. Forsyth, Jr., and the publisher, *MR&P* 25:38.

Figures 2-10, 12. Courtesy Dr. C. Behrens, Bethesda, Md.

Figure 2-13. Courtesy Dr. B. Epstein and the publisher, *MR&P* 34:60.

Figure 2-19. From *Fundamentals of Radiography*, pp. 48, 75, published by Eastman Kodak Co., Rochester, N.Y.

Figure 2-21. Courtesy Drs. A. Megibow and M. Bosniak, New York, N.Y.

Chapter 3

Figure 3-3. From *Fundamentals of Radiography*, p. 19, published by Eastman Kodak Co., Rochester, N.Y.

Figures 3-5, 6. Courtesy O. Alexander and the publisher *MR&P* 30:35, 36.

Figure 3-7. Courtesy R. Philips, Boston, Mass.

Figure 3-9. Courtesy S. Forczyk, Fall River, Mass.

Figures 3-11, 12. Courtesy Drs. J. Hope, E. O'Hara, T. Tristan, and J. Lyon, Jr., and the publisher, *MR&P* 33:30, 31.

Figure 3-13. Courtesy Dr. J. Atlee, Lancaster, Pa.

Figure 3-15. Courtesy A. Dini, Rochester, N.Y.

Figures 3-16, 17, 18. From *Fundamentals of Radiography*, pp. 25, 30, 95, published by Eastman Kodak Co., Rochester, N.Y.

Chapter 4

Figure 4-2. Courtesy R. Morrison and the publisher, *MR&P* 27:132.

Figures 4-4, 5. Courtesy Dr. J. Harris and the publisher, *MR&P* 39:2, 56.

Figures 4-9, 11. Courtesy Drs. B. Felson, F. Fleishner, J. McDonald, and C. Rabin, and the publisher, *Radiology* 73:744.

Figure 4-10. Courtesy Dr. C. Dotter and the publisher, *MR&P* 34:48, and Dr. J. Reed, Detroit, Mich.

Figures 4-12, 13, 42. Courtesy Dr. B. Epstein and the publisher, *MR&P* 34:58, 62, 66.

Figure 4-14. Courtesy Dr. B. Epstein, New Hyde Park, N.Y.

Figure 4-15. Courtesy Dr. W. Chamberlain, Washington, D.C.

Figures 4-16, 17, 18. Courtesy Drs. A. Bell, S. Shimomura, W. Guthrie, H. Hempel, H. Fitzpatrick, and C. Begg, and the publisher, *Radiology* 73:566.

Figure 4-19. Courtesy Dr. C. Dotter and the publisher, *MR&P* 32:48.

Figures 4-20B, 21E. Courtesy Dr. R. Sherman, New York, N.Y.

Figure 4-21F. Courtesy Dr. R. Weyher, Detroit, Mich.

Figure 4-22. Courtesy Dr. A. Bendick and the publisher, *MR&P* 34:76.

Figure 4-23. Courtesy Dr. J. Tollman, Omaha, Neb.

Chapter 5

Figures 5-4, 5. Courtesy Dr. M. Zariquiey and the publisher, *MR&P* 33:68–76.

Figures 5-10, 13. Courtesy Dr. G. Simon, London, England.

Figure 5-11. Courtesy Dr. B. Epstein and the publisher, *MR&P* 34:63, 66.

Chapter 6

Figure 6-2. Courtesy Dr. M. Strahl, Brooklyn, N.Y.

Figures 6-3, 4. Courtesy Dr. J. Hope et al., and the publisher, *MR&P* 33:26, 28.

Figure 6-5. Adapted from Sobotta-Uhlenhuth, *Atlas of Descriptive Human Anatomy*, 7th ed., 1957, Hafner Publishing Co., New York, N.Y.

Figure 6-6. Courtesy Dr. C. Dotter, Portland, Ore.

Figure 6-7. Courtesy C. Brownell and the publisher, *MR&P* 27:114.

Figure 6-9A. Courtesy Dr. W. Brosius, Detroit, Mich.

Figure 6-9B. Courtesy Drs. A. Fine and T. Steinhausen, and the publisher, *MR&P* 23:54–56.

Figures 6-12, 17. Courtesy Dr. J. Petersen and the publisher, *Radiology* 74:36, 40.

Figure 6-16. Courtesy Dr. E. Carpenter, Superior, Wis.

Figure 6-18. Courtesy Dr. G. Schwalbach, Rochester, N.Y.

Figure 6-19. Courtesy Dr. H. Forsyth, Jr., and the publisher, *MR&P* 31:129.

Figures 6-20, 21. Courtesy Dr. M. Fisher, and the publisher, *MR&P* 46:2.

Figures 6-22 through 26. Courtesy Dr. N. Solomon, Brooklyn, N.Y.

Chapter 7

Figure 7-1. Courtesy Drs. I. Harris and M. Stuecheli, and the publisher, *MR&P* 28:29.

Figures 7-2, 3, 8, 9. Courtesy Dr. J. Hope et al., and the publisher, *MR&P* 33:26–28, 30.

Figure 7-4. Courtesy Dr. W. Tuddenham et al., and the publisher, *MR&P* 33:60.

Figures 7-5, 6, 18–20, 23. Courtesy Dr. G. Simon, London, England.

Figure 7-10. Courtesy Dr. J. Mokrohisky and the publisher, *Radiology* 70:578.

Figure 7-12. Courtesy Dr. W. Crandall, Sulphur, Okla.

Figure 7-13. Courtesy Dr. H. Fulton and the publisher, *MR&P* 30:81, 82.

Figures 7-15, 16. Courtesy Drs. E. Uhlmann and J. Ovadia, and the publisher, *Radiology* 74:226, 269.

Figure 7-25. Courtesy Drs. V. Condon and E. Phillips, and the publisher, *Am. J. Roentgenol.* 88:548.

Chapter 8

Figures 8-3, 4. Courtesy Dr. C. Dotter and the publisher, *MR&P* 30:70.

Figure 8-5. Courtesy Dr. T. Newton and the publisher, *Am. J. Roentgenol.* 89:277.

Figures 8-6, 8. Courtesy Drs. P. Markovits and J. Desprez-Curely, and the publisher, *Radiology* 78:373, 377.

Figure 8-9. Courtesy Dr. W. Brosius, Detroit, Mich.

Figure 8-10. Courtesy Dr. G. Baron, Rochester, N.Y.

Figure 8-11. Courtesy Dr. G. McDonnell and the publisher, *MR&P* 30:84.

Figures 8-15, 17, 23. Courtesy Drs. A. Megibow and M. Bosniak, New York, N.Y.

Figure 8-16. Courtesy Drs. R. Ormond, A. Templeton, and J. Jaconette, and the publisher, *Radiology* 80:738.

Figure 8-18. Courtesy Dr. W. Irwin, Detroit, Mich.

Figure 8-19. Courtesy Dr. E. Carpenter, Superior, Wis.

Figure 8-20. Courtesy Dr. J. Hope et al., and the publisher, *MR&P* 33:35.

Figure 8-21. Courtesy Drs. K. Ellis and G. Renthal, and the publisher, *Am. J. Roentgenol.* 88:1072.

Figure 8-22. Courtesy Dr. B. Epstein and the publisher, *MR&P* 34:67

Chapter 9

Figure 9-3. Courtesy Dr. G. Schwalbach, Rochester, N.Y.

Figure 9-4. Courtesy Dr. G. Jacobson and the publisher, *MR&P* 44:21.

Figure 9-6. Courtesy R. Bottin, Indianapolis, Ind.

Figure 9-9. Courtesy Dr. G. Baron, Rochester, N.Y.

Figure 9-10. Courtesy Dr. W. Brosius and the publisher, *MR&P* 30:85, 86.

Figure 9-11. Courtesy Dr. W. Brosius, Detroit, Mich.

Chapter 10

Figures 10-1, 3. Courtesy Dr. H. Forsyth, Jr., Rochester, N.Y.

Figure 10-4. Courtesy Dr. J. Hope et al., and the publisher, *MR&P* 33:228.

Figures 10-5, 11. Courtesy Drs. W. MacIntyre, G. Crespo, and J. Christie, and the publisher, *Am. J. Roentgenol.* 89:317, 318.

Figure 10-6. Courtesy Dr. G. Simon, London, England.

Figure 10-8. Courtesy Drs. M. Klein and E. Walsh, and the publisher, *Radiology* 70:674.

Figure 10-10. Courtesy Dr. R. Barden and the publisher, *Radiology* 75:454.

Figure 10-12A. Courtesy Drs. H. Mellins, P. Kottmeier, and B. Keily, and the publisher, *Radiology* 73:15.

Figure 10-12B. Courtesy Dr. B. Gosink, San Diego, Calif.

Figures 10-13, 14. Courtesy Dr. B. Epstein and the publisher, *MR&P* 34:68, 69.

Figure 10-16. Courtesy Drs. A. Lieber and J. Jorgens, and the publisher, *Am. J. Roentgenol.* 86:1069–70.

Figure 10-22. Courtesy C. Bridgman, E. Holly, Dr. M. Zariquiey, and the publisher, *MR&P* 32:56.

Figure 10-23. Courtesy Dr. L. Cole, Blossburg, Pa.

Figures 10-24, 25. Courtesy Dr. B. Gasul et al., and the publisher, *MR&P* 35 (1959), supplement.

Figure 10-29. Courtesy Dr. W. Tuddenham et al., and the publisher, *MR&P* 33:61.

Figure 10-33. Courtesy Drs. R. Ormond and A. Poznanski, and the publisher, *Radiology* 74:548.

Figure 10-34. Courtesy Drs. R. Ormond and W. Eyler, and the publisher, *Radiology* 79:381, 382.

Figure 10-35. Courtesy Dr. S. Barton and the publisher, *MR&P* 28:109.

Figure 10-36. Courtesy Drs. J. Lehman, J. Debbas, and J. Boyle, Jr., and the publisher, *Am. J. Roentgenol.* 89:305.

Figure 10-37. Courtesy Drs. R. Kittredge, E. Arida, and N. Finby, and the publisher, *Radiology* 74:432.

Chapter 11

Figure 11-2. Courtesy Dr. J. Hope et al., and the publisher, *MR&P* 33:37.

Figures 11-3, 23. Courtesy Drs. J. Hope and C. Koop, and the publisher, *MR&P* 38:31, 49.

Figure 11-4. Courtesy Drs. B. Kalayjian and M. Sapula, and the publisher, *MR&P* 30:57.

Figure 11-5. Courtesy Dr. J. McGillivray and the publisher, *MR&P* 30:27.

Figure 11-7C. Courtesy Dr. C. Stevenson, Spokane, Wash.

Figure 11-8. Courtesy Dr. R. Alexander, Rochester, N.Y.

Figure 11-12. Courtesy G. Thompson and W. Cornwell, and the publisher, *MR&P* 25:43.

Figure 11-16. Courtesy V. Yamamoto and the publisher, *MR&P* 26:121.

Figure 11-19. Courtesy Drs. R. Salb and G. Burton, and the publisher, *MR&P* 33:106.

Figure 11-20. Courtesy Dr. F. Nelans, Wagner, Okla.

Figure 11-21. Courtesy Dr. J. Jiminez and the publisher, *MR&P* 25:53.

Figure 11-22. Courtesy Dr. L. Cole, Blossburg, Pa.

Figure 11-24. Courtesy Dr. J. Wainerdi, New York, N.Y.

Figure 11-30. Courtesy E. Holly and G. Weingartner, and the publisher, *MR&P* 29:91.

Figure 11-32. Courtesy Dr. W. Tuddenham and the publisher, *Radiology* 78:697.

Figure 11-33. Courtesy C. Bridgman and the publisher, *MR&P* 26:12.

Figure 11-36. Courtesy Dr. N. Solomon, Brooklyn, N.Y.

Figure 11-39. Courtesy Dr. W. Irwin, Detroit, Mich.

Figure 11-42. Courtesy Drs. G. Stein and A. Finkelstein, and the publisher, *MR&P* 31:5.

Figure 11-43. Courtesy Dr. G. Schwartz and the publisher, *MR&P* 30:55.

Figure 11-44. Courtesy Dr. A. Melamed, Milwaukee, Wis.

Figure 11-45. Courtesy Dr. H. Forsyth, Jr., and the publisher, *MR&P* 25:39.

Figure 11-46. Courtesy Dr. N. Alcock and the publisher, *MR&P* 23:27.

Figure 11-49. Courtesy Dr. W. Beacham and the publisher, *MR&P* 25:22.

Figure 11-50. Courtesy J. Hill, Lancaster, England.

Figure 11-53. Courtesy Drs. S. Larson and W. Madden, and the publisher, *MR&P* 24:27.

Figure 11-54. Courtesy Dr. G. Hutto, Columbus, Ga.

Figure 11-55. Courtesy Drs. W. Macklin, Jr., J. Bosland, and A. McCarthy, and the publisher, *MR&P* 31:91.

Figure 11-56. Courtesy J. Cahoon, Jr., Durham, N.C.

Chapter 12

Figure 12-1. Courtesy Dr. J. Hope et al., and the publisher, *MR&P* 33:49.

Figure 12-2. Courtesy Dr. D. Haff, Northampton, Pa.

Figure 12-4. Courtesy Dr. L. Love and the publisher, *Radiology* 75:394.

Figure 12-5. Courtesy Dr. E. Ahern and the publisher, *MR&P* 30:8.

Figure 12-6. Courtesy Dr. C. Nice and the publisher, *Radiology* 80:44.

Figure 12-8. Courtesy Dr. L. Hilt, Eugene, Ore.

Figures 12-9, 14. Courtesy Dr. B. Epstein and the publisher, *Radiology* 74:583, 585.

Figures 12-11, 12. Courtesy Dr. C. Meckstroth and the publisher, *MR&P* 26:125.

Figure 12-13. Courtesy Drs. F. Fleischner and P. Mandelstam, and the publisher, *Radiology* 70:474.

Figure 12-18. Courtesy Dr. J. McCort and the publisher, *Radiology* 78:51.

Figure 12-20. Courtesy Drs. J. Hope and C. Koop, and the publisher, *MR&P* 38:45.

Figures 12-24, 25. Courtesy Dr. E. Schultz and the publisher, *Radiology* 70:728, 729.

Figure 12-26. Courtesy Dr. H. Welsh, E. Fleming, and the publisher, *MR&P* 34:78.

Figure 12-27. Courtesy Dr. D. Robinson, Savannah, Ga.

Chapter 13

Figures 13-1, 30. Courtesy Dr. J. Hope et al., and the publisher, *MR&P* 33:38, 45.

Figure 13-5A. Courtesy Dr. E. Ahern and the publisher, *MR&P* 30:9.

Figure 13-6. Courtesy Dr. A. Templeton and the publisher, *Radiology* 75:240.

Figure 13-7. Courtesy Dr. G. Jaffrey, Santa Rosa, Calif.

Figures 13-8, 34. Courtesy T. Funke, Lorain, Ohio.

Figure 13-9. Courtesy Dr. C. Nice and the publisher, *Radiology* 80:43.

Figure 13-10. Courtesy Dr. R. Sherman, New York, N.Y. and the publisher, Eastman Kodak Co., Rochester, N.Y.

Figure 13-11. Courtesy Dr. J. Higgason and the publisher, *MR&P* 30:60.

Figure 13-12. Courtesy Dr. J. Dulin, Iowa City, Iowa.

Figures 13-13, 14. Courtesy Drs. J. Spencer and J. Schaeffer, and the publisher *MR&P* 29:22.

Figure 13-15. Courtesy Dr. G. Joffrey, Olean, N.Y.

Figure 13-16. Courtesy Dr. M. Kulick, Brooklyn, N.Y.

Figure 13-17. Courtesy Dr. J. Reed, Detroit, Mich.

Figure 13-18. Courtesy Dr. L. Cobbs and the publisher, *MR&P* 31:90.

Figure 13-20. Courtesy Dr. L. Cole, Blossburg, Pa.

Figure 13-21. From *Fundamentals of Radiography*, p. 6, published by Eastman Kodak Co., Rochester, N.Y.

Figure 13-22. Courtesy Dr. T. Orloff and the publisher, *MR&P* 35:53.

Figures 13-28, 29. Courtesy Dr. S. Prather, Jr., Augusta, Ga.

Figure 13-32. Courtesy Dr. E. Merrill, Rochester, N.Y.

Figure 13-35. Courtesy Dr. S. Wyman, Boston, Mass.

Figure 13-36. Courtesy Drs. M. Melamed, L. Steinberg, and A. Pavone, and the publisher, *Radiology* 70:405.

Figure 13-37. Courtesy Drs. W. McAllister, A. Margulis, P. Heinbecker, and H. Spjut, and the publisher, *Radiology* 79:780.

Figure 13-38. Courtesy Drs. W. Horrigan, H. Atkins, and N. Tapley, and the publisher, *Radiology* 78:440.

Figure 13-41. Courtesy Dr. C. Cimmino and the publisher, *MR&P* 30:45.

Figure 13-42. Courtesy Dr. R. Powers and the publisher, *MR&P* 30:43.

Figure 13-43. Courtesy Dr. F. H. Tyner, Houston, Texas.

Chapter 14

Figures 14-1 through 14-16. Courtesy Drs. G. Leopold and B. Gosink, San Diego, Calif.

Figures 14-17, 18. Courtesy Drs. A. Megibow and M. Bosniak, New York, N.Y.

Chapter 15

Figure 15-1. Courtesy Dr. W. Cole and the publisher, *J.A.M.A.* 82:613, 1924.

Figure 15-2. Courtesy Dr. E. Salzmann, Dr. R. Spurck, G. Mills, and the publisher, *MR&P* 37:2.

Figure 15-3. Courtesy Dr. A. Burlando, Buenos Aires, Argentina.

Figure 15-4. Courtesy Dr. J. Pepe, Brooklyn, N.Y.

Figures 15-5, 6. Courtesy Drs. G. Stein and A. Finkelstein, and the publisher, *MR&P* 31:10, 12.

Figure 15-7. Courtesy Dr. E. Pirkey, Louisville, Ky.

Figures 15-8, 9, 10. Courtesy Dr. T. Van Zandt, Rochester, N.Y., and Eastman Kodak Company.

Figures 15-11 through 14, 17, 18. Courtesy Drs. A. Megibow and M. Bosniak, New York, N.Y.

Figure 15-15. Courtesy Dr. S. Dallemand, Brooklyn, N.Y.

Figure 15-16. Courtesy Dr. N. Solomon, Brooklyn, N.Y.

Figures 15-20, 24, 25. Courtesy Dr. J. Hope et al., and the publisher, *MR&P* 33:49.

Figure 15-21. From *Fundamentals of Radiography*, p. 56, published by Eastman Kodak Co., Rochester, N.Y.

Figures 15-22, 27. Courtesy Dr. J. Becker, Brooklyn, N.Y.

Figure 15-23. Courtesy K. Fengler and the publisher, *J. Mt. Sinai Hosp.*, New York, N.Y.

Figure 15-26. Courtesy Dr. D. Gordon, Brooklyn, N.Y.

Figure 15-28. Courtesy F. Kent and the publisher, *MR&P* 24:3.

Figure 15-30. Courtesy Drs. G. Leopold and B. Gosink, San Diego, Calif.

Figure 15-31. Courtesy Dr. W. Foley and General Electric Company.

Figures 15-32, 33. Courtesy Drs. M. Bosniak and J. Becker, New York, N.Y.

Figure 15-34. Courtesy Drs. T. Tristan, J. Murphy, and H. Schoenberg, and the publisher, *Radiology* 79:733.

Figure 15-35. Courtesy Drs. J. Edeiken, G. Strong, and A. Khajavi, and the publisher, *Radiology* 79:88.

Figure 15-36. Courtesy Drs. J. Hope and C. Koop, and the publisher, *MR&P* 38:47.

Figure 15-37. Courtesy Dr. J. Dunlap, Waco, Texas.

Chapter 16

Figure 16-2. Courtesy Chicago Museum of Natural History, Chicago, Ill.

Figures 16-4, 10. Courtesy C. Bridgman and the publisher, *MR&P* 26:4, 9.

Figures 16-5, 38. Courtesy Dr. G. Mitchell and the publisher, *MR&P* 34:6, 7.

Figures 16-6, 15. Courtesy Dr. H. Isard, Dr. B. Ostrum, J. Cullinan, and the publisher, *MR&P* 38:97, 101.

Figure 16-8. Courtesy J. Cahoon and the publisher, *Radiography and Clinical Photography* 22:4, 6.

Figure 16-9. Courtesy C. Bridgman and the publisher, *MR&P* 27:72.

Figure 16-11. Courtesy Dr. L. Hilt, Eugene, Ore.

Figure 16-17 through 22. Courtesy T. Funke and the publisher, *MR&P* 36:9, 16, 17, 19, 20, 24, 29.

Figure 16-26. Courtesy Dr. W. Irwin, Detroit, Mich.

Figures 16-27, 46, 48. Courtesy Dr. D. Wilner, Atlantic City, N.J.

Figures 16-28 through 35. Courtesy Drs. G. Selin and H. Jaffe, and the publisher, *MR&P* 33:7–10, 12, 14–16.

Figure 16-36. Courtesy Drs. G. Wyatt and W. Randall, and the publisher, *MR&P* 24:30.

Figure 16-37. Adapted from A. W. Ham, *Histology*, 3rd ed., p. 295, published by J. B. Lippincott, Philadelphia, Pa.

Figure 16-39. Courtesy Dr. M. Urist, *Bone as a Tissue*, p. 37, and the publisher, McGraw-Hill Book Co., New York, N.Y.

Figure 16-40. Courtesy Dr. L. Luck, *Bone and Joint Diseases*, 1st ed., and the publisher, Charles C Thomas, Springfield, Ill.

Figure 16-41. Courtesy Dr. J. Feist, Pittsburgh, Pa.

Figure 16-42. Courtesy Dr. N. Solomon, Brooklyn, N.Y.

Figure 16-44. Courtesy Dr. J. Tollman, Omaha, Neb.

Figure 16-45. Courtesy Drs. D. Skarloff and N. Charkes, and the publisher, *Radiology 80:270.*

Figure 16-56. Courtesy Dr. W. Irwin and the publisher, Eastman Kodak Co., Rochester, N.Y.

Figures 16-58 through 61. Courtesy Dr. G. Hotson, Brooklyn, N.Y.

Figure 16-62. Courtesy Dr. B. Epstein, New Hyde Park, N.Y.

Figure 16-64. Courtesy Drs. R. Burnip, R. Cohen, and W. Yeider, and the publisher, *MR&P* 27:60.

Figure 16-65. Courtesy Drs. H. Hunt and R. Moore, and the publisher, *MR&P* 27:57.

Figure 16-66A. Courtesy R. Matthias and the publisher, *MR&P* 28:cover.

Figure 16-67. Courtesy Dr. J. Marsh and the publisher, *MR&P* 37:35.

Figure 16-69. Courtesy Dr. J. Edwin Habbe and the publisher, Eastman Kodak Co., Rochester, N.Y.

Figures 16-70, 71, 72. Drs. A. Megibow and M. Bosniak, New York, N.Y.

Figure 16-73. Courtesy Dr. C. Dotter and the publisher, *MR&P* 37:19

Appendix A

Figure A-1. Courtesy Dr. E. Emerson and the publisher, *MR&P* 33:112.

Figure A-2. Courtesy Dr. B. Epstein and the publisher, *MR&P* 34:66.

Figure A-3. Courtesy Drs. V. Condon and E. Phillips, and the publisher, *Am J. Roentgenol.* 88:551.

Figure A-4. Courtesy Drs. W. Macklin, H. Bosland, and A. McCarthy, and the publisher, *MR&P* 31:92.

INDEX